THE GIFT OF LIFE

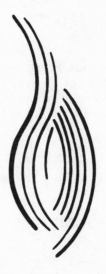

The Proceedings of a National Conference on the Vatican Instruction on Reproductive Ethics and Technology

D1264959

Marilyn Wallace, R.S.M., Ph.D.
Thomas W. Hilgers, M.D.

POPE PAUL VI INSTITUTE PRESS
Omaha, Nebraska 68106

This conference and the publication of its proceedings
was supported by a grant from
Our Sunday Visitor Institute

International Standard Book Number (ISBN): 0-9626485-0-7
Library of Congress Catalog Card Number: 90-61151

Cover design by
Susan Parrish

Published by
POPE PAUL VI INSTITUTE PRESS
6901 Mercy Road
Omaha, Nebraska 68106

THIS BOOK IS DEDICATED TO

THE BLESSED VIRGIN MARY
MOTHER OF GOD
MOTHER OF THE CHURCH

**"We believe in one Lord, Jesus Christ,
the only Son of God, eternally begotten of the Father,
God from God, Light from Light, true God from true God,**

BEGOTTEN, NOT MADE,

one in Being with the Father."

Nicene Creed

EDITORS

THOMAS W. HILGERS, M.D., Dip. ABOG, Dip, ABLS: Senior Medical Consultant in Obstetrics, Gynecology and Reproductive Medicine and director of the Pope Paul VI Institute for the Study of Human Reproduction, Omaha, Nebraska

SR. MARILYN WALLACE, R.S.M., Ph.D.: Assistant research consultant in bioethics, Pope Paul VI Institute for the Study of Human Reproduction, Omaha, Nebraska

CONTRIBUTORS

JOSEPH BOYLE, JR., Ph.D.: Professor of philosophy at St. Michael's College, University of Toronto

REV. ROMANUS CESSARIO, O.P., S.T.D.: Professor of systematic theology at the Dominican House of Studies and a Faculty Member at the Pope John Paul II Institute, Washington, D.C.

LORNA L. CVETKOVICH, M.D., Dip. ABOG: Associate Medical Consultant in Obstetrics, Gynecology and Reproductive Medicine, Pope Paul VI Institute for the Study of Human Reproduction, Omaha, Nebraska

GERMAIN GRISEZ, Ph.D.: Harry Flynn Chair in Christian Ethics, Mount St. Mary's College, Emmitsburg, Maryland

REV. RONALD LAWLER, O.F.M., Cap., S.T.D.: Professor of theology, Holy Cross Seminary, Cromwell, Connecticut

WILLIAM MAY, Ph.D.: Professor of theology, Catholic University of America, Washington, D.C.

REV. JOHN SHEETS, S.J., S.T.D.: Professor of theology, Creighton University, Omaha, Nebraska

JANET SMITH, Ph.D.: Associate professor of philosophy, University of Dallas, Dallas, Texas

WILLIAM WAGNER, J.D.: Associate professor of law, Columbus School of Law, Catholic University of America, Washington, D.C.

TABLE OF CONTENTS

PAGE

INTRODUCTION   1

CHAPTER ONE
The Reproductive Technologies: A Scientific Overview   5
Lorna L. Cvetkovich, M.D.

CHAPTER TWO
An Overview of the Vatican's Instruction on Reproductive Ethics   19
Joseph Boyle, Jr., Ph.D.

CHAPTER THREE
The Teaching Authority of the Church and Its
Relation to Reproductive Issues   27
Rev. Ronald Lawler, O.F.M., Cap.

CHAPTER FOUR
Expanding Our Human Sexual Horizons   41
Thomas W. Hilgers, M.D.

CHAPTER FIVE
The Vocation of Christian Marriage as an Approach
to the Bioethics of Human Reproduction   49
Janet Smith, Ph.D.

CHAPTER SIX
A Contemporary Natural Law Ethics   61
Germain Grisez, Ph.D.

CHAPTER SEVEN
Catholic Teaching on the Laboratory Generation of Human Life   77
William May, Ph.D.

CHAPTER EIGHT
The Ethical and Legal Implications of Surrogate Motherhood   93
William J. Wagner, J.D.

CHAPTER NINE
Recent Advances in Infertility Evaluation and Treatment   127
Thomas W. Hilgers, M.D.

CHAPTER TEN
The Christian Imperative to Follow the Teachings
of the Church: The Testimony of Couples   149
Pope Paul VI Institute Patient - Couples

CHAPTER ELEVEN
The Meaning of Virtue in the Christian Moral Life
and Its Significance to Bioethical Issues   161
Rev. Romanus Cessario, O.P.

CHAPTER TWELVE
Christian Anthropology as it Applies to
Reproductive and Sexual Morality   177
Rev. John Sheets, S.J.

CHAPTER THIRTEEN
The Gift of Life: An Inspiration for Our Time   193
Sr. Marilyn Wallace, R.S.M., Ph.D.

APPENDIX

Donum Vitae   205
Sacred Congregation for the Doctrine of the Faith

PERTINENT ARTICLES ON DONUM VITAE FROM
THE OFFICIAL TEACHING CHURCH

Diligent Search for Truth Requires the Teaching of the Magisterium   233
Pope John Paul II

On the Doctrinal Authority of "Donum Vitae"   239
Pope John Paul II

Easter's Gift of Life   245
Pope John Paul II

Health Care: Ministry in Transition   249
Pope John Paul II

Promote an Authentic Civilization of Life   255
Pope John Paul II

Departure Ceremony - Detroit, September 19, 1987   259
Pope John Paul II

GLOSSARY   263

FORWARD

I had a fine chat the other day with a first-year medical student who had just finished her final examination in Gross Anatomy.

She said she came away from the course with a greater appreciation of two things. First, even on the level of anatomy, human beings are far more complex than she ever thought or dreamed. In fact, she said that she could now understand for the first time why after creating Adam and Eve, God rested on the seventh day. She also said that her insights into the greater complexity of human life brought her also a greater appreciation of the beauty of human beings even on the biological level.

It is these two--namely the complexity and the beauty of the gift of life--which this conference will explore, addressing the fundamental values of life and human procreation.

As a young student I was greatly attracted by the truth of life. As I grew older, I became much more enamored of the goodness of the gift of life. And as the years go by, I am more and more in awe of the beauty of the gift of life.

This conference brought some of that beauty to the fore for me. I hope it will do the same for you.

Fr. Val J. Peter, JCD, STD
Executive Director
Boys Town, Nebraska

PREFACE

The Pope Paul VI Institute wishes to present to you the fruit of our labor: our conference *Donum vitae: The Gift of Life.* *Donum vitae*, the document of the Congregation for the Doctrine of the Faith, is an icon in word, written within cultural limitations of today. Like the true iconographer, the teaching Church relates the eternal as it touches upon the present. *Donum vitae situates scientific discoveries in human reproduction within the unchanging truth of the Tradition itself. Like rules for icon design down through the centuries, the Tradition frames the person as image of God within the divine order of Creation.*

Our conference wishes to draw attention, not to any one personality or theory, but rather to the beauty of the whole, to the religious symbol: to the icon of divine order which grounds the sanctity of human life in the Will of the Eternal Father.

We stand in awe before this divine goodness.

We reflect upon the perspective.

We find our freedom in being subject to this Truth.

Sr. Marilyn Wallace, RSM, Ph.D.

ACKNOWLEGEMENTS

We wish to acknowledge the following individuals for their contributions to the successful completion of this task: Jean Packard, Sr. Catherine Kenny, RSM, Sr. Michaele McGuire, RSM and the entire staff of the Pope Paul VI Institute for the Study of Human Reproduction. Without their help this conference and the publication of its proceedings would never have been accomplished. Thanks also to all of those who attended the conference and participated in its dynamic dialogue.

INTRODUCTION

On March 10, 1987, the Vatican Congregation for the Doctrine of the Faith released an *Instruction on the Respect for Human Life in its Origin and on the Dignity of Procreation (Donum vitae)*. This instruction examined such critical questions as *in vitro* fertilization, experimentation on human embryos, surrogate motherhood, prenatal diagnosis and therapeutic procedures for the human embryo, infertility in marriage and legislation related to procreation. A fundamental concern of the instruction was that human life be respected: the embryo must be treated as a person and defended in its integrity.

On October 28th, 29th and 30th, 1988, the Pope Paul VI Institute for the Study of Human Reproduction sponsored a national, interdisciplinary conference on this instruction on reproductive ethics and technology. This conference, entitled "The Gift of Life" reflected for three days on the "replies to certain questions of the day" which the Congregation for the Doctrine of the Faith was presenting.

The conference attempted to explore rational reflections on the fundamental values of life and of human procreation. The complex questions raised in *Donum vitae* and in our contemporary society were addressed by an internationally recognized faculty . . . indeed, it was perhaps the best faculty that had been brought together since the publication of the Vatican document. Catholic moral and ethical tradition was clearly enunciated, explained and supported. Clearly, it attracted clergy and religious, but it also attracted physicians, nurses, high school teachers, activists in the life issues, bioethicists, hospital administrators, natural family planning teachers, etc. The scholars who participated in the conference made formal presentations and the conference was designed to foster exchange between the audience and the speakers.

Today's world looks for "instant solutions". The massive dehumanization of human life which is so evident in the abortion holocaust has recently been referred to as "microwave abortion" . . . the instant solution to problem pregnancies. Indeed, the new reproductive technologies fall in line with our contemporary mode which says that we need a technological ("quick fix") solution to all problems confronting us.

Unfortunately, what has happened, from a medical point of view, is that there has been a huge void left in our basic understanding of infertility problems and the underlying causes of other reproductive abnormalities. In other words, with society's interest in a quick "technological fix", enormous energies have gone into the technological resolution of complex human problems. In the process, many talented researchers, large amounts of research funding and the time and energy of many talented physicians has gone into an exercise which has "leap frogged" vast areas of basic knowledge.

To the public, this is not so obvious. We hear everyday about "test tube babies" and the further development and application of this type of technology. Rarely do we ever see that basic questions such as, "Is the woman ovulating?", are going unanswered.

Perhaps the greatest tragedy of our current society, beyond the horrific loss of human life, is the basic intellectual dishonesty which has occurred and, with it, the trend toward making people feel like something positive and constructive is actually being done.

One of the unique features of this great conference, attended by over 170 people from over 35 states, was the interdisciplinary nature of its format. It was the first time when theologians, philosophers, bioethicists *and* medical consultants were able to sit down and discuss significant issues with regard to human reproduction and the technologies of procreation.

For far too long, Catholic philosophers and theologians have also worked within a vacuum. They have done a good deal of their basic theological and philosophical research in a void of medical input. This has led some to inadvertently support programs under the mistaken notion that there would be no other solutions forthcoming.

The chapter in this book which deals with the medical aspects of infertility and the new insights that have been gained out of basic research in this field should be of importance and significance to all of us. Not only the physician can gain new knowledge from this but the philosopher and the theologian as well. And, of course, in the long run those patients who so desperately seek help and who so much have a right to ethically sound medical services, will eventually be better served.

For those of you who might find reading the theologians, the philosophers and the physicians difficult, please read the chapter where the patient-couples give witness to their own situation. During the actual conference, when these three couples gave their witness to the conference participants, there were no less than four standing ovations given to them. Please read that chapter if you can't read any other chapter. Indeed, it is a great testimony to the will of the human spirit, the role of the Holy Spirit, and the ability of man and woman to act responsibly and together with God as their teacher and support. Indeed it is a great witness to the notion that pain and suffering can produce great joy and that patience is a virtue that leads us to the resolution of so many great difficulties.

This record of these proceedings obtains its richness from the integrated perspective which it presents. Taken as a whole, this collection of essays truly captures the dimensions of Catholic insight into these questions. For those searching for the truth, these proceedings should be immensely helpful. For those yearning for a loving, caring Church, these proceedings should be irreplaceable.

Thomas W. Hilgers, M.D., Dip. ABOG
Director
Pope Paul VI Institute
for the Study of Human Reproduction

4

1

The Reproductive Technologies: A Scientific Overview

Lorna L. Cvetkovich, M.D.

Prior to any discussion of the moral and ethical aspects of the new reproductive technologies, a basic understanding of the elements of each procedure, its medical consequences, and their ramifications for the couple must be obtained. It is the purpose of this presentation to describe and contrast from a moral medical point of view, the new reproductive technologies: *in vitro* fertilization-embryo transfer (IVF-ET), gamete intrafallopian transfer (GIFT), artificial insemination (AID, AIH), and low tubal ovum transfer (LTOT). In doing so, a sense of this technological experience, for both the couples and the physician/scientists involved will be gained.

IVF-ET, briefly, is the retrieval of the preovulatory ovum from the woman's ovary followed by fertilization in a culture dish and development of the conceptus to the 2 to 8 cell stage. It is then transferred into the woman's uterine cavity.

This complex procedure began in 1944 when John Rock and Miriam Menkin reported the first *in vitro* fertilization of a human ovum.[1] They described two ova which developed to the 2 cell stage and one which progressed to the 3 cell stage. Thirty four years later Louise Brown was born, a result of the first clinically successful IVF-ET pregnancy reported by Drs. Steptoe and Edwards in England.[2] In the ten years since 1978, IVF-ET programs have become available worldwide with over 100 IVF centers in the United States alone reporting on now over 3,000 births resulting from IVF-ET.[3]

CURRENT IVF-ET INDICATIONS

Initially used only to treat women with surgical loss of both tubes or irreparable tubal damage, the indications for IVF-ET have now been expanded to include all causes of infertility (except azospermia or total lack of sperm) after traditional medical and/or surgical therapy has failed. Thus, the indications

5

cited for the Norfolk IVF-ET program include: a generally healthy husband and wife, accessible ovaries, normally functioning uterus, normal or correctable menstrual function, maternal age under 40 and one of the following uncorrected problems: tubal factor, male factor (except azoospermia), endometriosis, unexplained infertility, DES exposure, cervical factor, immunologic factor or anovulation.[4]

IVF-ET consists of 4 major steps:

1. controlled ovarian hyperstimulation
2. oocyte retrieval
3. insemination and cleavage
4. embryo transfer

The first IVF-ET cycles used the woman's natural cycle but the success rates were poor. This was partially due to the production of only one oocyte per cycle making it possible to implant only one embryo, since later experience showed that *transfer of more than one embryo* improved pregnancy rates.[5] The natural cycle also proved to be inconvenient since oocyte retrieval had to be timed to the woman's natural LH surge necessitating surgical and laboratory teams to be available at all hours.[6] The concept of controlled ovarian hyperstimulation was thus developed in which multiple preovulatory oocytes were produced and the timing of oocyte retrieval could be manipulated to occur during normal surgery hours.

The most common protocols utilize clomiphene citrate (CC), human menopausal gonadotropin (HMG), or follicle stimulating hormone (FSH) alone or in combination to override the normal mechanism by which only one dominant follicle is selected for ovulation each cycle. Human chorionic gonadotropin (HCG) is then used as a substitute for the luteinizing hormone (LH) surge which ordinarily causes follicular rupture.

Follicular growth is tracked in most protocols by daily ultrasound examinations starting about day six to nine of the cycle and serum estradiol levels measured daily beginning somewhere between day 3 and 9 of the cycle. Some protocols also call for daily monitoring of vaginal and cervical changes, the so-called "biological shift".

The objective in the hyperstimulation protocols is the development of two or more follicles to a preovulatory size (approx. 1.8 cm.) with adequately rising estrogen levels. When adequate hyperstimulation is thus attained, the HMG is discontinued and 10,000 units of HCG is given 48 hours later. Follicular development is adequate in about 65-75% of stimulated cycles.[2] If the estradiol levels and/or follicular growth are not adequate, that stimulated cycle can be cancelled (prior to laparoscopy) and a different regimen of controlled ovarian hyperstimulation used for the next cycle.

If adequate follicular stimulation does occur, the woman then enters the second major step: *oocyte retrieval*. This is done via laparoscopy which is scheduled 34-36 hours after the HCG trigger is given. At laparoscopy, the ovary is stabilized with a grasping forceps and a long stainless steel beveled needle is introduced through a third small incision or the operating laparoscope itself. The follicles are punctured and the follicular fluid along with the ovum and cumulus mass is aspirated into a trap. The fluid is immediately examined in the lab for the presence of a preovulatory oocyte. Oocytes are retrieved over 95 percent of the time.[6] Most centers aspirate all possible follicles, particularly if they have the availability for oocyte or embryo cryopreservation. If excess oocytes cannot be frozen for later use, some authors have advised stopping when six oocytes are obtained.[6] While most oocyte retrievals are accomplished via laparoscopy, some programs have now initiated the use of ultrasound directed oocyte retrieval through the abdominal wall, bladder, or vagina. Ultrasonic methods of oocyte retrieval avoid surgery and anesthesia, and are applicable even when the ovaries are inaccessible by laparoscopy.

The third stage of IVF-ET is the fertilization process. After the maturity of the oocytes is evaluated, they are incubated in Hams F-10 media + 7.5% fetal cord serum in 5% CO_2 for 3-8 hours.[4] However, immature oocytes may be incubated longer, up to 24 hours. The degree of maturation is important because fertilization rates have been shown to be higher with more mature oocytes.[4] The embryologist is looking for a well dispersed corona radiata and the presence of the first polar body (evidence that the first meiotic division of the oocyte has occurred and the oocyte is at the proper stage for insemination).

During the incubation period, the husband produces by masturbation, a semen specimen which is washed, centrifuged, and allowed to "swim up". This process removes sperm antibodies, decapacitation factors, bacteria and abnormal sperm, concentrating the progressively motile, normal sperm in the supernatant. Capacitation, a biochemical change in the sperm necessary before it is able to fertilize the oocyte, is thought to occur during this preparation time.

The concentration of sperm is then adjusted and a total of 50,000 to 100,000 sperm are added to the oocytes and allowed to incubate for 12-18 hours. When the sperm enters the oocyte, the second polar body is extruded and two pronuclei are formed. If it appears that fertilization has occurred, the pronuclear oocyte is transferred to another culture dish and allowed to incubate another 24 hours at which point a two cell embryo should be noted if development is progressing normally.

The final step in IVF-ET is *embryo transfer* which is accomplished 48-72 hours after fertilization. The woman is placed in the supine or knee-chest position. After the embryos are loaded into a transfer catheter, the tip is inserted into the uterus within 1-2 cms. of the fundus and the embryos are injected. After the catheter is reexamined to ensure that the embryos are not still in it, the woman remains at rest for the next six hours. She is then discharged and told to stay in bed as much as possible over the next two to three days.

It is at the transfer stage where most IVF-ET cycles fail. The percentage of embryos implanting is reported to be 8 to 12 percent.[7,8] Many reasons have been given to explain the inefficiency of embryo transfer, one being the inability to assess the quality or viability of the embryo. Many embryos which appear to be normal do not implant while some thought to be abnormal result in normal infants.[8] The timing of transfer may also contribute. In IVF-ET, the embryo arrives in the uterine cavity several days before it would arrive in a natural cycle and so the synchrony between embryo and uterine lining may not be optimal. In stimulated cycles, the high estrogen levels may also contribute to an abnormal development of the uterine lining. And, finally, the transfer procedure itself may be traumatic or stimulate uterine activity which would expel the embryo. One study using embryo-like microspheres showed that only 45% remained in the uterus at one hour.[8]

IVF - PREGNANCY RATES AND OUTCOMES

Pregnancy rates with IVF-ET have been the subject of much discussion and controversy. One problem lies in the difficulty of comparing results among studies. *There are so many variables* - patient selection, stimulation protocol, technique of oocyte retrieval, embryo culture and transfer, to name just a few - that one is often comparing apples and oranges. Secondly, the method of reporting pregnancy rates varies. A pregnancy rate is a percentage consisting of a numerator and a denominator. In a report of IVF pregnancies, the numerator may be the number of positive pregnancy tests, the number of clinically detectable pregnancies, the number of pregnancies beyond 20 weeks gestation or the number of babies taken home from the hospital. The denominator may be the number of couples beginning a treatment cycle, the number of stimulated cycles, the number of laparoscopies, or the number of embryo transfers. Obviously, the number of positive pregnancy tests per embryo transfer will be much higher than the number of term infants per stimulation cycle.

Although pregnancy rates vary widely from center to center, it is possible to obtain an overall figure by looking at collaborative reports. The National IVF Registry of the Society of Assisted Alternative Reproduction reported on 41 of 160 United States centers for the year 1986. The pregnancy rate per embryo transfer was 16.9% (13.8% per oocyte retrieval and 9.9% per stimulation cycle). The "take home baby rate" per oocyte retrieval was 8.9 percent.[3] Other data is presented in Table 1.

Twenty to thirty percent of the clinically recognizable IVF pregnancies will end in spontaneous miscarriage. This rate is higher than the 15 percent which is quoted for the normal population but not higher than that seen in the infertile population treated medically or surgically.

Ectopic pregnancies were reported in 1.6% of pregnancies at the Third World Congress and 4.6% at the Fourth World Congress.

TABLE 1

ANALYSIS OF DATA FOLLOWING CONTROLLED
OVARIAN HYPERSTIMULATION USING HMG-HCG FOR IVF-ET
FROM FEBRUARY 1983 TO APRIL 1986[a]

Number of patients	296
Number of laparoscopies	443
Number of oocytes recovered	1595 (3.6/patient)
Number of oocytes fertilized	1356 (85%)
Number of embryo transfers	409
Number of embryos transferred	1372 (3.2/patient)
Clinical pregnancies	151 (11.0%)
Multiple pregnancies	17 twins
	2 triplets
Total	19 (12.6%)
Miscarriages	32 (21.2%)
Ectopic pregnancies	1 (0.7%)
Congenital anomalies	1 (0.7%)
Total live births to date	81
Livebirths: embryo transfers ratio	19.8
Livebirths: embryos transferred ratio	5.9
Embryo loss ratio	9.1

a. Data from: Frederick CM, Paulson JD, DeCherney AH: *Foundations of In Vitro Fertilization.* Hemisphere Publishing Corp., Washington, DC, 1987.

Multiple pregnancies are reported in 10-20% of cases and are related to the number of embryos transferred, especially when that number is greater than four.

Congenital abnormalities in IVF pregnancies are, in general, lower than in spontaneous pregnancies with the U.S. Centers reporting 1.7% and the Australians reporting 2.6% at the Fourth World Congress.

Obstetrically, these pregnancies have a higher rate of prematurity and low birth weight which are related to the increased incidence of multiple pregnancies. The Cesarean section rate is 36-55%. The high rate is in part due to the higher maternal age and poor obstetrical history seen in these patients and in part due to the desire of the obstetrician to avoid any possibility of fetal risk during labor.

Caution should be exhibited when looking at or evaluating any of the success data on the reproductive technologies. For example, no one has yet pointed out the highly embryocidal effects of IVF-ET, resulting in well over 90 percent of all embryos conceived *in vitro* eventually dying in the subsequent development process.

GIFT - DEFINITION/HISTORY

The GIFT (gamete intrafallopian transfer) procedure and its variations are the most recently developed of the new reproductive technologies. GIFT is the "direct transfer of preovulatory oocytes and washed sperm into the fallopian tube in an attempt to mimic the early physiologic processes that lead to gestation in humans."[9] Thus, the major difference between GIFT and IVF is that in GIFT, both sperm and ovum are placed at the normal site of fertilization in the woman and fertilization is allowed to occur *in vivo* or within the woman's fallopian tube rather than in an *in vitro* culture dish. Because the fertilization process does not occur extracorporeally, many authors have commented that GIFT is considered morally licit by the Church.[10,11] A more definitive commentary on that very issue occurs later in these proceedings (see Chapter 7).

The history of GIFT is short, dating only from 1984 when the first pregnancy resulting from this technique was described by Asch. Since that time, there has been a rapid expansion of its application. In 1985, eight clinics reported three pregnancies from 56 treatment cycles in 47 patients. By 1986, there were 25 clinics reporting 108 pregnancies resulting from 466 treatment cycles in 47 patients. [12]At this point, some centers now offer GIFT to all couples without tubal infertility as a first choice instead of IVF-ET.[13,14]

CURRENT MEDICAL INDICATIONS FOR GIFT

GIFT is thought to be effective by virtue of being able to bypass deficiencies in transport of the oocyte or sperm to the site of fertilization.[15] Thus, it has been utilized in patients with unexplained infertility and endometriosis where it is thought that deficient oocyte pickup and/or oocyte entrapment (the "luteinized unruptured follicle syndrome") are preventing pregnancy, as well as in male factor, cervical factor and immunologic factor infertility where deficient numbers of sperm at the site of fertilization are implicated.

GIFT has also been used in premature ovarian failure in conjunction with donated oocytes.[16] In short, the only absolute contraindication is the absence or total occlusion of both fallopian tubes for which IVF-ET remains the only form of treatment. The use of GIFT in more minor degrees of tubal damage is avoided in some studies for fear of ectopic pregnancies,[17,18] but is included in others.[12,19,20]

GIFT - THE PROCEDURE

A GIFT treatment cycle begins with one of the ovarian hyperstimulation protocols as in IVF-ET. Superovulation is necessary, because, as with IVF, pregnancy rates are improved if more than one oocyte is transferred up to a maximum of 3-4.[18,20] Daily hormone assessment and ultrasonic tracking of follicular growth are also carried out as in an IVF-ET cycle. Finally, oocyte retrieval is accomplished 36 hours after the LH surge or HCG pulse via laparoscopy with direct puncture and aspiration of the follicles. The oocytes obtained are then taken to the embryology lab and their maturity is evaluated according to a grading system established by Veeck.[21] The embryologist is looking for a second polar body and a well expanded corona radiata. Two hours prior to the oocyte retrieval, semen is obtained by *masturbation*. The sample is washed, re-suspended, allowed to "swim up" and then adjusted to a concentration of approximately 100,000 motile sperm per 25 microliters.[23] It is at this point that the procedure differs from IVF-ET. Instead of inseminating the oocytes in a culture dish, the most mature ova and 25-50 microliters of the prepared sperm are loaded into a 50 cm 16 gauge Teflon catheter. The catheter is prepared under sterile conditions and brought to the surgeon who lifts the tube atraumatically and after advancing the catheter 1.5-4 cms. into the fimbrial end of the tube, the gametes are injected. The Teflon catheter is taken back to the lab to assure that the oocytes and sperm have indeed been expelled. The process is usually repeated with the other fallopian tube as well, transferring up to four ova at a time. Once the woman recovers from the anesthetic, she is discharged from the hospital. Following the transfer procedure, progesterone supplementation is usually used to support the luteal phase of the cycle and a pregnancy test is done 11-16 days later.

The factors which have made GIFT a rapidly expanding technology are several. Most importantly, pregnancy rates seem to be higher than in IVF-ET in the range of 30 percent per transfer.[11] This is thought to result from (1) a decreased manipulation of the gametes, (2) an undefined beneficial effect of the tubal environment on the conceptus, and (3) a better synchrony between the endometrium and the arrival of the embryo in the uterus.[12,25] GIFT is also seen as a technically simpler procedure which requires less of both the lab and the embryologist's time. Because it is simpler and does not require embryo transfer, GIFT cycles are about 25 percent less expensive than the estimated $6,000 per cycle cost of IVF-ET.[11] However, this difference would be minimal if ultrasound, rather than laparoscopy, were used for oocyte retrieval in IVF-ET cycles.

As one can see in the list of major GIFT studies, the pregnancy rates vary widely as in IVF, and even though some quote rates as high as 40 percent,[18] when Leeton[10] compared GIFT to IVF-ET in unexplained and male factor infertility, the rates were similar for both procedures. Further, the results of a multinational cooperative study showed an overall success rate of 29 percent per GIFT procedure (with as many as one in three such pregnancies failing to go to term). In male factor and immunologic factor infertility the rates were much lower at 15 percent and 10 percent respectively (see Table 2).

Finally, outcomes of GIFT pregnancies reveal a 20-25 percent[10,16] spontaneous abortion rate as in IVF. Ectopic pregnancies account for 4.4 percent[19] to 7.5 percent[12] of fetal wastage, most cases occurring in patients with mild tubal adhesions. A large cooperative study of 800 GIFT procedures reported an ectopic rate of 2.9%, a figure not significantly higher

TABLE 2

CLINICAL PREGNANCIES FOLLOWING GIFT[a]

ETIOLOGY	NUMBER OF STIMULATION CYCLES	NUMBER OF CLINICAL PREGNANCIES	SUCCESS RATE[b] (PERCENT)
Unexplained infertility	796	247	31
Endometriosis	413	132	32
Male factor	397	61	15
Tubo-peritoneal	210	61	29
Failed artificial insemination by donor	160	66	41
Cervical	68	19	28
Immunological	30	5	10
Premature ovarian failure	18	10	56
Total	2,092	601	29[b]

a. Results of a multinational cooperative study.

b. Percent of stimulation cycles leading to a clinical pregnancy. *As many as one in three such clinical pregnancies fails to go to term.*

SOURCE: R.H. Asch, UCI/AMI Center for Reproductive Health, Garden Grove, CA, personal communication, December 1987.

DATA FROM: U.S. Congress, Office of Technology Assessment, *Infertility: Medical and Social Choices,* OTA-BA-358 Washington, DC: U.S. Government Printing Office, May 1988.

than that for IVF-ET. So whether GIFT will supersede IVF-ET based on improved pregnancy rates and similar complication rates remains to be seen.

GIFT	**IVF-ET**

INDICATIONS

All indications except tubal factor (severe oligospermia relatively contraindicated)	All indications failing medical and surgical treatment

SURGICAL PROCEDURE

Laparoscopy for oocyte retrieval and gamete placement	Laparoscopic or sonographic oocyte retrieval followed by embryo transfer

PREGNANCY RATES

Pregnancy rates approximately 30% per ovum retrieval	Pregnancy rates 15-20% transfer in best centers (approx. 10% overall)

12

SITE OF CONCEPTION

Fertilization *in vivo*   Fertilization *in vitro*

TECHNOLOGICAL ADVANTAGES/DISADVANTAGES

Unable to assess whether fertilization occurs and select "best oocyte/conception"	Able to determine fertilization and perform embryo selection
Decreased manipulation of gametes; simpler procedure; decreased amount of laboratory work and personnel	Requires *in vitro* insemination and oocyte/embryo culture for up to 72 hours prior to embryo transfer

LOW TUBAL OVUM TRANSFER (LTOT)

Low tubal ovum transfer (LTOT) was first described by Kreitman and Hodgen in 1980.[26] In their animal study, they monitored mature rhesus and cynomolgus monkeys for the estimated time of ovulation, performed oocyte retrieval in 31 cases and then transferred the oocytes to the proximal portion of the fallopian tube. The monkeys were mated before and after the procedure. Five pregnancies were obtained.

In LTOT, insemination and fertilization are the results of *normal coitus.* Because of this, in 1983, Dr. David McLaughlin set up a clinical trial with Archbishop Daniel Pilarczyk's approval at St. Elizabeth's Medical Center in Dayton, Ohio.[27,28] Seven women underwent ovarian hyperstimulation, laparoscopic oocyte retrieval and transfer of the oocytes to the proximal portion of the fallopian tubes. Insemination was by a normal act of coitus. No pregnancies ensued from the initial trial but one pregnancy has subsequently been reported.

Dr. McLaughlin has since left St. Elizabeth's and is presently at the Indianapolis Fertility Center. According to information from his staff, the original LTOT procedure is no longer being offered. He now does essentially the GIFT procedure where both ova and sperm are transferred by catheter into the distal fallopian tube, the sperm having been obtained by masturbation. However, if a couple requests or has "scruples" regarding seminal fluid collection in this way, they are offered "TOT." This is a GIFT procedure but the seminal fluid is obtained using a Milex Seminal Fluid Collection Device during a normal act of coitus. Thus, continuing work on LTOT is not currently being done.

ARTIFICIAL INSEMINATION

Artificial insemination (AI), though not really new, is one of the reproductive technologies to which many infertile couples are exposed.

Generically, AI refers to any procedure in which semen or a sperm preparation from the husband or a donor is introduced into the woman's vagina, cervix, or uterus. Thus, one may have intravaginal, intracervical or intrauterine inseminations. In addition, the source of the sperm may be either the husband (artificial insemination by Husband - AIH) or a donor (artificial insemination by Donor - AID).

The indications for artificial insemination include, physiologic or psychologic dysfunction (such as severe hypospadias, vaginismus, retrograde ejaculation, neurologic/psychogenic or drug related impotence), oligoasthenospermia, hostile cervical mucus, immunologic infertility, unexplained infertility, and in the case of AID, azoospermia or genetic abnormalities. Sims, who in the mid-1800's performed one of the earliest studies on AIH stated, "Before undertaking this (AIH) we must satisfy ourselves that the semen is perfectly normal and that it does not and cannot enter the canal of the cervix in the usual way."[29] Although AIH began as a treatment in cases where normal deposition of semen near the cervix could not occur, its present clinical application is primarily to couples with oligoasthenospermia (male factor).

Artificial insemination requires timing ovulation in the woman either by Basal Body Temperature (BBT), cervical mucus, LH surge, estradiol levels, or ultrasound. Inseminations are carried out a variable number of times (from 1 to 9) around the time of ovulation. This timing is obviously important.

The semen preparation depends on the type of insemination and the problem being treated. Fresh, whole ejaculates or frozen specimens are used for AID, whereas, AIH may be done with a split ejaculate if the husband's semen volume is high or with a specimen that has been fractionated on an albumin column to increase motility. In AID, the semen is normally screened for sexually transmitted diseases but in many centers, the screening is very lax.[30] And presently, because of AIDS, some states have outlawed the use of fresh donor semen. Once the semen is prepared, it is loaded into a syringe, cannula, or tubing and injected either intracervically or intravaginally. If a cap is used, the semen is placed in the cap which is then applied to the cervix and allowed to remain in place for 6-12 hours. With intrauterine insemination (IUI), a very small amount (0.1-1.0 cc) of washed sperm that have been allowed to "swim up" are injected past the cervix into the intrauterine cavity. The preparation concen- trates the motile sperm and removes the seminal fluid which contains prostaglan- dins and may cause severe cramping.[31]

The mean number of cycles to achieve pregnancy with AIH is 3.5 and few pregnancies occur after five cycles. Therefore, couples are advised to continue treatment for at least three cycles but not beyond six cycles.

The early spontaneous abortion rate in AIH is reported as 25 percent which may reflect the basic abnormality causing the infertility, or, in IUI, might be due to the bypassing of the cervical mucus which usually filters out abnormal sperm.

Aside from AIH in normospermic males where a physiologic or psychologic factor prevents proper deposition of semen (in which the pregnancy rate is reported to be 60-90 percent), the pregnancy rates for AIH are very low. Nachtigall summarized 15 studies of the use of AIH in oligospermia and found a combined pregnancy rate of 18 percent.[29] This is compared to a spontaneous pregnancy rate of 14 percent seen in six series totaling 416 couples. In two of the studies, the spontaneous pregnancy rate exceeded the rate with treatment. It becomes clear, then, that except for specific indications, AI does not overcome the difficulty it is most commonly used to treat.[29-31]

SUMMARY

In summary, the technologies of assisted reproduction have evolved as a means to overcome the many factors which may cause infertility. They are complex and technically demanding procedures because they are attempting to reproduce and manipulate the delicate and complex processes of oocyte maturation, follicular development, spermatogenesis, fertilization, and implantation. They are also expensive, and physically and emotionally taxing for the couple. That so many couples willingly submit to this expense and effort, not to mention the handing over of this intimate aspect of their relationship to a laboratory, serves clearly to demonstrate the extreme vulnerability present whenever a couple cannot achieve a much desired pregnancy.

REFERENCES

[1]Menkin, M and Rock, J: In Vitro Fertilization and Cleavage of Human Ovarian Eggs. Am. J. Obstet. Gyn. 55:440, 1948.

[2]Edwards, R.G., Steptoe, PC and Purdy, JM: Establishing Full-Term Human Pregnancies Using Cleaving Embryos Grown In Vitro. Br. J. Obstet. Gynaecol. 87:737, 1980.

[3]Medical Research International: In Vitro Fertilization/Embryo Transfer in the United States: 1985 and 1986 Results from the National IVF-ET Registry. Fertil. Steril. 49:826, 1984.

[4]Jones, HW Jr., Jones, GS, Hodgen, GD, et al. Eds: In Vitro Fertilization, Norfolk, Williams and Wilkins, Baltimore, 1986.

[5]Jones, HW Jr., Acosta, AA, Andreas, MC, et al: Three Years of In Vitro Fertilization at Norfolk. Fertil, Steril. 49:826, 1984.

[6]Frederick, CM, Paulson, JD, DeCherney, AH: Foundations of In Vitro Fertilization, Hemisphere Publishing Corp., Washington, D.C., 1987.

[7]Yovich, JL: Embryo Quality and Pregnancy Rates in IVF. Lancet II:283, 1985.

[8]Cohen, J: Pregnancy, Abortion and Birth After In Vitro Fertilization. In: In Vitro Fertilization, Past, Present, Future, Eds. Fishel, S, Symonds, EM, IRL Press, Oxford, 1986.

[9]Asch, RH, Ellsworth, LR, Balmaceda, JP: Pregnancy Following Translaparoscopic Gamete Intrafallopian Transfer (GIFT). Lancet 2: 1034, 1984.

[10]Leeton, J, Rogers, P, Caro, C: A Controlled Study Between the Use of Gamete Intra-fallopian (GIFT) and In Vitro Fertilization and Embryo Transfer in the Management of Idiopathic and Male infertility. Fertil. Steril. 48:605, 1987.

[11]Seibel, MM: A New Era in Reproductive Technology. In Vitro Fertilization, Gamete Intrafallopian Transfer, and Donated Gametes and Embryos. NEJM 318:828, 1988.

[12]Yovich, JL, Yovich, JM, Edirisinghe, WR: The Relative Chance of Pregnancy Following Tubal or Uterine Transfer Procedures. Fertil. Steril. 49:858, 1988.

[13]Medical Research International: In Vitro Fertilization/embryo Transfer in the United States: 1985 and 1986 Results from the National IVF/ET Registry. Fertil. Steril. 49:212, 1988.

[14]Quigley, MM, Sokoloski, JE, Withers, DM, Richards, SI, Reis, JM: Simultaneous In Vitro Fertilization and Gamete Intrafallopian Transfer (GIFT). Fertil. Steril. 47:797, 1987.

[15]Asch, RH, Balmaceda, JP, Ellsworth, PA, Wong, PC: Preliminary Experiences with Gamete Intrafallopian Transfer (GIFT). Fertil. Steril. 45:366, 1986.

[16]Asch, RH, Balmaceda, JP, Ord, T, et al: Oocyte Donation and Gamete Intrafallopian Transfer in Premature Ovarian Failure. Fertil. Steril. 49:263, 1987.

[17]Corson, SL, Batzer, F, Eisenberg, E, English, ME, White, SM, Laberge, Y, Go, KJ: Early Experience with the GIFT Procedure. J. Reprod. Med. 31:219, 1986.

[18]Molloy, D and Spiers, A: A Laparoscopic Approach to a Program of Gamete Intrafallopian Transfer. Fertil. Steril. 47:289, 1987.

[19]Matson, PL, Yovich, JM, Bootsma, BD, Spittle, JW, Yovich, JL: The In Vitro Fertilization of Supernumerary Oocytes in a Gamete Intrafallopian Transfer (GIFT) Program. Fertil. Steril. 47:802, 1987.

[20]McGaughey, RW and Nemiro, JS: Correlation of Estrogen Levels with Oocytes Aspirated and with Pregnancy in a Program of Clinical Tubal Transfer. Fertil. Steril. 48:98, 1987.

[21]Veeck, LL: Morphological Estimation of Mature Oocytes and Their Preparation for Insemination. In: In Vitro Fertilization, Norfolk, Eds. Jones, HW, Jones, GS, Williams and Wilkins, Baltimore, 1986.

[22]Yovich, JL, Matson, PL, Blackledge, DG, Turner, SR, Richardson, PA, Yovich, JM, Edirisinghe, WR: The Treatment of Normospermic Infertility by Gamete Intrafallopian Transfer (GIFT). British J. Obstet. Gynaecol. In press.

[23]Frederick, CM, Paulson, JD, DeCherney, AH: Foundations of In Vitro Fertilization. Hemisphere Publishing Corporation, Washington, 1987.

[24]Guastella, G, Romparetto, G, Palermo, R, et al: Gamete Intrafallopian Transfer in the Treatment of Infertility: The First Series at the University of Palermo. Fertil. Steril. 46:417, 1986.

[25]Martinez, F and Trounson, A: An Analysis of Factors Associated with Ectopic Pregnancy in a Human IVF Program. Fertil. Steril. 45:79, 1986.

[26]Kreitman, O and Hodgen, GD: Low Tubal Ovum Transfer: An Alternative to In Vitro Fertilization. Fertil. Steril. 34:375, 1980.

[27]Hospital Progress: Program Offers Alternatives to In Vitro Fertilization. October, 1983.

[28]Hospital Progress: Should Catholic Hospitals Encourage Low Tubal Ovum Transfer? March, 1984.

[29]Nachtigall, RD, Faure, N, Glass, RH: Artificial Insemination of Husband's Sperm. Fertil. Steril. 23:141, 1979.

[30]Andrews, LB: Ethical and Legal Aspects of In Vitro Fertilization and Artificial Insemination by Donor. In: Urologic Clinics, Male Infertility. Eds. Howards, SS, Lipschultz, LI, W.B. Saunders, Philadelphia, 1987.

[31]Allen, NC, Herbert, CM, Maxson, WS, et al: Intrauterine Insemination: A Critical Review. Fertil. Steril. 44:569, 1985.

2

An Overview of the Vatican's Instruction on Reproductive Ethics

Joseph Boyle, Jr., Ph.D.

I. THE PURPOSE OF THE INSTRUCTION

On Feb. 22, 1987, the Sacred Congregation for the Doctrine of the Faith issued a moral evaluation of various widely discussed reproductive procedures and related activities.[1] The name of this document is *Instruction on Respect for Human Life in its Origin and on the Dignity of Procreation: Replies to Certain Questions of the Day*. This Instruction is often referred to by the first two words in the official Latin text, *Donum vitae:* Gift of Life.

As its title suggests, the purpose of the *Instruction* is to answer certain "questions of the day" concerning such matters as *in vitro* fertilization, artificial insemination, and the medical treatments of the unborn. Thus, the instruction is not concerned directly with questions of science, nor even with the underlying technological possibilities created by the developments of modern biological science, but is concerned with certain human actions, those in which scientific knowledge and technological possibilities are used to solve problems of infertility, treat the diseases of the unborn, and so on. Such uses of scientific knowledge and technology raise serious moral questions, as virtually everyone admits. It is these moral questions which the *Instruction* addresses.

In fact, the *Instruction* exhibits a welcoming and grateful attitude not only toward the great advances in scientific understanding of human beings, but also toward the technological potential which these advances create. Properly used, this technology can be a great help to human beings in carrying out their vocations in this world. So there is no suspicion of the technological or the artificial, just as such, and no nostalgia for natural ways of, say, reproduction, just because they are natural. If certain medical procedures are evaluated negatively, it is not because they are artificial, but because they fail to properly respect all the persons and human goods involved.

Moral evaluation of the kind found in the *Instruction* is common enough in human life. When carried out by the authorized teachers of the Church, it has the distinctive character of Christian moral teaching. As teaching by those especially empowered by Christ to teach, it differs from ordinary moral evaluation in being more than simply the opinion of one person or group to be accepted only on the basis of one's estimate of the merits of the arguments presented. Still, Christian moral teaching is teaching. It is not giving orders or handing down decrees. It is not, in other words, like the exercise of legitimate political or legal authority in which legislators or judges make decisions which others have some duty to obey. In the case of such decisions, which must be made within the Church as well as in political society, the issue is not the truth of the decision, but its wisdom and legitimacy. In the case of moral teaching, by contrast, the issue is fundamentally one of truth.

That is why the authors of the *Instruction* proceed as they do. Like Christian teachers generally, they do not simply issue edicts, but present moral reasons. They appeal to the vision of human life which is found in the Scriptures and has been constantly taught within the Church, and apply it to questions which trouble the faithful and people generally. This application involves highlighting especially relevant aspects of this vision, and considering carefully how certain human actions are to be evaluated in light of them.

So the *Instruction* is literally that: instruction, teaching. Contrary to the impressions created by the way the media often characterize Church teaching, especially about moral questions, the Instruction is not upholding a ban or issuing a condemnation, but providing a reasoned evaluation. As such, it is meant to invite reflection. Indeed, in its closing paragraphs, the Instruction makes explicit this invitation. Proper orders are to be obeyed, but teaching is to be pondered, understood, and personally appropriated.

II. THE PRINCIPLES UNDERLYING THE INSTRUCTION'S TEACHING

The elements of the Christian vision of human life highlighted in the *Instruction* are those relating to the conception of the human person, the nature of marriage and sexuality, and the sacredness of human life. The most important of these can be expressed as five propositions which function as principles for the evaluation of the particular concerns of the *Instruction*. First, God makes human individuals in His own image and likeness, and He is directly involved in the coming-to-be of each new person. Second, the human person is one being, bodily as well as spiritual, so bodily life and sexuality may not be treated as mere means to more fundamental purposes. Third, every living human individual, from the moment of conception, should be treated with the full respect due a person and so is inviolable. A human being is always a he or a she, an I or a you, never an object, a mere something. Fourth, sexual activity and procreation can be morally good only if they are part of marital intercourse. Fifth, in marital intercourse, love-making and life-giving should not be separated.

These principles underlie the Church's teaching concerning all the issues in sexual morality, bioethics, and respect for human life. Not surprisingly, therefore, the moral outlook of the Instruction is identical to that of *Humanae Vitae* the *Decree on Procured Abortion* and *Familiaris Consortio.* In fact, the *Instruction* explicitly relies on these and other recent magisterial statements, especially those of John Paul II and Pius XII. All the principles used in the *Instruction* are to be found in these earlier magisterial statements where they are much more fully articulated and defended.

What is distinctive about the *Instruction* is that it applies these principles to a related set of current questions which have not been evaluated before in a systematic and unified manner. Thus, the *Instruction* makes use of these principles, but generally does not seek to establish their truth or demonstrate their special place within the Christian view of human life. Rather, their truth is reasonably taken for granted as fixed within the teaching of the Church, knowable by the natural moral law, and amply explained and defended in recent Church teaching.

It is a mistake, therefore, to suppose that one can find in the *Instruction* an attempt to persuade those who reject its principles. Since dissenting theologians and many outside the Church reject at least some of these principles, it is not surprising that the *Instruction* has been found unpersuasive by many. But that is no criticism of the *Instruction*. Its task is to deal with certain questions of the day, not defend, from the ground up, the entire fabric of Christian ethics as understood within the Church. A fairer question, then, is whether the *Instruction's* evaluation of various procedures is justified by these principles, and by the larger vision of human life of which they are part. As will become clear, even in this short overview of the *Instruction*, the *Instruction's* evaluations clearly are justified by this standard.

This is not to suggest that there are no difficulties in understanding the precise ways in which these principles are applied to the specific actions evaluated. For example, there is considerable unclarity about how the principle of the inseparability of the love-making and life-giving aspects of marital intercourse actually applies to such things as artificial insemination by husband and *in vitro* fertilization within marriage.

Further, the *Instruction* does contain some argumentation in support of at least some of its principles, in particular the principle requiring that all living human individuals be treated as persons from the moment of conception. *The Instruction's* argument emphasizes the continuity of the development of human life from the moment of conception, and, while recognizing that science cannot by itself resolve all the problems in this area, and that purely speculative questions about the moment of ensoulment cannot be definitively settled, concludes that there is an indefeasible presumption in favor of the personhood of every living individual. "How could a human individual not be a human person?"

This argumentation seems sound as far as it goes, but given the importance of this principle, not only for the Church's overall sanctity of life stance, but also for the immediately relevant question of the status of the embryo immediately after conception, one might reasonably expect a more extended and analytical treatment. It seems to me that the following considerations might reasonably be added to what the *Instruction* actually says. First, the only thing all those whom we consider persons have in common is that they are all human individuals. By what non-arbitrary criterion could the newly conceived human individual be excluded from personal status? Second, there is no doubt that the newly conceived is a human individual. The possibilities of twinning and mosaics do not show that the individuals who can divide or combine are not living human individuals. Third, medieval theorizing about the beginning of life supposed that life came from non-living materials. Unhampered by this false view, we have no such reason for thinking that the developing individual cannot be a person from the outset.

III. ACTS JUDGED MORALLY PERMISSIBLE

The *Instruction* considers carefully a number of perplexing questions concerning the treatment of the unborn. The basic principle used to evaluate these matters is that as persons, the unborn deserve the same moral consideration as other persons. Thus prenatal diagnosis and treatment, including experimental treatment if that is the best one can do, are permissible if done for the child's benefit under the same conditions as would apply for children already born. Likewise, research, (that is, observation), upon the unborn is permissible if it is harmless and done with parental consent.

The same principle is extended to deal with the question of the handling of the corpses of the unborn. They are to be treated with the same respect due, any human corpse. Thus, experimentation upon the corpses of the unborn may be permissible, although under stringent conditions. Experimentation may be permissible upon the corpses of those deliberately aborted if the conditions are met. Those conditions are the following: first, that one be certain that the individual is dead; that it is a corpse and not a living person; second, that the consent of the parents or at least the mother be obtained; third, that there be no complicity in deliberate abortion; fourth, that scandal be avoided; and fifth, that human remains not be bought and sold.

Closely related to the questions of the treatment of the unborn are attempts to influence inheritance. Such efforts are justified if done for therapeutic benefit of the person treated, if the usual conditions for therapy apply, and if the special character of the risks is properly taken into account.

The *Instruction* also deals with technical interventions in the reproductive process. It finds some of the most familiar of these unacceptable, but judges morally acceptable those interventions which facilitate the performance of the marital act and those which enable the marital act to be fruitful. The *Instruction* does not say exactly what these procedures are, but the general idea is both important and clear: interventions which do not replace or substitute for the marital act as the human activity which brings forth new life, but assist the act in having this result, are morally permissible. How this distinction is to be applied to such procedures as Gamete Interfallopian Transfer (GIFT), or Tubal Ovum Transfer (TOT) is not addressed in the Instruction and is in dispute among moralists who accept its teaching.

IV. ACTS JUDGED MORALLY IMPERMISSIBLE

Experimentation upon the unborn, at any stage of development, is categorically rejected. "Experimentation", here, refers to nontherapeutic experimentation, and seems to include any kind of research which has even slightly adverse effects on the subject. I say "seems", because the explanation of the distinction between experimentation and research is perhaps the least perspicuous explanation in the *Instruction*. The *Instruction's* concern, however, is in no way obscure. No human being is to be treated as if he/she were a mere means for the satisfaction of the needs of others. Every person is to be loved and respected for his or her own sake.

Similarly rejected as incompatible with the human dignity of the unborn is the production of embryos to be used as experimental materials, or to be wasted incidentally to *in vitro* fertilization.

A variety of other techniques, actual and possible, are also rejected, both because they fail to respect the personal dignity of the subject, and because they fail to respect every person's right to be born in and from marriage. Thus, asexual reproduction, combining human and animal gametes, the gestation of humans in animal or artificial uteruses, the freezing of human embryos, even to save their lives, and non-therapeutic attempts to influence inheritance are all rejected as immoral. The *Instruction's* treatment of these questions is very brief, and will, no doubt, have to be spelled out as these procedures become more available.

The freezing of embryos is already being done, so it is worth considering the *Instruction's* briefly stated reason for rejecting it. This procedure is wrong because it exposes the embryo to grave risks of death and bodily harm as well as placing it in a situation in which further manipulation and offense is possible. It also deprives the embryo of maternal shelter and gestation. This account needs amplification. Clearly it shows that it is absolutely wrong to bring a person into existence with the intention of freezing him/her. But once the individual is brought into being outside his/her mother's body, the risk to life and health of not freezing may be as great as that of freezing, and the mother's womb may be simply unavailable. Amplification of the argument is needed to show that in this situation the threat of future offense and manipulation is sufficient to absolutely exclude freezing.

The *Instruction's* concern that very young and vulnerable individuals not be put unreasonably at risk, manipulated, abused or "wasted", underlies its specific judgment on the morality of *in vitro* fertilization. As actually practiced, IVF involves all of these harms to the embryo. All of them are made possible by the fact that the embryo comes to be and lives for a time outside of his or her mother's body.

But the *Instruction's* evaluation of IVF and other technological interventions used to cope with infertility is not based on concerns about the welfare of the newly conceived individual. Concerns about the relationship between

23

procreation, marriage and the marital act are also operative. These two types of concern are closely connected. The Church's conviction that procreation should take place within marriage is based on the belief that the family provides the only context within which a child can come to be and develop in a way compatible with his or her human dignity. The unity and fidelity of husband and wife are essential for the communion of the family, and have their special character because of the family's orientation toward procreation and the nurturing of children. The goods of marriage, the goods of spouses and their children, are inextricably woven together. Acts which seek some of these goods outside marriage, or seek some of them while disregarding others, cannot, in the end, fail to harm them all. That is at least part of the sense of the principle of the inseparability of the various meanings of the marital act.

Thus the *Instruction* rejects all extramarital uses of procedures like IVF and artificial insemination, simply because they are extramarital. The clearest examples of such uses are those in which non-married people use them to have children outside the context of marriage. The most notorious are the well known, if misnamed, cases of surrogate motherhood in which a woman conceives and carries a child for a couple whose husband provides the sperm. The commonest are those in which sperm is obtained from a donor for use by way of artificial insemination. A similar situation would arise if ova were donated for use by way of *in vitro* fertilization.

The degree and character of the separation of procreation and marriage vary considerably among these procedures. But they are all extramarital in the relevant sense, for even in those cases in which the reproductive activities take place within the context of marriage, the child does not come to be *from* the marriage. When third parties provide the gametes, it is impossible to meet what the *Instruction* regards as a necessary condition for responsible procreation that the child be "the fruit and the sign of the mutual self-giving of the spouses, of their love, and of their fidelity" (Section II, A).

Many balk at this reason. They note that in many cases the use of donor sperm, for example, is done for the most loving of motives. The very fact that a couple is willing to undertake such measures shows real love and self-giving. The *Instruction* does not deny this. Its point is more precise. It is pretense to tell oneself that reproduction using donated gametes is literally the fruit of a couple's marital acts. It is, strictly speaking, the result of the technological intervention in which the donor's gametes are joined to those of one of the spouses.

Many, however, do not see why this should be morally objectionable. Why should procreation be so tightly tied to marital intercourse as the quoted condition requires? The *Instruction's* emphasis on the inseparability of the unitive and procreative meanings of the marital act is not sufficient to answer this question because, in effect, it asks for the rationale behind this principle's application to reproductive technologies. The reason seems to lie in a conviction which is stated in the *Instruction,* but does not emerge as a full-fledged argument--namely, that in reproductive activities which do not meet its condition, the child in its coming-to-be is treated as an object, a thing and not a person.

The sign and the fruit of an action of mutual self-giving are not products made, but are a gift and blessing welcomed. By contrast, the results of productive activities cannot but be regarded as things having a status inferior to those who make them. The communion of the family must always be a communion among persons, all of whose equal personal dignity is to be respected. It hardly needs saying, therefore, ,that the babies brought into being by procedures rejected by the *Instruction* are in no way condemned or disvalued. It is because these procedures require that the babies be treated in a way incompatible with their true human status that the procedures must be rejected.

The *Instruction* provides, therefore, a rationale for excluding not only the separation of procreation from marriage by the use of donor gametes, but also the kind of separation of procreation from marital intercourse which occurs even within marriage when the gametes of the spouses are joined by technological procedures which replace the marital act. These activities are excluded, in other words, not only because in IVF they place the newly conceived individual at risk, and because in IVF and artificial insemination using the husband's sperm they involve masturbation to obtain the sperm, but because they separate procreation from marital intercourse. The masturbation, as the *Instruction* observes, is a sign of this separation.

V. IMPLICATIONS OF THESE JUDGMENTS FOR VARIOUS PERSONS

The substantive moral judgments of the *Instruction* have implications for various persons having diverse responsibilities. The implications for infertile couples and those who advise and assist them are plain. They may, of course, seek legitimate therapies to overcome infertility, but they must recognize that no one has a right to a child. A child is a person, not a thing, and one cannot have rights to persons. One may desire a child as one desires a blessing or a gift; one does not have a right to a blessing. Sterility, therefore, is a cross, often a terrible one, which some people must bear, and others must help them bear.

It seems to me that the alternative to this understanding of sterility is to suppose that couples may do anything to have a child, but the willingness to do anything to have a child suggests a possessiveness although at odds with the attitude of service required of those who would be good parents. Supporting possessive desires towards other persons hardly qualifies as Christian compassion.

The desire of a couple to have children is natural. It can be quite exigent and can cause terrible suffering if unfulfilled. Yet there is no desire which an upright person will not carefully scrutinize, particularly when its fulfillment affects central human relationships. The desire to have children is, therefore, not beyond moral scrutiny. Indeed, human life abounds with examples in which is provided unworthy motivation, for example, cases in which people seek children simply to continue a dynasty or family name, or cases in which people seek children simply as an insurance policy for old age. The *Instruction*, in effect, asks us to consider the motivations behind decisions to use artificial insemination and *in vitro* fertilization, and in particular, to ask whether the child so desperately wanted is desired simply to fulfill the couple's emotional needs. If that is why they want a child, then it is hard to see the difference between wanting a child and wanting a thing one finds very desirable. But children are not things, and being a parent is not having possession, but serving life, cooperating with God in a marvelous activity which is profaned by reduction to the categories of production and desire satisfaction.

The special implications of the *Instruction's* judgments for physicians are closely related: the basis for medical ethics should be service to people's lives and health, and respect for the values of human sexuality. Thus, physicians have no business disposing of people, and they should not take over the reproductive function. Catholic physicians, scientists and health care facilities should bear witness by carefully observing the relevant norms. The Instruction acknowledges the great good which has been accomplished by scientific and medical efforts to deal with infertility. Physicians and scientists are urgently requested to continue this work to find ways of dealing with infertility which are both effective and fully respectful of the dignity of marriage, of spouses and of their offspring.

The implications of the Instructions' judgments for legislators and civil authorities are based on the principle that civil law should protect human rights, in particular the right of every person to life from the moment of conception, and should protect the family and marriage. Thus, there should be laws forbidding all killing of innocent human beings, all genesis of human life in which the materials are not from a married couple, surrogate motherhood, embryo banks, and post-mortem insemination. The *Instruction* does not say that all its moral judgments should be legally enforced.

The *Instruction* closes with a plea for further study of the issues it considers, especially by moralists. This plea is not a suggestion that its specific conclusions are tentative or revisable, but rather is a recognition of how difficult these issues are, and how hard it is to adequately understand them. This reflection is called for because of the importance of correctly understanding the reasons for and the validity of the *Instruction's* teaching. It is to be carried out "in unrenounceable fidelity to the teaching of the Church".

ENDNOTE

[1] Reprinted with permission from the article "An Introduction to the Vatican Instruction on Reproductive Technologies," Linacre Quarterly 55 (July 1988): 20-28.

3

The Teaching Authority of the Church and Its Relation to Reproductive Issues

Rev. Ronald Lawler, O.F.M., Cap.

Reflecting on the magnificent technological advances of our age, and on our frequently manifested inability to make wise and good choices about how to live with them and use them, the Second Vatican Council declared: "Our era needs more wisdom than bygone ages if the discoveries made by man are to be truly human. For the future of the world stands in peril unless wiser men are forthcoming."[1]

In our era we have grasped atomic power and we have created astonishing weapons. We have created communications media with mighty powers to affect the minds and hearts of men. We have even crafted new ways to bring human beings into existence, and we foresee arts of shaping radically the new persons we have acquired the power to make.

It is exhilarating to have great power. But we know also that it is dangerous; for while we have much power, we do not know how to use well the power we have. We are very unsure about whether it is good to do the things we have power to do. In too many ways we risk destroying ourselves and our hopes.

I. FAITH GIVES LIGHT ON NEW QUESTIONS

The Catholic Church believes that she has a duty to reflect on new questions about the generation of human life in the light of Gospel teachings about man, and in the light of moral principles. These moral principles she knows both from that natural law that lies within the heart of every man, and also from the Gospel.

It is most true that one cannot find in the Gospel the assertion that *"in vitro* fertilization is unacceptable" or that "amniocentesis is in some circumstances immoral." Nowhere does the New Testament assert that homologous artificial insemination is forbidden by the Lord.

But faith does know many principles that cast light on these subjects. How to enable apparently sterile spouses to become parents in the safest and most promising ways is a scientific question. But the question whether it is right and good to adopt one of the possible procedures for doing this is a moral question. And right answers to moral questions depend on right visions about man and moral conduct--about what it is to be a human person, and how human persons should live to be faithful to what they are. Hence the most central teachings of Catholic faith cast light on how we are to respond to questions never raised in New Testament days.

One must have some clear idea of what it is to be a human being to know securely what one is doing when one terminates the life of a fertilized ovum: is one then killing a human being, or simply keeping some genetic material from becoming a human being? Could one actually be a human being when one by no means looks like a human being? Is it permissible to end the life of such a small thing, about which many debates rage, and concerning which many calm and contradictory dogmas are erected, if being willing to do so might enable us to accomplish wonderful things, even to make new babies, for other people?

These questions are not scientific questions, but moral and human questions: answers to them depend largely on what a human being is, and on the ways of acting that become the dignity of persons. Principles of such moral thinking are not new to the Church. The Church does not claim a special scientific expertise, but she professes to be an "expert in humanity,"[2] because she reflects faithfully on the teaching of Christ.

If every human being is a determined being, whose choices and acts will necessarily serve his most pressing needs and desires; if a human being is so shaped by his culture that he must act in accord with the pressures of that culture; if man is a technological animal, if his central meaning is technological progress ... If these or other secular visions of man are true, then the right decision on how to act in our new questions will be of one form.

But Catholic faith has a different vision of what the human person is, and what he can become, and of the grandeur God made every human being to share.[3] Her vision is one that she professes to be entirely certain of. In Christ, faith begins to understand the *mystery of man*. In faith we begin to understand the mystery of our own humanity, and how we are to live freely in ways that become human persons and children of God.

This vision of man: in which each human being, however poor and useless, has a worth and dignity beyond the sun and all the stars; this vision, that the most trivial human being, the youngest and the weakest and the most helpless, has the same human rights that the greatest human persons have--is one shared by much of human civilization, west and east. And indeed it is to all men that the Church wishes to speak of matters important to every man. To all she speaks in the light of the Gospel which is graspable to every human intelligence: in dealing with matters of such elemental importance as bringing human persons into being, we must consult not only the powers and skills of men, but also our central moral principles.

First I shall speak of what the Catholic Church actually teaches about new technologies of bringing human beings into existence, and about the duty to treat every human being as a person.

II. CHURCH TEACHING ON THE ARTIFICIAL GENERATION OF CHILDREN

In the nineteeth century, when technologies of artificial generation were first commended for human use, the Church spoke of the need to provide moral guidance for this most sensitive of human applications of technology. Already in 1887, the Church insisted that artificial insemination of a woman is immoral.[4] Subsequent papal teaching consistently expounded and developed her teaching about distinguishing ways in which scientific and medical ways of helping parents have children were human, wise, and good, and ways which involved failure to give minimal respect to basic human goods in the pursuit of attractive goals. Until the last two decades of dissent there was almost universal Catholic support for this teaching.[5]

But in the last few decades the situation has changed dramatically. This has been a time of moral confusion everywhere: a time of straining at the moral roots of mankind generally in a time of wrenching change; and for Catholics it has been a time of painful disorder and dissent in the Church. At the same time, it has been a time in which there have been many specific problems that have deeply intensified the longing for scientific help in providing children for those who could not otherwise have them. For a variety of reasons the rates of infertility have risen sharply. There has been a greater demand for scientific help to have children. And there has been great technological progress: there are brilliant new methods that fascinate the imagination, even if they may run counter to principles that Catholic faith and natural human morality ought not abandon.

In 1987, a century after its first judgment on artificial insemination, the Holy See published its *Instruction on Respect for Human Life in its Origin and on the Dignity of Procreation (Donum vitae).* This document is far richer in content than earlier papal teachings on the artificial generation of children, and presents a surprisingly large number of specific teachings related to artificial generation. These are not just the opinions of Cardinal Ratzinger or Pope John Paul II on the questions at hand. They are the *teachings* of the Catholic Church on these matters. Still the document is a very brief pamphlet. Its chief purpose is to state the teaching of Catholic faith in an important area: it does not present in any detail vigorous arguments for each of its positions. It does offer brief accounts of why the various teachings are judged to be right: but the document is addressed primarily to Church leaders and scholars who know the history and context of the questions addressed.

Rather than provide a persuasive account of all its teaching, the document leaves to scholars the task of drawing upon all the sources of Church teaching in this area in order to make the teaching appear clearly to be true and good. Those who read this sketchy document (from a position of firm commitment to other stances in this area) have often protested that the document is "unpersuasive." Such a judgment exhibits a misunderstanding of the nature of the document: it is not an effort to persuade people that Catholic teaching is right, but an effort to present that teaching briefly, and to invite the Christian and human community to share in the task of making persuasive positions of whose truth and goodness the Church is certain both by faith and by reflective thinking.

Meaning of "Catholic Teaching"

Let us offer here a brief account of the basic idea of *teachings of the Church*. "Teachings" are not commands, laws, or orders. When one teaches, he is not issuing imperatives, but making known what is true or truly good. When the Church *teaches* she is not offering opinions. Rather she is handing on what she has learned from Christ, what she knows with certainty, and presents to others for their confident assent. What she teaches here she claims to have learned from Christ, not in the sense that he has been personally perceived applying his principles directly to these questions that have arisen only in our time. Rather, he has given to his Church resources, in the vision of man he gives, in the values that he has taught, in the moral forms of teaching; and he has been present to his Church, guiding those who teach in his name, keeping secure the proclamation of his word. As they apply his teaching to new questions, he and his Holy Spirit guard them in the truth, giving them the sure charism of truth. To his faithful he gives the gifts that lead to recognizing Christ's teaching in those he has sent; leading them to assent with freedom and joy to what he himself teaches in the midst of those he has sent.[6]

The Church *teaches* only that which she is certain of in faith. She has long known and taught that it is wrong to speak of grave duties to believe and to act, if one is not certain that these are real duties.

And when the Church *teaches* she is not uttering statements from without, and demanding assent from people who are humiliated by requirements to hold what they themselves find wrong or evil. To teach has always been a service aimed at leading into freedom and truth. One does not teach another mathematics by making a student mechanically assert what he or she does not see or know because the teacher demands that the student conform to the teacher's will. To teach is, in ordinary and natural things, to draw knowledge out of a student rather than forcing opinions in. The teacher seeks to enable the learner to see for himself, from things that the student already knew, that something he once did not know is in fact so. The mathematics teacher enables the learner to see personally, to be set free from every error, and to grasp securely with his own intellect what the teacher guides the hearer to grasp.

Teaching faith is very much like this. The believer does not naturally know the mysteries of faith, nor does he naturally know with the firmness of faith the natural truths (such as, that God is, that the moral requirements of Christian living are good, that the human person does not fully die at death); that they are part of the gift of faith. But the believer, just as he has been given natural intelligence that makes a teaching toward truth possible, has also a gift of faith. When one sent by Christ, as the apostles and their successors, teaches in his name and by the power of his grace, the revealed word of God, the believer,

in the light of his own faith, knows in faith that this message is true.[7]
One might say, rather, certainty that this saying is true is accessible to him.
Just as the teacher cannot teach mathematics to one who resists and will not see,
the teacher of faith cannot lead into its light one who will not come. The
Catholic believer knows out of his own faith, out of a gift he personally
possesses, that when the leaders of the family of faith teach as certain, in the
name of Christ, matters of faith and morals, that it is good and right for him to
give religious and free assent to this teaching.

When the Church teaches matters that can be known to be true both by reason
and by the gift of faith, it appeals both to the natural intelligence and to
motives proper to faith. Those who have faith are invited to share the truths
proclaimed first of all as believers, as people who have found that Christ teaches
in his Church when his spokesmen teach in his name as surely as he baptizes when
one baptizes in his name; and knowing that he teaches, they accept his word, just
as they acknowledge the power of baptism, because they recognize that he baptizes
when a mere human being baptizes. Christ teaches in various ways in the Church;
when the Church teaches infallibly, by its ordinary or extraordinary magisterium,
the baptized hearer is able to recognize that Christ gives an unshakable warrant:
this he may firmly hold to the very word of God, and most certainly true. When
the teaching is less absolute, when the Church teaches authoritatively (as having
a confident certainty rooted in the Gospel, but not proclaiming the word as one
proposed definitively), she does not unconditionally assert the word so proclaimed
as simply God's word and entirely irreformable. Rather, she teaches that this is
to be held, and securely, as taught by those Christ has sent, in whom Christ calls
all to unity of faith; a teaching that Christ will not allow to do harm to those
who seek to find his word and do his will.

Teachings of the Church not infallibly proposed (teaching proposed by the
Church as certain, but not as now infallibly proposed) may indeed be subject to
further reflection; problems not now envisaged may later lead to revisions that
make it more faithful to and expressive of the whole Gospel.[8] But though
one does not have an infallible warrant for truths not infallibly taught, one does
have a real certainty of another kind: a certainty that Christ now wants me to
hear and heed his Church, and to assent to what the Church insistently teaches,
because his presence in and his gifts to the Church give me a better ground for
holding to her teaching, than to the uncertain arguments that a culture or an
individual can raise against it.[9] (Whenever there would be a certain knowledge on a hearer's part that what the Church has taught in a non-infallible way
is not in fact true, the hearer would not, of course, have a duty to hold it.
This certainty can be had, but only in unusual cases: e.g., when a bishop might
teach insistently something that the hearer knows certainly to be in contradiction
to what the Church has infallibly taught.)[10]

But when one is "certain" that the Church is wrong, because it contradicts
when the hearer--influenced by an unbelieving culture--finds in plain contradiction to "truths" or values to which he has committed himself, this is no real
certainty. One has a better reason to believe what the Church speaks in the name
of Christ, than what one holds because of manifestly uncertain grounds. One who

has come to an intelligent faith has excellent reasons for believing what the Church teaches, even when she is bearing witness to Christ's teaching with her ordinary God-given authority, and not in the most definitive and even infallible way in which she teaches at times.

Survey of Church Teachings

Let us survey quickly the range of teachings found in *Donum vitae*. Here I wish merely to provide a brief picture of the broad scope of the document. It teaches with a clearness and specificity more positions in this area than the Church had previously taught: yet there is a clear consistency with her past teaching, and with the moral principles that have guided all Catholic moral teachings in its efforts to assist people to live in the light of faith and in accord with the demands of every human value.

The first set of teachings in *Donum vitae* is concerned with respect for every human being, and rejects whatever would treat some human beings as if they were not persons. (1) First it states a basic principle: every human being must be respected as a person. Every human being: without excluding those whom it might be convenient to withdraw acknowledgment of humanity and the rights that cme with being a human being. Every human being: from the very first moment of his or her existence, from fertilization (I,1). (2) Hence, while prenatal diagnoses (as amniocentesis) are permissible if they are aimed simply at healing detectable disorders, it would be illicit to engage in them if one intends to eliminate defective fetuses that are detected (I,2,3). (3) There must be no research on live embryos (for these are young living human beings) unless there is both a moral certainty that it will not harm the child, and the parents have given free and informed consent (I,4). (4) Embryos obtained by fertilization *in vitro* are also living human beings; to use them as disposable biological material, or to kill them, is immoral (I,5). (5) The manipulation of embryos in acts such as gestation of them in the uterus of animals, freezing them, or the non-therapeutic manipulation of genes, is immoral (I,6).

Another set of teachings is aimed at defending the essential nature and dignity of human procreative acts. The Church draws this teaching from her long history of reflecting on what the Gospel teaches about love, and life, and of how reverently life is to be brought into this world. One should have reverence and awe, and protective concern, for acts that summon a new human person into being. Every human being is of great concern to God. Even if a scientist (rightly or wrongly) unites the gametes, it is God who creates the soul. God calls each person into being with great love, and the human beings who call others into being should also act through acts of love. Here the Church teaches (1) that human procreation must take place within marriage (II,1). (2) Heterologous artificial fertilization--obtaining a human conception by using sperm or ovum coming from at least one donor other than the spouses--is illicit (II,2). (3) Surrogate motherhood is morally illicit (II,3). (4) Effecting procreation by acts which are not acts of human love, the result of the act of sexual intercourse in marriage, are immoral (II,4). Hence homologous IVF is always morally illicit, even if it involves no killing of surplus embryos and no masturbation (i.e., even the "simple case" is wrong (II,5). (5) Homologous artificial insemination, in which the implanting of the semen by artificial means in fact replaces the conjugal act, is immoral (II,6). (6) A child is a gift; no one has a right to a child. Similarly, no one has a right to procure a child by these kinds of acts.

In all this the Church does not at all reject scientific assistance to parents who long for children. The Church favors efforts to help the apparently sterile conceive;[11] and there are many ways of progressing in this area without utilizing means that suffer from moral disorders. Efforts to restore fertility to prospective parents, so that they may conceive their own children (as in microsurgery) have no moral objections, and often have higher success rates than using artificial technologies in cases in which microsurgery is also applicable. Methods in which the physician does not replace the parents as the one actively bringing about the actual origin of life, but rather assists parents in their acts of marital love so that the generative act they themselves perform may be made fruitful with skilled assistance.

The Church here also teaches certain points touching civil law, and the way in which civil law should protect life and the family in the light of the truths taught in this document.

All these positions the Church teaches to be true, and to be good. It teaches that they flow from essential elements of the teaching she has received from Christ. She teaches that all who have the gift of Catholic faith have the duty to adhere to these teachings that are needed to defend the human person and to guard the integrity and goodness of acts that summon persons into being.

III. REACTIONS TO THE TEACHING OF DONUM VITAE

Reactions to the 1987 Instruction were varied. Many Catholics and many outside the faith welcomed the document warmly. The bringing into being of new human persons is one of the deepest concerns of the human race. There is a certain manifest beauty in the ordinary and normal way of generating children. How suitable it is that a child should be born out of an act of love between its parents, that the child should be a gift of God's love to the parents' love. This means much more than technological and other acts extrinsically motivated by love: it means acts that are of their very nature and inner meaning essential acts of love. Memories of *A Brave New World* and fears that eugenic dreams should be rekindled as technologies became more powerful led many to be grateful to stern cautions about placing the generating of children into the hands of technicians. The document appeared at a time when the mass media in the United States was revealing the tragic consequences of a New Jersey case of surrogate motherhood.

But many others reacted angrily to the Church document. They saw it as breath-taking blunt. Certainly, some replied, cautions are needed in the use of these new technologies. But surely (they argued) we must respect also the brilliant mastery of the world that these new methods reveal. There is a great need for these technologies. In an age of tragic increases in sterility, when science has given hope to those who long for children they cannot have in ordinary ways; the Church ought not flatly condemn almost every new way to restore hope to many.

Many who rejected the Church's teaching seemed to suppose that because good things are achieved by IVF and artificial insemination, the practices themselves must be good. This is obviously false. Many good things are achieved by evil means. It is of course obvious that the artificial technologies of conception lead to many good results: to wonderful babies, to astonishing advances in human skills, to a rich growth in human knowledge. But most of all, it gives to those who long for them wonderful babies. "The last time I saw her," Dr. Robert Edwards said of the newly born Louise Brown, the first test tube baby, "she was just eight cells in a test tube. She was beautiful then, and she's beautiful now."[12]

Unfortunately, it is also true that the worst moments in medical morality can come when--precisely because we are in pursuit of important goals--we neglect adequate ethical reflection. It is especially easy to make major moral errors when questionable behavior seems to pay off so well. When we seem to have grand reasons for rushing forward, we are most likely to refuse to take sufficiently into account every important moral consideration.

The most severe criticisms of *Donum vitae* came, as was expected, from Catholics who disagree with very basic moral teachings of the Church, or from groups influenced by such dissenting Catholics.[13] For example, the Ethics Committee of the American Fertility Society published a very severe critique of *Donum vitae* in a supplement to the February, 1988 issue of *Fertility and Sterility*. (Jesuit Father Richard McCormick is a member of that committee.) This critique of the Holy See's teaching argued that there is a "very broad ecumenical and scientific consensus" that disagrees with much of what the document says. "No other national committee or other religious body" has rejected certain of the procedures this document rejects. The critique continues with a stinging rebuke: "The Committee believes that such consensus reflects *basic known human experience and intuition* about the morally appropriate and inappropriate. The *Instruction* seems to take no account of this consensus, but to rely exclusively (sic!) on previous ecclesiastical pronouncements."[14] Refusing to recognize that this brief document is to be studied in the context of all Catholic teaching, or to consider it possible that "official" Catholic teaching might have an intelligent defense, the critique testily claims that the Catholic position on the sacredness of every life at every stage of its being is "set forth without any rational basis".[15] Again it complains that the document does not rely solely on biological evidence to establish a certain point, has recourse to "a predetermined position (revelation) that is not persuasive." Obviously so gross a critique reveals no understanding of the logic and pattern of Catholic thinking, and contributes almost nothing to serious discussion of the important issues at hand.

IV. AUTHORITY OF THIS DOCUMENT'S TEACHING:

Why so many Catholics rightly accept it

It is not surprising, in this time of hostility to authority and to institutions, that many Catholics profess a right to reject teachings of the Church for very broad reasons. But great numbers of Catholics welcomed all the teaching of this document gladly, and judge that they had excellent reasons to accept it: the whole array of reasons that have led them to Catholic faith, and the special reasons they see imminent in the Church teaching here, join in giving the reasons to accept the teachings of Catholic faith in this matter.

For Catholics have commonly believed that acceptance of papal teaching is not mere acceptance of a certain man's opinions. It is acceptance of the teaching of the Church: and so it is accepting the teaching of Christ. For the Church is a place in which Christ himself teaches. Because through the gift of faith they have found Christ in his Catholic Church, they are not embarrassed to believe what the Church teaches in his name. They must indeed, to be coherent, have good reasons for believing who Christ is and that he teaches now in his Church. The Catholic believes the teachings of the Church because he has come to believe that it is Christ himself who assures him of the wisdom of accepting what the Church teaches. Catholics regularly have believed: Christ is the teacher of life. He has taught, and he causes to be taught in his Church, a way of life that is wise and good. The moral teaching of the Church is held to be a natural law teaching, that is, a teaching that can be grasped by intelligent reflection: even if we had no faith, it is in principle possible to see the solid reasons for this teaching. But the teaching is in fact also revealed. Most Catholics are not skilled ethicians; they can be confused by the complex moral debates of the time. And it is important if they are to have a good life that they have a sure grasp on what really is good and pleasing to God. One can know truth in moral matters not only by argument, but also by faith: for the way of Christ is taught in the Church, and He promises to remain with the Church until the end of the age.[16]

An immediate objection arises, one we have noted before. How can one say that Christ teaches such new and specific things as *Donum vitae* treats? Does Christ himself teach that heterologous conception is immoral or that *in vitro* fertilization is wrong? Many of the teachings in this document are new teachings; and no one pretends that Christ whispered into the ears of Church officials the correct answers to difficult contemporary questions.

Even in this document the Church suggests the answer to this question.[17] Christ does not answer new questions that arise in the Church by whispering answers. But he does teach us by his quiet presence, guarding in the Church the saving truth that the Gospel has given. The whole message of faith once given to the Church has resources for illuminating problems of every age. But it is a serious responsibility for the Church to face these questions with honest resolve: to say what must be said about *in vitro* fertilization in the light of what the Gospel teaches us about the dignity of persons, and sexual love, and the values we must guard always.

But in saying what *Donum vitae* says of Church teaching in this area, that it flows from central teaching of faith about man, about love, and life, are we suggesting that everything the Church taught in *Donum vitae* is infallible? The brief answer to this is no: while the Church has an intelligent, faith-grounded basis for what she teaches here, she does not present teachings about all these new questions as infallible.

Catholic faith indeed believes that the Church teaches infallibly at times in matters of faith and morals. She believes that Christ is with the family of faith and leads her securely to right answers to pressing questions; and he is able to mark teaching in some cases with signs that show that what is taught is indeed his word, and worthy of our unconditional belief. Faith holds that what is taught in certain ways by bishops scattered over the whole world, or in solemn definitions of councils and popes, must be recognized as declaring the word of the Lord, and is most certainly true.[18]

Some things in the document on the dignity of life and procreation are, I am convinced, infallible teachings of the Church: as the teaching that it is always gravely wrong to directly kill an innocent human being (however young) for any reason whatever.

But many teachings here seem clearly not to be infallibly taught. The Holy Father obliges all to apply Gospel teaching to new questions. Christ, who is quietly with the Church, and is grasped by faith, not immediate experience, guards his flock in these times of development of doctrine. The Gospel portrays him as requiring his disciples to believe and heed what those whom he has sent declare, in proclaiming the Gospel and in applying it to life. Hence he guards the Church in the truth; but not in such a way that all Church teaching is infallible.

How sure are we that every principle in this document is absolutely true? We are not absolutely sure. Many of these teachings have not been taught with moral unanimity by all bishops everywhere, and certainly they have not been solemnly defined. For example, the teaching that no research may be done on embryos if there is a risk of any injury at all, however slight;[19] this could conceivably later be judged in need of more precise formulation, even correction. Nothing in Church teaching urges that such a teaching be counted as infallibly proposed.

But how sure is the Church teaching that all Catholics must not reject these teachings, and must not publicly assail them? This is a most certain Church teaching: from the first days of the early Church the canonical writers, the first fathers, have spoken of the duty to attend to, to accept and live by, the teaching of the bishops of the Church.

The teaching of the bishop of Rome has had a special authority: for he is the center of unity for faith, the successor of Peter, and the vicar of Christ in a most special way. For centuries Church teaching and practice have proclaimed the duty not to contradict the firm judgment of the Holy Father in matters of faith and morals, even when he is not teaching in an infallible manner. The teachings of the last two ecumenical councils on this point have helped make clear the firmness of Catholic teaching. It may well be argued that when the pope speaks simply in an authoritative mode, what he teaches may not be irreformable, but it is infallibly certain that we have a duty not to contradict and seek to persuade others to reject his teaching. For the Church everywhere, in the morally unanimous voice of its bishops (and even of its theologians) has taught for centuries (in a way that surely seems to fulfill the conditions spelled out by Vatican II for infallibility in the ordinary magisterium)[20] that one owes reverent assent to papal teaching in such matters (with a rare exception to be noted below), and that no Catholic is to seek to persuade others to reject insistent papal teaching.

To say that authentic teachings are not infallible, and in some cases could even prove to be flawed, in need of correction, *and* at the same time say that it is entirely certain that one must not dissent from it--defends both proper freedom within the Church and also the unity and peace of faith. In teachings like that of *Donum vitae* scholars certainly have the right to continue probing, to test whether what the Church proposes authentically fits entirely all the data of the question, and is in full conformity with all the faith principles related to it. It is possible that there may yet be further development of these positions. Scholars study these questions as really noninfallible ones. But they too must guard the unity and obedience of faith There is no conflict between scrutinizing authentic teachings and testing them with care, and at the same time adhering to them willingly.

This is not at all to say that a scholar who knows that a teaching of the Church not infallibly proposed is false is still obliged to treat it as if it were true. Of course, if a scholar really knew that some teaching of the Church, not infallibly proposed, were false, he would not be obliged to accept it.[21] But it is most rare for one to *know* that a Church teaching is false. If, for example, a bishop or other Church teacher were to proclaim as true something that opposes an infallible teaching of the Church, or that contradicts the plain sense of a Scripture saying, in the sense in which the Church has always understood it; then clearly one who knows of the error is in no way obliged to accept it, or cease teaching what the Church has so firmly taught. If one had really an absolute certainty about a natural truth, and the Church were, in a noninfallible way, come to teach the opposite, one would of course not be bound to hold what he knows to be false.

But in the actual contemporary disputes, no dissenter has ever proved any moral teaching of the Church wrong. The real pattern of dissent is more like this. A scholar adopts philosophical or other cultural presuppositions, perhaps because they are so popular or attractive at a given time.[22] Church positions may begin to appear flawed to him when he studies them in the light of certain special presuppositions. But, if he is intelligent, he knows that he cannot simply prove those presuppositions. Or a scholar may adopt certain popular value positions (e.g., that a woman has an absolute right to have a child; or that she has a firm right to terminate a pregnancy for certain reasons). In the light of these commitments, the Catholic positions will not appear to be clearly a good one. But those who adopt such values really know that other intelligent people agree with the Church in the matter in question, and that they are not absolutely certain of their own position.

When philosophical or pastoral or other cultural reasons dear to one, incline him to perceive a moral teaching of the Church as "unacceptable," he is indeed facing a difficult spiritual decision. But from the Fathers, saints, doctors and authentic pastors of the Church, a firm answer to this question has been given over the centuries. When one has uncertain arguments from natural sources against a *teaching* of the Church, even one not infallibly proposed, the faithful person will adhere to Church teaching. For the reasons to assent are far more solid than those urging dissent. For they know that Christ dwells with the Church even in its noninfallible teaching; and in the Church he teaches that we must assent even when our favored visions urge us to protest. He may study it, probe it, examine it and report difficulties in it: but he must never flatly declare it false, and seek to persuade others to count it as false.

V. AUTHORITY OF THIS DOCUMENT:

Why many outside the faith honor it

When St. Justin Martyr became a Christian, he reports in his *Apology*, he did so because he had long been seeking answers to the deep riddles of life. After hearing the positions of a great array of pagan thinkers, he heard the teaching of Christ. "I found this philosophy (Christianity) alone to be safe and profitable. Thus, and for this reason, I am a philosopher."[23]

The believer has no difficulty in seeing why those without faith are attracted by its teaching, and learn to love it, in part or entirely. Those who have lived in faith taste the truth and goodness of what faith proclaims.

From certain perspectives, it is true, the teaching of the Church in its life ethic and in its teachings on procreation can seem absurd. When one absolutizes certain societal commitments or values, it seems absurd to argue that an adult person must be willing to suffer to avoid doing harm to a non-conscious little entity that does not yet even look human. When one's focus is on a longing for "one's own child," it may seem absurd to say that acts of generating children must always be acts of love, not merely acts motivated by love.

When one's concerns are focused on pressing near-term goals, whatever impedes these goals is intolerable. But the human heart longs to find not only what is good from the point of view of this personal or cultural interest. Lurking within it always is a longing for that which is good altogether.

In reading the American Fertility Society's critique of one teaching of *Donum vitae* it seems clear to me why they adopt a position that is undoubtedly fundamentally antithical to some of their own beliefs. The Church teaches the profoundly democratic position that human beings have certain rights precisely because they are human. Different human beings may be unequal in a vast number of ways: one may be wiser, nobler, stronger, more beautiful, more skilled, in every way superior to another. Yet they are equally human beings, and what they have a right to precisely because they are human, they have an equal right to.

But to apply this to the case of the youngest humans would be unsettling to broad cultural interests. People want the freedom to have abortions when that becomes necessary. Some researchers have good things they think they can achieve, things that please great masses of people, if they can experiment on surplus embryos, or dispose of unneeded embryos after one has been implanted. In this case it is necessary to argue, as the critique does: "The degree and nature of respect and moral value accorded to the human pre-embryo or fetus rises continuously until birth."[24] That is, the more developed, the more excel- lent these young humans are, the more respect is to be given to their claimed rights. We cannot say they are equally human, and so equally have an equal right with all other men. So we must say: they are not equally human. The born baby (no reason is given for saying it has full humanity, but that is culturally acceptable) is human, as is the adult. But the not yet born baby is not yet human simply: it is human to a degree. But all this is clearly unacceptable. Substan- tive traits are spoken of in qualitative terms, as if a thing could be in only a partial degree the kind of reality it is. Some predicates are had or they are not had: one is dead or not dead, he is not somewhat dead. A woman is pregnant or not pregnant; she is not somewhat pregnant but simply pregnant. And a young fetus is either a living human being or it is not. It is not "somewhat" a human being.

Half the nation favors abortion; half favors right to life. But the approach- es are different. There are many reasons to take a pro-choice stance. But one is never protected from the danger of encountering one day a sharp question: but what *is* it that we are killing? If they are happy enough, as Justin Martyr was, to find those who will teach them how Christian faith faces the riddles of life, there will be a moment of decision. One has had a host of sophisticated reasons to defend the prejudices of a special school. But they are reasons not calculated to catch the truth of things, but to provide a perspective from which people may do what they crave to do. When one is given instead a chance to catch a vision of the truth of things, the opportunity is a precious one. There may be great disadvantages: one may have to lose much, even one's life, to pursue not what is good from this or that interest perspective, but what is simply good. But it is an opportunity that the human heart longs to have. We need a vision and a morality that does not serve our intense interests, but the deepest longings of our hearts. Because so many people long not for rationalizations and relative visions, but the truth of things, there are many who long for what *Donum vitae* says of the sacredness of life and of the acts that summon persons into being.

ENDNOTES

[1] Second Vatican Council, <u>Pastoral Constitution on the Church in the Modern World, Gaudium et spes</u>, n. 15.

[2] The expression is from Paul VI, "Discourses to the General Assembly of the United Nations" (Oct. 4, 1965), <u>Acta Apostolicae Sedis</u> 57 (1967), 878.

[3] Congregation for the Doctrine of the Faith, <u>Instruction on Respect for Human Life in its Origin and on the Dignity of Procreation</u>, (Feb. 22, 1987), Introduction, n. 1; (hereinafter <u>Donum vitae</u>).

[4] <u>Decree</u> of the Holy Office, March 17, 1887 (DS 3954).

[5] For evidence of the virtually unanimous Catholic consent to this teaching in the mid-1960's, cf. P. McKeever, "Artificial Insemination," <u>New Catholic Encyclopedia</u>, vol. 1. New York: McGraw-Hill, 922-24.

[6]Second Vatican Council, <u>Dogmatic Constitution on the Church</u>, n. 21; (hereinafter <u>Lumen Gentium</u>).

[7]On the personalism of faith and the reverence the faith as teacher has for the believer, cf. International Theology Commission, <u>Apostolicity and Apostolic Succession</u>, (April 17, 1974), IV: "The Spiritual Aspect of Apostolic Succession."

[8]G. Grisez, <u>The Way of the Lord Jesus</u>, Vol. 1: <u>Christian Moral Principles</u>, (Chicago: Franciscan Herald Press, 1983,) 851; (hereinafter <u>Christian Moral Principles</u>).

[9]R. Lawler, "The Magisterium and Catholic Teaching," in <u>Persona, Verita e Morale. Atti del Congresso Internazionale di Teologia Morale</u> (Rome, April 7-12, 1986), Rome: Citta Nuova Editrice, 1987, 232; (hereinafter "The Magesterium").

[10]Grisez, <u>Christian Moral Principles</u>, 854.

[11]<u>Donum vitae</u>, II, n. 8: "The Suffering Caused by Infertility in Marriage."

[12]Edwards is quoted in P. Gynne, "Was the Birth of Louise Brown Only a Happy Accident?", <u>Science Digest</u>, (Oct. 1970) 7.

[13]See the critiques of Richard McCormick, S.J., and Lisa Cahill, "The Vatican Document on Bioethics: Two Responses," <u>America</u>, (March 28, 1987) 246-48. Also the stinging critique in the American Fertility Society's Report of the Ethics Committee, Supplement (February 1988); <u>Fertility and Sterility</u>; (hereinafter "Report"). Richard McCormick, S.J., was a member of that committee.

[14]Ibid., p. 18.

[15]Ibid., p. 38

[16]That the natural law is not only accessible to reason, but is also confirmed by revelation, see R. Lawler "The Magesterium," 222-23.

[17]<u>Donum vitae</u>, Introduction, part I.

[18]<u>Lumen Gentium</u>, n. 25.

[19]<u>Donum vitae</u>. I, n. 4.

[20]<u>Lumen Gentium</u>, n. 25.

[21]R. Lawler, "The Magesterium," 232.

[22]F.A. Sullivan, <u>Magisterium. Teaching Authority in the Catholic Church</u>. (New York: Paulist, 1983), 163. Here Sullivan points out that it is "rare" for a dissenting scholar to have evidence by which he "is compelled to reject" a teaching of the Church that is not infallibly proposed.

[23]St. Justin Martyr, <u>Apologia</u>, 8. Quoted in E. Gilson, <u>History of Christian Philosophy in the Middle Ages</u>, (New York: Random House, 1955), 12.

[24]"Report" (n. 13 above), 38.

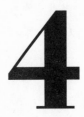

Expanding Our Human
Sexual Horizons

Thomas W. Hilgers, M.D.

When *in vitro* fertilization was first promoted, it was promoted as a therapeutic approach for infertile women with *scarred fallopian tubes.* Physicians were under pressure to find an approach for treating this major cause of infertility which was clearly on the increase. But few people asked the relatively simple question: *Why was it on the increase?*

Fallopian tube obstruction had increased because of a significant increase in sexually transmitted diseases (STDS), especially gonorrhea. But why was venereal disease on the increase? The "permissive sexuality" of the 50's and 60's was beginning to take its toll. Sexually transmitted diseases were out of control.

One must wonder why a conference, which aims to look at the questions of artificial reproduction, would be interested in also looking at the horizons of our human sexuality. It might just be that *at the very foundations of our current dilemmas* might be a truly distorted view of human sexuality. It might also be that within the context of a healthy view of human sexuality lies a number of the ultimate, if not penultimate, solutions to these problems.

At the bottom line, the justification for such things as *in vitro* fertilization, other forms of artificial reproduction and surrogate motherhood rests at the end of a chain of events that started several years ago as a cascading set of immoral dominoes began to fall. Now, as the last dominoes are falling, they are falling because the preceding domino fell. We seem to have forgotten that it all had to start somewhere.

Over the past 30 years, in response to the call for sexual freedom, we have seen major sociological and cultural changes. Most of these have resulted in a significant denigration of the human person and his or her family. We have seen a number of the dominoes fall. There has been a rapid increase in the use of contraception and abortion, but with a socially paradoxical increase in out-of-wedlock pregnancies. The divorce rate has been exponentially on the increase; there has been an increase in the exploitation of both men and women through graphic pornography; an increase in physical child abuse; sexual child abuse; drug abuse; teenage suicide; homosexuality; *and* artificial reproduction through artificial insemination by husband, donor and *in vitro* fertilization. The overall increase in family violence is well recognized by most investigators.

It is tempting to suggest that it was the massive introduction of contraceptive agents which was mostly responsible for setting the falling dominoes in motion. But I am more likely to suggest that the family was in great difficulty before the introduction of contraception and was *highly vulnerable* to its influences. The family was highly vulnerable because of an inadequate view of human sexuality. The introduction of contraceptive agents was more of a *trigger* to the developing social trends rather than their primary cause. But the social changes of the last one to two generations have become so dangerous that they threaten the very fabric of our society and they undermine all efforts to promote human rights and social justice.

The contemporary emphasis on the view that our sexuality is only physical and only genital actually *inhibits rather than enhances* our true sexual development and freedom. We live in a *hypererotic genital culture* which is powerfully inhibiting to the development of true sexual freedom and meaningful relationships at all levels.

If we are to have healing and wholeness, we must, as Mary Joyce suggests, begin to recognize our *intuitive intellectual potential*. We must reveal that the body is manifestly sexual in *all* that it is - not just in its parts! All of the good will in the world will not make us more fulfilled sexually if we begin with false precepts. We must reach the truth, for *sharing the truth* is what *compassion* is all about and it is in the truth that healing can occur.

Let us ask the question: *"What does it mean to be sexually active?"*[5] Our answer to this can be any one of the four following statements:

1. One can be sexually active while at the same time being genitally active;
2. One can be sexually active while at the same time *not* being genitally active;
3. In the same way, one can be sexually inactive while being genitally active, and;
4. One can be sexually inactive while being genitally inactive.

Thus, the meaning of being "sexually active" is not dependent upon our being genitally active. While our genital activity may be a more dramatic expression of our sexual activity, it is *no more dynamic* than other non-genital forms of sexual interaction.

We can *choose* from two basic forms or concepts of our human sexuality. These two forms are important to understand because they allow us to "center" ourselves within the other dimensions of our sexuality. These two forms can be referred to as . . .
1. *The genitocentric form*
2. *The cerebrocentric form*

In the *genitocentric* form, our genital organs and their various forms of expression become the primary focus of our sexual expression. In this form, barriers are placed which markedly inhibit the non-genital expression of our sexuality. The genital organs become our primary sexual organs.

In the *cerebrocentric* form, the focus is on the multidimensional nature of our human sexuality - the spiritual, physical, intellectual, creative/communicative and emotional/psychological. In this form, the brain becomes the primary sexual organ.

In this presentation, I will be challenging you to choose the cerebrocentric form because to do so allows the human person to once again become *whole* - and as you will see later - *holy*.

Choosing the cerebrocentric form is also *revolutionary* - revolutionary in a *Copernican sense*. Just as people thought that the sun revolved around the earth prior to Copernicus, they came to realize that, after Copernicus, the earth revolved around the sun. In human sexuality, we will also come to realize that our sexuality does not revolve around our genital organs but rather around our mind.

To understand this further, we must know what it means to be male and female. Many today are familiar with the descriptions of the *animus* and the *anima* which were described for us by Dr. Carl Jung.[1]

The *animus* is the male, the giver, the co-creator, the speaker having the expressive, assertive tendencies.

The *anima* is the female, the receiver, the listener, the intimate one.

Within each man there is a feminine quality and within each woman there is a masculine quality. While the male is *emphatically* animus, he is also very much *anima*. But he needs to integrate his anima into his animus. A man weak in anima is too "macho" and egotistical, always wanting to prove himself, lacking tenderness, sensitivity and warmth. When the man represses his anima he finds it hard to understand and feel with, and have compassion for, a woman.

Men are *intensely feeling* human persons. But all too often they have been led to believe that they should not or cannot express those feelings. It is one of the great tragedies of our time and it makes them *particularly vulnerable* to the genitocentric development of their sexuality.

While the female is *emphatically* anima she is also very much animus. But she needs to integrate her animus into her anima. When a woman lacks animus she is emotionally insecure and dependent, possessive. Without the animus, she finds it difficult to fully love and appreciate her husband. Thus women must work toward inner independence, the cultivation of their talents, the ability to think and be objective.

It is vitally important for the man and the woman to cultivate an inward friendship between their own animus (their masculine tendencies) and their anima (their feminine tendencies). When these two forces are out of balance, we repress the wholeness of our natural and inherent sexuality. This repression is at the root of our current sexual ineptitudes.

While these are being integrated within each man and each woman, they will always be expressed *differently* within the context of their own unique masculinity and femininity. Thus, we need not fear that "sameness" will ever result - nor should it ever be our goal.

By broadening our concepts of sexuality, we seek the challenge of *integrating* it. This integration is the *foundation* of a long lasting, *bonded* relationship. This type of relationship spreads joy within the family.

The intimacy of the mind and the heart is both the best part of love and the best part of sexual fulfillment. In other words, genital intercourse is not the best part of sexual intercourse.

Genitality is part of our sexuality just as reason is part of, but not all of, our intellect. In a similar way, the largest portion of our sexuality goes beyond the genital.

The heart of sexuality is *sharing*. Genitality, if it is engaged in well, is sharing. It is not just giving and taking. True *genital sharing* is a form of *communion* not just communication (communication can be one of dislike, indifference, exploitation, etc., as well as, love).

All that is genital is sexual, but everything that is sexual is not genital. Authentic and fulfilling expressions of our sexuality include such things as shared work, shared sensitivities, shared parenting and shared prayer.

When one sees that a close friendship with a person of the other sex need not lead to physical, genital intimacy, one becomes less fearful of friendship. When one feels less fear, one uses up less energy exercising the necessary physical restraint. When one sees that affection can be expressed, but in a limited fashion, without necessarily leading to physical sexual arousal, *one receives a whole new freedom* to give and receive through touch.

When one begins thinking about his or her sexuality in an integrated and cerebro-centric fashion, then one's emotions tend to follow in a natural and harmonious way. One can experience touch as deeply life giving and yet it is remarkably easy to contain within appropriate limits.

When our emotions have room in which to expand and relax, then our sense of touch can also be more expansive and relaxed.

In looking at physical touching, one must learn to distinguish between the *affirming touch* and the *arousal touch*.

The *affirming touch* says that "It is good for you to be you". The *arousal touch* says "Give yourself to me" or "I want you". The arousal touch tends to be more "me" oriented. We need to work on and develop our ability to express the affirming way of touching.

When we change our concept of our sexuality to the broader, affirming notions, it has a healing, liberating effect on our emotional life and our relationships.

Affirmation is the most basic aspect of the loving presence. You need to be affirmed, to feel good about yourself, if you are going to be able to affirm others in a feeling or affectionate way.

Affirmation starts in the family and is transmitted from the parents to their children. This process begins prior to the child's conception with the parents' affirmation and appreciation of themselves and their fertility. It continues for each child from the womb onward and each child needs to be treated as a person who is unique and special.

When we have an affirming relationship with our emotional life, we receive these emotions as energy for creative relationships, communication, giving and receiving. Thus, the importance of affirming all of our sexual emotions and not denying them.

When our sexual feelings are affirmed in this way, they stimulate us to grow in self-knowledge, to intensify our sexuality and to grow in our male and female personalities. *Sharing feelings, thoughts and values* is a form of *sexual intercourse* and it leads to *true sexual fulfillment* although it is physical on ly in an indirect sense.

Once we are able to relate with our own sexual feelings and share our feelings, thoughts and values in a non-genital way, then we can consider the expression of the genital component of our sexuality. But this latter must be done *only* in the context of marriage, for that is where it is properly ordained.

Only when we are able to integrate, or attempt to integrate, the spiritual, physical, intellectual, creative and emotional aspects of our personalities are we then able to come into balance with our sexuality. This requires a life-long commitment to a willingness to continue one's growth and development - to be forever enriched.

This type of sexual balance can be achieved in married couples only with the use of natural family planning because this provides the opportunity for the couples' human sexuality to be placed into a balanced, cerebrocentric perspective. During those times when the couple chooses genital absence, the couple is given the opportunity to broaden their sexual horizons. This time is used to expand the non-genital aspects of the couple's sexual interaction.

With this approach, one can expect *true marital bonding* to occur. This is a bonding which is based in an authentic love, filled with trust and appreciation of the other as a whole person. A form of bonding which gives security and affirmation to the children of the family and ultimately can be expected to make a major impact on the family violence of our day.

Our culture teaches people to be concerned about *functioning genitally* but not about *being genital.* Everyone, married or celibate, fertile or infertile, can be genital without necessarily functioning genitally. There is a difference between *being genital* and thinking that in order to be genital you *have to function genitally.* Being genital means that you are affirming your genitality. Everything in your sexuality that is oriented toward genital intercourse and procreation *must be affirmed!* You must integrate your genital feelings within the whole of your sexual being. But you must also affirm that none of these feelings, impulses or urges have to be expressed in a genital action.

The foundations of *any* relationship, married or celibate, fertile or infertile, are *not* primarily genital. *No marriage has stood strong and bonded, in growth and holiness, when based primarily in the genital union.* It is the non-genital expression of our human sexuality, *the integration of our animus and anima,* and the full sexual sharing that is at the foundation of such relationships.

As you grow and mature, you begin to see individuals as human persons regardless of their sex, and you don't need to make a special effort in your mind to relate the attractive qualities of the "sexual other" to anything other than that of a human person with his or her own dignity and worth.

While this will become natural and spontaneous eventually, I must point out that it is a *learned* phenomenon. It is something that each person must *acquire* during their lives.

The very beautiful, powerful, erotic and genital emotion is a tremendous energy that one is allowing to transform oneself and bring one more deeply and intimately into relationship with the other person. The genital energy becomes *a sharing energy.* This *sharing* enriches the feeling, develops it and gives it dimension and life.

It is no longer a "raw" feeling but a developed, enriched feeling that is then given the opportunity to proliferate itself in many creative ways. One is actually *being* genital without *functioning* in a genital way.

Such transformations are essential to the married couple and their practical use of natural family planning and it allows the celibate to reach a fully enriched sexual life. There is an important complementariness between the celibate clergy and religious and the married couple using natural family planning. They give powerful witness to each other.

The type of sexual concepts that I have presented relate to people of the same sex as well as to those of the opposite sex.

What is popularly referred to as homosexuality is more properly called *homo-genitality*. It is not healing to say that homosexuality is just an alternate lifestyle to heterosexuality. In fact, it is fundamentally dehumanizing not to recognize it as a disorientation.

At the same time, it is not healing to assume that heterosexuals cannot also be disoriented in their sexuality, when, in fact, their relationship is distortedly genitocentric.

Prayer is vitally important to the development of our sexuality. In prayer, we especially exercise our *anima - the side of our sexuality that is receptive. Everytime we pray well--and that means contemplatively and in communion with God--our capacity for being in communion with a sexual other is deepened and strengthened.*

Prayer is a way of receiving the affirming touch of God. Prayer is very healing for our sexuality.

When a man balances his sexuality by integrating more receptivity, he becomes more able to share with a woman, to receive what she gives. The reverse is also true for a woman. The integration of prayer and the sacramental life is essential if we are to have a healthy, growing, dynamic relationship.

We are taught that in marriage "two become one flesh". This can be expressed in the equation $1 + 1 = 1$. However, in order for this to be truly fulfilled, the equation must be $1 + 1 + 1 = 1$. In this equation, we have a trinity, with the man, the woman and God coming together to form a oneness or unity.

In human procreation, the human person, man and woman, are given a *very special privilege.* Through their bodies, they become co-creators with God of an "absolutely unique singular" human life.[6] But human life is *not just life, it is eternal life!* Thus, the married couple becomes a *co-creator* with God at the only moment in their earthly existence when this is possible. The couple participates in the physical and physiological act of conception, while God intervenes to create the new person's eternal soul. If we sincerely understand this principle, then we cannot help but understand the sacramentality of the genital union and the co-creative and very sacred powers of the human person in human pro- creation.

I work with infertile couples day-in and day-out. The pain they feel is real! But to provide therapies which go contrary to the true nature of their human sexuality (in all of its dimensions) is to add pain where such pain is already enormous. *Compassion in the absence of truth is not compassion at all. True caring comes with a willingness to share and sustain truth!*

The concepts of human sexuality I have discussed here are universal and apply to us all. For the infertile, their infertility is truly burdensome. But their burden can be a "source of *spiritual fruitfulness*".[6] Their sexuality is not demeaned within this fuller concept of human sexuality as it is so easily demeaned by the more limited, genitocentric, view of the artificial reproduction clinics.

Physical sterility, if permanent, can become *a source of service* to others. Once the grieving for this loss subsides, or comes under control, then the couple is able to reach out to others: *to others who are infertile, to the child who needs adoptive parents, to the assistance of other families, through the foster care of children in need,* and/or *in service to poor or handicapped children.*

The extension of ourselves in this way, or ways similiar to it, is a response to the call of Christ Jesus, "Love one another as I have loved you." Please understand that we *must not* stand around to catch the last domino! We *must,* for our sake and the sake of our children and their children, start re-setting and probably re-assembling the dominoes. We must start now a *Copernican-like* revolution in our understanding of our human sexuality.

ACKNOWLEDGMENTS

A very special thanks to my wife, Susan, and our five children for helping me continue my pursuits of these major questions.

An additional very special thanks to Robert and Mary Joyce who have shared with Sue and I the richness of their insights into our human sexuality. A richness which, we believe, carries insights beyond those of most contemporary philosophers. A richness which is liberally reflected in this paper and to which they deserve primary credit.

REFERENCES

[1] Fabricant, S.: Understanding our Sexuality: An Interview with Robert and Mary Joyce. Journal of Christian Healing. 6:6-13, 1983.

[2] Joyce, M.R.: The Meaning of Contraception. New York: Alba House, 1970. Republished by Liturgical Press, Collegeville, Minnesota, 1975.

[3] Joyce, M.R. and Joyce, R.E.: New Dynamics in Sexual Love. St. John's University Press, Collegeville, Minnesota, 1970.

[4] Joyce, R.E.: Human Sexual Ecology: A Philosophy and Ethics of Man and Woman. University Press of America, Washington, DC, 1980.

[5] Joyce, M.R.: "The Sexual Revolution is yet to Begin." In: Hilgers, T.W. and Horan, D.J.: Abortion and Social Justice. Sheed and Ward, New York, New York, 1972, pp. 221-230.

[6] "Instruction on Respect for Human Life in its Origin and on the Dignity of Procreation." Vatican Congregation for the Doctrine of the Faith. Origins. 16:687, March 19, 1987.

5

The Vocation of Christian Marriage as an Approach to the Bioethics of Human Reproduction

Janet Smith, Ph.D.

Marriage is an institution that has been around as long as mankind.[1] One would think, then, that we would know a lot more about marriage than we do. If anything, current statistics on divorce and infidelity would seem to indicate that we are regressing rather than progressing in our understanding of marriage. Here is not the place to rehearse the misunderstandings of the nature of marriage that are rampant in contemporary society. The challenge here is to determine what truth or truths about the objective reality of marriage need to be heard by our contemporaries and to explore how we might get them to see and accept the objective reality of marriage. The intent here is to use this information to understand better the Vatican teaching that *in vitro* fertilization (IVF) and embryo transfer (ET) are morally impermissible even for spouses.[2]

There are truths about marriage that are so at odds with the way a society thinks that to insist upon them only discredits the prophetic voice that promotes them. Many of the truths about the differences between men and women, the appropriateness of different roles for men and women, the notion that, for the most part, the husband should be the head of the household, are all messages that simply enrage rather than enlighten so many living in our times. For my part, I think it is best to promote other truths and hope that these insights concerning men and women will follow.

In each age there are truths that society is aching to hear since it suffers so greatly from the rejection or neglect of these truths. Our age is belatedly becoming aware of the damage done to individuals and to society through sex outside of marriage, through broken marriages, through broken families. Our society is still oblivious to the extent of the damage done through these evils; it does not yet realize how connected are the evils of broken homes, alcoholism, drug abuse, poverty, and homelessness--indeed, careful reflection suggests that the evil of broken families may well have a contributing influence to most of the troubles that our society faces. Nor do broken families tend to produce the healthy and sane human beings we need to guide us out of our problems. That we have such problems, however, may make us more receptive to the saving truth. Voices that purport to offer some kind of solution to these miseries have a chance of being heard. For instance, the voices that proclaim it is more important and more effective to teach teenagers to be chaste than to provide them with easy access to contraceptives are starting to be heard in some quarters.

There are also truths that a society desperately needs to hear, truths to which it may be most resistent, but that are its only hope for extricating itself from its miseries. The truths about the evils of abortion, contraception, and technological manipulation of human reproduction are among these truths that our society needs to hear.

REALITY OF MARRIAGE

One suggested way of leading people to see the objective reality of marriage is to draw their attention to marriage, to have them reflect upon good and faithful marriages--marriages open to the transmission of life--and through these observations to draw conclusions about the nature of true and authentic marriage. Although much of my understanding of marriage has come through such a process, I have found that it is difficult to guide others through this sort of analysis. It is my good fortune to know an uncommon number of good marriages, to have had the opportunity to observe them closely, and to learn from them how marvelous is the love that flows within these marriages, how steady is the growth of the spouses in maturity and love for each other, how beautiful is the development of the children. Yet, when I speak to others of such marriages, I find they have no experience of these; many of their parents have been divorced, many if not most of their friends have been divorced, and they are virtually unaware of marriages in which the spouses do not practice contraception. They may have met someone from a large family, but they have not seen an intact, large family up close. When I do draw such families to their attention, what they see are the scruffy and tacky toys on the front lawn, the scruffy and tacky furniture in the living room, the somewhat unfashionable attire worn by family members, the used station wagon in the driveway, the constant clamoring of the kids and the corresponding testiness of the parents. Features such as a wife not working and the lack of money, time, or freedom for European travel (by the spouses) also have their impact. Many cannot and do not see the strong bonds of love being formed and the generous spirits being developed in these families. They cannot see the compelling sense of meaning and purpose to life experienced by the parents as the underlying wellspring keeping them committed in the midst of their daily hassles. They cannot see the benefits of the steady generosity, sometimes verging on the heroic, that individuals in these marriages eventually develop. They cannot see the deep and nearly inexpressible happiness that comes from caring so much and working so hard for others. Marriages that are not simply arrangements for the mutual self-indulgence of the spouses have an inner reality which is not always easy to see. This reality is revealed only to those who have eyes to see.

CHRISTIAN COMMITMENT

So were do we start in explaining the nature of marriage? I believe we need to start with a more general explanation of the Christian commitment. In *Familiaris Consortio*, Pope John Paul II states:

The Church is deeply convinced that only by the acceptance of the Gospel are the hopes that man legitimately places in marriage and in the family capable of being fulfilled.

Willed by God in the very act of creation, marriage and the family are interiorly ordained in fulfillment in Christ and have need of his grace in order to be healed from the wounds of sin and restored to their "beginning", that is, to full understanding and the full realization of God's plan.[3]

It seems to me that before the larger society can be reformed in its understanding and practice of marriage, Christians must first make full use of the resources of their faith and Church and work to form marriages and families out of which will come those who have eyes to see and who will be articulate and persuasive proponents of true marriage. Christians understand that marriage is a part of God's plan, and it is this objective reality of marriage that I believe must be more deeply understood.

MARRIAGE: A NATURAL INSTITUTION

Certainly marriage is not an institution exclusive to Christians. It is an institution natural to man, which satisfies some of his deeper yearnings, meets some of his most pressing needs, and enables him to live his life in a more purposeful fashion. The Church has long taught that natural law reveals to man that marriage is monogamous and indissoluble and ordained to the bringing forth of new life. I suspect that many recognize these as essential features of marriage; when young people get married, they intend to be monogamous, married for a lifetime, and open to bringing forth children--if only a few well-planned children. But too few are able to be true to these intentions. It is not easy to have this kind of marriage, especially in our times when the social and political supports for such marriages are few and the forces against such marriages are powerful and pervasive. Spouses need tremendous graces to live true marriages, and they simply are not getting them. It must be acknowledged that few are actively seeking graces, and most engage in practices that are obstacles to growth in grace. One of the most devastating obstacles to grace and most insidious forces against marriage is the contraceptive mentality stemming from contraceptive practice. It corrodes marriages in ways that are not wholly visible but very damaging. Only a few in our society seem able to see this truth about marriage. What might reveal it to others?

I am going to enunciate four principles that I think might lead us to an understanding of marriage and that will aid us in seeing the vision of the Church on the issues that concern us here. First, we need to deepen our sense that our existence in this world is a gift. Second, we need to understand that marriage is a vocation that commits the spouses to a certain apostolate. Third, we need to understand better what it means to say that God is the Creator of all life and that each human life is the result of a special act of creation by God. And fourth, we need to understand what role spouses have in the transmission of human life. Let me elaborate on these principles.

THE GIFT OF EXISTENCE

The opening paragraph of the *Instruction on Respect for Human Life* states, perhaps all too briefly, that God is the Creator and Father of the gift of life:

> *The gift of life which God the Creator and Father has entrusted to man calls him to appreciate the inestimable value of what he has given and to take responsibility for it: this fundamental principle must be placed at the centre of one's reflection in order to clarify and solve the moral problems raised by artificial interventions on life as it originates and on the processes of procreation.*[4]

This passage, which should be expanded into a book, suggests that the teaching of the *Instruction* will not be understood unless we understand that God is the Creator and Father of the gift of life. This is just about all that the Instruction says about creation as a gift, but it serves to establish that unless we follow its direction to make this truth the center of our reflection we will not fully appreciate the wisdom of the document. We must come to appreciate that all of creation is a gift and that we are greatly privileged to share in the splendor of this gift. Among other benefits, a stance of gratitude towards the world aids anyone in perceiving more correctly the meaning of life and creation. We must gain a deeper understanding of God as a loving Creator who created out of his love. We must get a surer grasp of the connection between love and creation and especially the creation of new life. Too few Christians have a sufficient sense of what it means to say that God is the Creator of human life and thereby fail to grasp precisely what role spouses have in the transmission of that life. More will be said about this point in a moment; here I want to stress that we have too weak a sense of the fundamental Christian truth that our life in this world is a sojourn and that our time here is time in preparation for eternal union with our Father. Too few of us have a sense that such actions as marrying and having children are a part of the vital role we have to play in the history of salvation.

MARRIAGE AS A VOCATION

Donum vitae speaks of marriage and the transmission of life as a vocation. It states that "God, who is love and life, has inscribed in man and woman the vocation to share in a special way in this mystery of personal communion and in his work as Creator and Father".[5] *Humanae Vitae* has a similar passage:

> *Married love particularly reveals its true nature and nobility when we realize that it derives from God and finds its supreme origin in him who "is love", the Father "from whom every family in heaven and on earth is named."*

> *Marriage, then, is far from being the effect of chance or the result of the blind evolution of natural forces. It is in reality the wise and provident institution of God the Creator, whose purpose was to establish in man his loving design. As a consequence, husband and wife, through that mutual gift of themselves, which is specific and exclusive to them alone, seek to develop that kind of personal union in which they complement one another in order to co-operate with God in the generation and education of new lives.*[6]

These short passages speak a truth that again deserves a volume of elaboration. They speak the truth that all spouses have a special vocation to share God's loving and creative work. Unless we come to understand that all Christians have a vocation and that marriage is a well-defined vocation, we will not understand the Church's teaching on marriage and related bioethical problems. This vocation is a calling, a calling that flows out of the spouses' Christian commitment. A passage from the *Second Vatican Council's Decree on the Apostolate of Lay People* describes the perspective on vocation and apostolate that all Christians must hold:

> *The Church was founded to spread the kingdom of Christ over all the earth for the glory of God the Father, to make all men partakers in redemption and salvation, and through them to establish the right relationship of the entire world to Christ. Every activity of the Mystical Body with this in view goes by the name of "apostolate"; the Church exercises it through all its members, though in various ways. In fact, the Christian vocation is, of its nature, a vocation to the apostolate as well. In the organism of a living body no member plays a purely passive part, sharing in the life of the body it shares at the same time in its activity. The same is true for the Body of Christ, the Church: "the whole Body achieves full growth in dependence on the full functioning of each part" (Eph. 4:16). Between the members of this body there exists further, such a unity and solidarity (cf. Eph. 4;16) that a member who does not work at the growth of the body to the extent of his possibilities must be considered useless both to the Church and to himself.*[7]

To be a Christian is to be called and to be sent, that is, it is to have both a vocation and an apostolate. (The word "vocation" comes from the Latin *vocare*, meaning "to call," and the word "apostolate" comes from the Greek word *apostello*, meaning "to be sent out.") It is a part of God's plan that people marry. Marrying is both part of their calling and part of their apostolate. Those who marry must come to appreciate this more deeply: they are marrying not only for each other, but they are marrying as an answer to a call which God gives them, and this call entails certain responsibilities and duties.

Marriage, like other vocations, is remarkably various, but it is also true that it has a nature and has responsibilities that are independent of the wishes of those who answer the call to this vocation. It is good to note that although the priesthood is a vocation with many possible manifestations--priests are teachers, counselors, college presidents, accountants, and lawyers for the Church-- nonetheless, there are certain actions that are obligatory for priests and certain actions that are forbidden to priests by the very virtue of their priesthood. Like the priesthood, the marriage relationship takes on certain dimensions because of the personalities, temperaments, talents, and opportunities of the spouses; but it also has a nature to which the spouses must submit themselves. Married couples, in fact, need to study the nature of marriage; they need to learn about their vocation in the same way a priest needs to learn about his. One engagement encounter weekend will not suffice. Christians must not assume that they can learn what marriage is from the society around them.

CREATION OF HUMAN LIFE

Much could and probably should be said here about the personalist values of marriage, but the element of marriage that I believe needs greatest elucidation is marriage as a relationship ordained to the bringing forth of new life. Older marriage manuals used to explain that just as sex in the animal kingdom is ordained to bring forth new life, so too is human sex. Thus it is concluded, sex is for the propagation of the species and contraception a violation of what is good for the species. Undoubtedly there is some truth in these statements, but they can also be misleading. As *Donum vitae* asserts:

> *Marriage possesses specific goods and values in its union and in procreation which cannot be likened to those existing in lower forms of life. Such values and meanings are of the personal order and determine from the moral point of view the meaning and limits of artificial interventions on procreation and on the origin of human life.*[8]

What needs to be kept in mind is that procedures that are acceptable for the treatment of other animals are not acceptable for human beings; we may sterilize animals, cross-breed them, and create new life in test tubes, but we may not do these things to human life. This principle shows the falsity of the claim that the Church has a "physicalistic" or "biologistic" view of sex; truly, it has a personalist view of sex, or it would allow all these procedures for human beings.

It is good to understand clearly why we may not do these things to human beings, that is, why the processes of the generation of human life are not to be manipulated in the same way as those of other animals. The chief and inestimably great difference between the bringing forth of animal life and the bringing forth of human life is, as seen above, that each and every human life is the result of a special act of creation by God. This is necessary because human life is immortal, and only God can bring immortal life into existence. Although God is the true creator of each and every human life, the role of spouses is neither unimportant nor simply mechanical. As *Donum vitae* teaches, the creation of human life should be the result of a deliberate and willing act of sexual intercourse between two spouses.

> *By comparison with the transmission of other forms of life in the universe, the transmission of human life has a special character of its own, which derives from the special nature of the human person. "The transmission of human life is entrusted by nature to a personal and conscious act and as such is subject to the all-holy laws of God: immutable and inviolable laws which must be recognized and observed. For this reason one cannot use means and follow methods which could be licit in the transmission of the life of plants and animals."*[9]

Since the creation of life on the part of God is a loving and free act, the creation of life on the part of spouses should also be the result of a loving and free act. Again, human life is not created by chance, it is not the result of the simple physical uniting of male and female gametes; it involves a special act of creation by God. This crucial claim, explicitly stated in the Instruction on Respect for Human Life, is at the center of the teaching of that document and of *Humanae Vitae*. As *Humanae Vitae* states at the outset, spouses *collaborate* with God in the transmission of human life.

THE ROLE OF SPOUSES

In Church documents there is a word which cannot be translated easily into English, that captures well the nature of marriage as a vocation and defines well the place of having children within this vocation. This is the Latin word *munus*. I have done a rather lengthy philological review of the meaning of this word, which I shall only summarize here.[10] This review may seem to take us far afield from the "objective reality of marriage," but I think this word and the concepts it conveys singularly illuminate the relation of marriage and procreation.

What drew the word to my attention was its appearance in the first line of *Humanae Vitae* which reads, *"Humanae vitae tradendae munus gravissimum,"* and is usually translated, "the most serious duty of transmitting human life." My classical language training however would have led me to translate *munus,* here translated as "duty," as "gift." This led me to trace the word in several works, most notably the documents of Vatican II where it appears 248 times.

A variety of words are used in the English translations of the Council for *munus;* "duty," "role," "task," "mission," "office," "vocation," and "function" are all used. In classical Latin, this word is not uncommonly used for an appointment made by a public official to his subordinate. Selection to a public office would be considered an honor. Certainly, the appointment would entail duties, sometimes onerous duties, but the recipient would willingly embrace them. In Church documents, the word carries a similar meaning; it seems most often to refer to a solemn assignment that God has given to an agent to accomplish an extremely important task for the kingdom.

Lumen Gentium lays out the *munera* of many of the participants in the Christian mission.[11] This document, by no means uniquely, has as a theme the distribution of characteristic participation of different members of the Church in the "priestly, prophetic and kingly office *(munera)* of Christ"(LG, 31). Christians, in their various callings, participate in this threefold *munus* of Christ by fulfilling other *munera* specifically entrusted to them. For instance, Mary's *munus* (office) is to be the Mother of God (LG, 53); this also confers on her a maternal *munus* (function) as mother of all men (LG, 60). Christ gave Peter several *munera:* for instance, Peter was given the *munus* (office) of binding and loosening (LG, 22) and the *grande munus* (noble task), which was also granted to the apostles, of spreading the Christian name (LG, 23). The apostles were assigned the *munera* (exalted functions) of "affirming the Gospel of the grace of God, and of gloriously promulgating the Spirit and proclaiming justification"(LG, 21). To help them fulfill these *munera,* they were granted a special outpouring of the Holy Spirit (LG, 21). By virtue of his *munus* (office) as Vicar of Christ, the Roman Pontiff has "full, supreme and universal power over the whole Church" (LG, 22) and also by virtue of his *munus* (office) he is endowed with infallibility (LG, 25). Bishops, by virtue of their episcopal consecration, have the *munus* (office) of sanctifying and also the *munus* (duty) of teaching and ruling (LG, 21). The laity also share in the priestly, prophetic, and kingly *munus* of Christ. Living in the world, "they are called by God that, being led by the spirit to the Gospel, they may contribute to the sanctification of the world, as from within like leaven, by fulfilling their own particular duties *(munera)"* (LG, 31). *Munera* are conferred by one superior in power upon another; it is important to note that in each instance Christ is acknowledged as the source of the *munera*. *Munera* are not man-made, but God-given.

Vatican Council II issued specific documents to clarify further the nature of the *munera* of different groups. For instance, *Christus Dominus* has as its subtitle, "Decree on the Pastoral Office *(munere)* of Bishops in the Church." This practice continues after the Council: the subtitle of *Familiaris Consortio* is "Regarding the Role *(muneribus)* of the Christian Family in the Modern World."

Forms of *munus* appear ten times in the six sections of *Gaudium et Spes* that speak about the role of married people in the Church.[12] There we learn that spouses and parents have a *praecellens munus* (lofty calling) (GS, 47); that married love leads spouses to God and aids and strengthens them in their *sublimis munus* (lofty role) of being a mother and father (GS, 48); that the sacrament of marriage helps them fulfill their conjugal and familial *munus* (role) (GS, 48); that spouses are blessed with the dignity and *munus* (role) of fatherhood and motherhood, which helps them achieve their duties *(officium)* of educating their children (GS, 48); that young people should be properly and in good time instructed about the dignity, *munus* (role), and exercise of married love (GS, 49). *Gaudium et Spes* further speaks of the *munus* (duties) of procreation and notes that "among the married couples who thus fulfill their God-given mission *(munere a Deo Commisso)*, special mention should be made of those who after prudent reflection and common decision courageously undertake the proper upbringing of a large number of children" (GS, 50). We are told that "human life and its transmission *(munus eam transmittendi)* are realities whose meaning is not limited by the horizons of this life only: their true evaluation and full meaning can only be understood in reference to man's eternal destiny" (GS, 51).

Forms of the word *munus* appear twenty-one times in *Humanae Vitae*. It is used four times in reference to the *munus* of transmitting human life, three times to the *munus* of responsible parenthood, and once to the apostolic *munus* that spouses have to other married couples. It seems fair to say that the *munus* of "transmitting human life" and the *munus* of "responsible parenthood" are one and the same *munus;* the second phrase specifies and clarifies the first. Indeed, the Church has always linked together the begetting of life with the obligation to educate and guide the life begotten. *Casti Connubii*, for instance, explicitly connects the begetting of children with the obligation to educate the children--not just for prosperity in this life, but with a view to their eternal destiny:

> Christian parents should understand that they are destined not only to propagate and conserve the human race, nor even to educate just any worshippers of the true God, but to bring forth offspring for the Church of Christ, to procreate fellow citizens for the Saints and servants of God, so that the worshippers devoted to our God and Savior might daily increase.[13]

Gaudium et Spes also adopts the customary linking of procreation and education when it states that "marriage and married love are by nature ordered to the procreation and education of children".[14] The encyclical *Humanae vitae*, then, has as it purpose the clarification of the Christian *munus* that belongs to spouses, the *munus* of bringing forth, and being responsible to children with a view to guiding children to be worthy of eternal union with God.

Raising children is a *munus;* it is an honor conferred upon spouses that brings with it certain obligations; it is the assignment that God gives to spouses so that his kingdom of love might begin to prevail in this world. By freely and deliberately accepting the calling of marriage, spouses also freely and deliberately accept the *munera* that go along with that calling, in the same way that a priest, in responding to the calling of the priesthood, accepts the *munera* of his assignment. To be married but not to accept the *munus* of transmitting life is like taking on an assignment, but not taking on the full responsibilities of that assignment and not realizing the full goods of that assignment both for one's self and for others. For instance, a man may wish to be a priest but not wish to perform some of the sacraments; that would be a repudiation of his calling and its *munera*.

MUNUS AND ARTIFICIAL FERTILIZATION

Elsewhere I have applied this analysis to the teaching of *Humanae Vitae* that the unitive and procreative meanings of conjugal union are truly inseparable.[15] Here I wish to explore what light it might shed on the teaching in *Donum vitae* that married couples may not have recourse to *in vitro* fertilization or embryo transfer, a teaching that is most difficult for many to accept.

Suppose a married couple were to accept the Church's understanding of the objective reality of marriage. Suppose they were truly grateful for the gift of life that God shared with them, were thrilled to be called to the vocation of marriage, and were eager to embrace their *munus* of transmitting human life. And suppose they were to discover that theirs was an infertile marriage. Do they not have an obligation or at least a right to fulfill their *munus*?

There are other instances where, although one cannot carry out one's assignment, one ought not then to manipulate things so that one can fulfill that assignment. For instance, soldiers may go through years of training and years of watchfulness and never fight; if war has not been duly declared, they have neither an obligation to fight nor a right to fight. Soldiers ought not to start wars so that they may fulfill their assignment. Their assignment is not so much to fight as it is to be willing to fight. Similarly, a wife may wish to bear her husband's child but if the husband is in a prison camp in a foreign land, she would not be able to fulfill that wish. Simply because one has a *munus* does not mean that one has failed if one does not actualize the full reality of that *munus*, nor does it mean that one has a right to actualize one's *munus*.

But some will ask, if it is the *munus* of spouses to have children, why could they not use the assistance of technology to help them have a child? As *Donum vitae* makes clear, some kinds of assistance are moral and some kinds are not. Those which serve to make the child the direct product of someone else's act, of the doctor's or the technician's act, are immoral. It states:

> *In reality, the origin of a human person is the result of an act of giving. The one conceived must be the fruit of his parents' love. He cannot be desired or conceived as the product of an intervention of medical or biological techniques; that would be equivalent to reducing him to an object of scientific technology (DV, II, B, 4, C,).*

And further,

> *Homologous IVF and ET is brought about outside the bodies of the couple through actions of the third parties whose competence and technical activity determine the success of the procedure. Such fertilization entrusts the life and identity of the embryo into the power of doctors and biologists and establishes the domination of technology over the origin and destiny of the human person (DV, II, B, 5).*

And still further,

> *Conception in vitro is the result of the technical action which presides over fertilization. Such fertilization is neither in fact achieved nor positively willed as the expression and fruit of a specific act of the conjugal union. In homologous IVF and ET, therefore, even if it is considered in the context of 'de facto' existing sexual relations, the generation of the human person is objectively deprived of its proper perfection: namely, that of being the result and fruit of a conjugal act in which the spouses can become "cooperators with God for giving life to a new person" (DV, II, B, 5).*

We are all aware that there are actions appropriately done only by the individual, actions that one ought never to delegate to others. A famous and apt example is that of Christian in *Cyrano de Bergerac;* his story makes it clear that we ought to write our own love letters. We ought to be the ones to kiss our spouses and take them out to dinner on anniversaries; this ought not be delegated to others. We ought not to buy machines that might do a fairly good job of writing our love letters or kissing our spouses. We ought not to hire robots to take our spouses out to a wedding anniversary dinner. A priest cannot delegate or hire someone else to say his daily mass for him; mass may get said, but it is not his mass. Children are very sensitive to the difference between a personal action that truly represents the agent and one that is inappropriately delegated. A child does not want his father's secretary to attend his school play in his father's place; it is just not the same if Dad is not there. Attending a school play is a marginally "non-delegatable" human action, but parenting one's own children through a bodily act of loving human intercourse is essentially such an action. There are some actions that are so integrally bound up with our person- hood, with our personal vocation, with our personal responsibilities, that if we cannot do these things, no one ought to do them for us.

Let me elaborate briefly on the claim that producing children through *in vitro* fertilization amounts to delegating others to perform an action that is appropriately performed only by one's self. Suppose the spouses had the skill to perform the techniques of fertilizing the egg and sperm *in vitro;* would this not be a personal act of procreation? It would not. Rather, this is just the sort of action that one can delegate to others; it makes little real difference who performs this action. It would be indeed curious to think *in vitro* fertilization moral only if the technique were performed by the spouses themselves. But we do not find it curious to think making love to one's spouse moral only when performed by one's self. One action is "delegatable"; the other is not.

What makes the child produced by *in vitro* fertilization the child of particular spouses is that egg and sperm biologically belong to them; it is not that they have performed the action of conjoining the egg and sperm. Let us also consider that it is possible for babies to be reproduced *in vitro* contrary to the wishes of a spouse; a technician, without permission, could unite the frozen sperm and eggs of any two individuals. Who then are the parents of the reproduced child? The donors or the technicians? Who has legal responsibility for a child conceived in such a manner? A child conceived through loving sexual intercourse, however, is manifestly the result of the loving action of his or her parents, an action that would have been inappropriate for anyone else to have performed.

CONCLUSION

These reflections have grown out of the attempt to articulate some of what we know about the objective reality of marriage. Individuals called to the vocation of marriage are called to vowing a lifetime union with another, a union appropriate for the task of parenting. Marrying and begetting children are intimately personal actions, actions that to be performed appropriately must conform to certain demands and responsibilities. The above reflections attempt to shed some light on the teaching of *Donum vitae* that the techniques of *in vitro* fertilization and embryo transfer are not in keeping with the dignity of the spouses nor with the dignity appropriate for the transmission of human life. It attempts to show that they remove the begetting of children from the realm of proper personal and spousal action. Whether these insights bear fruit remains to be tested, but the principle remains that a true understanding of the nature of marriage is essential to an understanding of the Church's teaching in *Humanae Vitae* and in *Donum vitae*.

ENDNOTES

[1]The original version of this paper can be found in the International Review of Natural Family Planning 11.3 (Fall, 1987).

[2]Congregation for the Doctrine of the Faith, Instruction on Respect for Human Life in Its Origin and the Dignity of Procreation, (22 February 1987), Part II; (hereinafter Donum vitae).

[3]John Paul II, Familiaris Consortio (22 November 1981), n. 3.

[4]Donum vitae, Intro., n. 1.

[5]Ibid., n. 3.

[6]Paul VI, Humanae Vitae (25 July 1968), n. 8 reprinted in Vatican II: More Post Conciliar Documents, Vatican Collection, Vol. 2 ed. Austin Flannery (Boston: St. Paul Editions, 1982), p. 400.

[7]Second Vatican Council Decree on the Apostolate of Lay People, Apostolicam Actuositatem, n. 2, reprinted in Vatican Council II: The Conciliar and Post Conciliar Documents, 2nd ed., ed. Austin Flannery (Collegeville, Minn.: Liturgical Press, 1980), 767-68. (All quotations are from this edition.)

[8]Donum vitae, Intro., n. 3.

[9]Ibid., n. 4, the internal quotation is from John XXIII, Mater et Magistra (15 May 1961), II.

[10]See my forthcoming book on Humanae Vitae to be published by Catholic University of America Press.

[11]Second Vatican Council, Dogmatic Constitution on the Church in the Modern World, Lumen Gentium reprinted in Vatican Council II: The Conciliar and Post Conciliar Documents, 2nd ed. Austin Flannery (Collegeville, Minn.: Liturgical Press, 1980).

[12]Second Vatican Council, Pastoral Constitution on the Church in the Modern World, reprinted in Vatican Council II: Flannery (Collegeville, Minn.: Liturgical Press, 1980); all quotations are from this edition; (hereinafter Gaudium et spes).

[13]Pius XI, Casti Connubii (31 December 1930), I, n. 13.

[14]Gaudium et spes, n. 50.

[15]See note #10 above.

6

A Contemporary Natural Law Ethics

Germain Grisez, Ph.D.

ABSTRACT

This paper summarizes the natural-law theory I have been developing with the help of other philosophers. This ethical theory is a cognitivist, nonintuitionist, personalist alternative to consequentialism, Kantianism, and virtue ethics. The idea of *basic human goods* is explained, and the basic goods listed. The first principle of morality is proposed and clarified. The idea of *modes of responsibility* is explained, and a few of them articulated. Some elements of action theory are presented, especially to clarify the distinction between choosing and accepting side effects. The manner in which moral norms are derived from principles is summarized, and the idea of moral absolutes explained. Free choice, personal identity, and character are treated, and the notion of *virtue* clarified. A theological epilogue states the relationship between this ethical theory and Christian faith. Finally, a selected, annotated bibliography points readers interested in the theory to other works which further explain and defend it.

1. Introduction

In 1959, I began working on ethical theory by studying St. Thomas on natural law.[1] Over the years, I made the modifications required by modern and contemporary problems, phenomenological descriptions of moral realities, linguistic clarifications of relevant expressions, and a constant effort at critical reflection and systematization. Other philosophers, especially Joseph M. Boyle, Jr., and John Finnis, have been helping with this work. The theory we are developing is *a*--not *the*--contemporary natural-law ethics.

This paper only summarizes the theory. For its further explanation and defense, those interested may look into works listed in the bibliography.

Like consequentialist, Kantian, and other natural-law theories of morality, ours is cognitivist but not intuitionist. We think there are true moral principles from which the most specific moral norms can be deduced and by which judgments of conscience can be criticized. The theory we propose is less familiar than its consequentialist and Kantian alternatives, and can be initially situated by reference to them.

Consequentialist theories are teleological; they try to ground moral judgments in human well-being. Kantian theories are deontological; they try to ground moral judgments in the rational nature of the moral subject, whose inherent dignity they emphasize. Teleology appeals to many because it does not absolutize morality but subordinates it to a wider human flourishing. But deontology also has its appeal, for it tries to defend the absolute dignity of human persons, especially against any attempt to justify using some as mere means to the goals of others.

Our theory tries to combine the strengths and avoid the weaknesses of teleology and deontology. Morality, we hold, is grounded in human goods--the goods of real people living in the world of experience. Still, each person's dignity is protected by moral absolutes, and it never is right to treat anyone as a mere means.

2. The idea of basic human goods

In the widest sense in which the word "good" is applied to human actions and their principles it refers to anything a person can in any way desire. But people desire many things--e.g., pleasure, wealth, and power--whose very pursuit seems to empty a person and to divide persons from one another. However, there are other goods--e.g., knowledge of the truth and living in friendship--whose pursuit of itself seems to promote persons and bring them together. Goods like these are real parts of the integral fulfillment of persons. We call them "basic human goods"--*basic* not to survival but to fulfillment.

Some goods are definite objectives, desired states of affairs--e.g., losing twenty pounds, getting an enemy to surrender, or successfully completing a research project. But in themselves the basic human goods--e.g., health, peace, or knowledge of the truth--are not definite objectives. Pursuit of these goods never ends, for they cannot be attained finally and completely. Interest in them goes beyond particular objectives sought for their sake, for they transcend states of affairs which instantiate them. It follows that persons acting alone and in various forms of community can contribute to the realization of such goods and share in them, but can never become wholly identified with them.

But if the basic human goods are not definite objectives, how do they guide action? By providing the reasons to consider some possibilities choiceworthy opportunities. An enemy's surrender becomes an objective to be pursued because of the belief that it will contribute to peace; the loss of twenty pounds is sought, perhaps, for the sake of health; particular projects of theoretical research are carried out in the hope that their results will advance knowledge. These reasons for choosing and acting provided by basic human goods do not require any prior reasons. The prospects of human fulfillment held out by peace, health, knowledge, and so on, naturally generate corresponding interests in human persons as potential agents.

Thus, human practical reflection begins from the basic human goods. They are expanding fields of possibility which underlie all the reasons one has for choosing and carrying out one's choices. This fact gives human life both its constant and universal features, and its diversity and open-endedness. The basic human goods explain the creativity characteristic, in our experience, only of human beings. They provide the framework of ideals necessary for the unfolding in history of human cultures.

3. Which are the basic human goods?

Some goods, though important, are not basic, for they are not intrinsic to personal fulfillment. No external good--nothing a person makes or has, considered as distinct from the person--can be basic. Individuals and communities always seek such goods for ulterior reasons, which culminate within persons.

Even goods of a more personal and interpersonal character are not yet basic if they can be desired only for their instrumental value. Liberty, for example, is a great good, but not basic; by itself it does not fulfill persons, but only enables them to pursue various forms of fulfillment. Thus, people want liberty to pursue the truth, to worship as they believe right, to live in friendship, and so on.

"Enjoyment" refers to a variety of states of consciousness, which have in common only that they are preferred to their alternatives. A preferred state of consciousness is at best part of a person's sharing in some good; in other words, it is part of the instantiation of a good. Thus enjoyment is not basic. But since "enjoy" refers to conscious participation in one or more of the basic goods, one needs no ulterior reason to enjoy oneself.

Both reflection on one's own deliberation and observation of the diverse ways in which people organize their lives make it clear that there are several basic human goods. For example, truth and friendship plainly mark out distinct fields of concern. Neither is reducible to the other nor to any more fundamental concern. This diversity of basic human goods is no mere contingent fact. Rather, since such goods are aspects of the integral fulfillment of persons, they correspond to the inherent complexity of human nature, both in individuals and in various forms of association.

As *bodily beings*, human persons are living animals. Life itself--its maintenance and transmission--health, and safety are one category of basic human good. As *rational*, human beings can know reality and appreciate beauty and whatever intensely engages their capacities to know and feel. Knowledge and esthetic experience are another category of basic good. As simultaneously *rational* and *animal*, human persons can transform the material world by using realities, beginning with their own bodily selves, to express meanings and/or serve purposes within human cultures. The fullness of such meaning-giving and value-creation is still another category of basic good--excellence in work and play.

Everyone shares to some extent in the preceding goods prior to any deliberate pursuit of them. Life, knowledge, and various skills are first received as gifts of nature and as parts of a cultural heritage. But children quickly come to see these goods as fields in which they can care for, expand, and improve upon what they have received. Life, knowledge, and excellence in performance are basic human goods insofar as they can be cherished, enhanced, and handed on to others.

There is another dimension of human persons. As *agents through deliberation and choice,* they can strive to avoid or overcome various forms of conflict and alienation, and can seek after harmony, integration, and fellowship. Choices themselves are essential parts of this relational dimension of persons. The already given aspects of personal unity and interpersonal relationship provide grounds for this dimension, yet it goes beyond what is given.

Most obvious among the basic human goods of this relational dimension are various forms of harmony between and among persons and groups of persons: friendship, peace, fraternity, and so on. Within individuals, similar goods can be realized: inner peace, self-integration, authenticity. And beyond human relationships, there can be harmony between humans and the wider reaches of reality and its principles. Concern for this last good underlies such diverse activities as believers' worship and environmentalists' work to save endangered species.

The relational goods are instantiated by a synthesis of elements--feelings, experiences, beliefs, choices, performances, persons, and wider realities. Ideally, harmony enhances its diverse elements, but, in fact, conflict is seldom overcome without loss to the elements synthesized. Defective forms of harmony often are built upon a significant level of conflict. For example, established, working relationships between exploiters and exploited are a sort of peace, yet radically defective. Such defective harmonies, as harmonies, are intelligible goods; they can serve as principles of practical reasoning and action. Yet they are mutilated forms of the basic human goods.

4. The first moral principle

To understand right and wrong, one must bear two things in mind. First, the possibilities of human fulfillment are indefinite and always unfolding, for there are several basic human goods, and endless ways of serving and sharing in them. Second, human beings, even when they work together, can only do so much. No one can undertake every project and serve in every possible way. Nor can any community. Choices must be made.

Compulsive behavior, ineptitude, and the unwelcome results of mistakes and bad luck are not moral wrongs. Only in choosing can people go wrong morally. On any ethical theory, moral norms tell people how to choose.

On the account of human goods outlined above, it might seem hard to see how anyone can choose badly. Without reasons for choosing grounded in basic human goods, there would be no options; yet the choice of an option is never rationally necessary--otherwise, there would not be two or more real options. Thus, on the preceding account, every choice is grounded in some intelligible good, and to that extent is rational, yet no choice has a monopoly on rationality. Moreover, virtually every choice has some negative impact on some good or other. Thus, no choice can be made without setting aside some reason for not making it.

Partly in response to this real complexity, consequentialists try to distinguish good from bad choices by their effectiveness in maximizing good and minimizing evil. But consequentialism is unworkable, for although one may be able to commensurate the measurable value and disvalue promised by different instantiations of goods, one cannot commensurate the goods and bads which make diverse possibilities choiceworthy opportunities, for these goods and bads go beyond what is definite at any moment of choice.

But if consequentialism is unworkable, how can basic human goods mark the moral distinction between choosing well and choosing badly?

There are two ways of choosing. First, one can accept the inevitable limitations of choosing and regard any particular good one chooses as a mere participation in the wider good; choosing thus, one sees the good one chooses as part of a larger and ever-expanding whole, and chooses it in a way which allows for its harmonious integration with other elements of that whole. Second, one can choose in a way which unnecessarily forecloses some further possibilities of fulfillment; one treats the particular good one is realizing here and now as if it were by itself more complete than one knows it to be.

Choices made in the first way are well made, for they are entirely in accord with reality; choices made in the second way are badly made, for they are partly at odds with reality. This distinction between choosing well and choosing badly is the first moral principle. It can be formulated: In voluntarily acting for human goods and avoiding what is opposed to them, one ought to choose and otherwise will those and only those possibilities whose willing is compatible with integral human fulfillment.

This formulation can be misunderstood. "Integral human fulfillment" does not refer to individualistic self-fulfillment. Rather, it refers to the good of all persons and communities. All the goods in which any person can share also can fulfill others, and individuals can share in goods such as friendship only with others.

Nor is integral human fulfillment some gigantic synthesis of the instantiations of goods in a vast state of affairs which might be projected as the goal of a U.N.O. billion-year plan. Ethics cannot be an architectonic art in that way; there can be no plan to bring about integral human fulfillment. It is a guiding ideal rather than a realizable idea, for the goods are open-ended.

Moreover, integral human fulfillment is not a supreme good, beyond basic goods such as truth and friendship. It does not provide reasons for acting as the basic goods do. Integral human fulfillment only moderates the interplay of such reasons so that deliberation will be thoroughly reasonable.

5. Specifications of the first moral principle

One might like the ideal of integral human fulfillment but still ask: How can the formula proposed above be a serviceable first moral principle? How can any specific moral norm be derived from it?

None can be derived directly, but the first principle does imply intermediate principles from which norms can be deduced. Among these intermediate principles is the Golden Rule (or universalizability principle), for a will marked by egoism or partiality cannot be open to integral human fulfillment. And this intermediate principle leads to some specific moral judgments--e.g., Jane who wants her husband Jack to be faithful plainly violates it by sleeping with Sam.

Thus, there is a route from the first moral principle to specific moral norms. This route can be clarified by reflection on a case such as the intuitively obvious relationship between the first principle and the Golden Rule, and between the Golden Rule and specific norms of fairness.

Human choices are limited in diverse ways. Some limits are inevitable, others not. Among inevitable limits are those on people's insight into the basic goods, ideas of how to serve them, and available resources. Insofar as such limits are outside people's control, morality cannot require that they be transcended.

But some limits on choices are avoidable; one can voluntarily narrow the range of people and goods one cares about. Sometimes this voluntary narrowing has an intelligible basis, as when a person of many gifts chooses a profession and allows other talents to lie fallow. But sometimes avoidable limitations are voluntarily set or accepted without such a reason.

Sources of limitations of this last kind thus meet two conditions: (1) they are effective only by one's own choices; and (2) they are nonrational motives, not intelligible requirements of the basic human goods. Normally, the acting person either can allow these nonrational limiting factors to operate or can transcend them. For they are one's own feelings or emotions, insofar as these are not integrated with the rational appeal of the basic goods and communal fulfillment in them. Such nonintegrated feelings offer motives for behavior yet are not in themselves reasons for choosing.

The first principle of morality rationally prescribes that nonintegrated feelings be transcended. The Golden Rule forbids one to narrow interests and concerns by a certain set of such feelings--one's preference for oneself and those who are near and dear. It does not forbid differential treatment when required by inevitable limits or by intelligible requirements of shared goods.

Nonrational preferences among persons are not the only feelings which incline people to prefer limited to integral human fulfillment. Hostile feelings such as anger and hatred toward oneself or others lead intelligent, sane, adult persons to choices which are often called "stupid," "irrational," and "childish." Self-destructive and spiteful actions destroy, damage, or block some instantiations of basic human goods; willing such actions obviously is not in line with a will to integral human fulfillment.

Behavior motivated by hostility need not violate the Golden Rule. People sometimes act self-destructively without being unfair to others. Moreover, revenge can be fair: An eye for an eye. But fairness does not eliminate the unreasonableness of acting on hostile feelings in ways that intelligibly benefit no one. Thus, the Golden Rule is not the only intermediate principle which specifies the first principle of morality. It follows that an ethics of a Kantian type is mistaken if it claims that universalizability is the only principle of morality. Respect for persons--treating them always as ends and never as mere means--must mean more than treating others fairly.

Not only hostile feelings, but positive ones, can motivate people to do evil --i.e., to destroy, damage, or impede an instantiation of some basic human good. One can choose to bring about evil as a means. One does evil to avoid some other evil or to attain some ulterior good. In such cases, the choice can seem entirely rational, and consequentialists might commend it. But, as I explained above, the appearance of complete rationality is based on a false assumption: that human goods do not matter except insofar as they are instantiated and can be commensurated.

Thus, it is unreasonable to choose to destroy, damage, or impede some instance of a basic good for the sake of an ulterior end. If one makes such a choice, one does not have the reason of maximizing good or minimizing evil--there is no such reason, for the goods are noncommensurable. Rather, one is motivated by different feelings toward different instances of good. In this sort of case, one plays favorites among instantiations of goods, just as in violating the Golden Rule one plays favorites among persons.

And so, in addition to the Golden Rule and the principle which excludes acting on hostile feelings, there is another intermediate principle: Do not do evil that good may come.

Because this principle generates moral absolutes, it often is considered a threat to people's vital concrete interests. But while this principle may be a threat to interests, the moral absolutes it generates also protect real human goods which are parts of the fulfillment of actual persons; and it is reasonable to sacrifice important concrete interests to the integral fulfillment of persons.

The Golden Rule and the other principles just enunciated shape the rational prescription of the first principle of morality into definite responsibilities. Hence, we call such intermediate principles "modes of responsibility." In all, we distinguish eight of them.

6. Human action

Specific moral norms are deduced from the modes of responsibility. But one cannot explain this process without first saying something about human action.

Many people, including philosophers, unreflectively assume a rather simple model of human action, involving three elements: (1) a possible state of affairs which a potential agent wants to realize; (2) a plan to realize it by causal factors in the agent's power; and (3) the carrying out of a more or less complex set of bodily performances to bring about the desired state of affairs.

This model of action is inadequate, yet it does refer to something: to what Aristotle called *making* as distinct from *doing*. Kant saw the inadequacy of this model; he knew there is more to moral life than the pursuit of one goal after another. But because he separated the noumenal realm from the world of experience, Kant did not challenge at its own level the oversimplified account of human action. Yet reflection upon our experience as persons living our own lives will verify a more complex model.

As explained above, the basic human goods are broad fields of human possibility. Interest in these goods underlies the desire to realize any particular goal. For persons, whether acting as individuals or in groups, projects first appear as interesting possibilities, worthy of deliberation and perhaps of choice, because they seem to offer ways of uniting persons as open to fulfillment with goods which are intrinsic aspects of that fulfillment. For instance, beyond the specific objectives of any course, dedicated teachers want their students to become mature and cultured persons; beyond all his strategic objectives, a statesmanlike military commander hopes to contribute to a more peaceful and just world.

Thus, from a moral point of view, actions primarily are voluntary syntheses of acting persons or communities with basic human goods. There are at least three ways to make such a synthesis. These constitute three senses of "doing" which, from the moral point of view, are irreducibly diverse.

First, one acts when one chooses something by which one directly participates in a good. For example, when one gives a gift as an act of friendship, one chooses to realize a certain state of affairs--giving the gift--as a way of serving the good of friendship, the very fulfillment of self and other in this form of harmony, which is instantiated by giving and receiving the gift.

Second, one acts in a different way when one chooses something not for itself but as a means to an ulterior end. What is chosen is not willed as an instantiation of a basic good, but as something through which one expects to bring about an instantiation of a good. For example, many people work only to get their pay. The chosen means need not be such that it would never be chosen for its inherent value: For business purposes one sometimes makes a trip one might also take as a vacation.

Third, one acts in a still different way when one voluntarily accepts side effects incidental to acting in either of the two prior ways. Here one is aware that executing one's choice will affect, for good or ill, instances of goods other than those on which one's interest directly bears. Although one does not choose this impact on other goods, one foresees it and accepts it--sometimes reluctantly (e.g., when one accepts the loss of a diseased organ to save one's life), sometimes gladly (e.g., when one accepts the bonus of making new friends when one agrees to participate in a philosophy workshop).

Because the three sorts of willing distinguished here relate acting persons to goods in different ways, they ground three distinct meanings of "doing." The significance of the distinction emerges most clearly in negative cases. One may reveal shameful truths about another out of spite, or to arouse shame and provide an occasion for repentance, or as a side-effect of preventing harm to some other, innocent person. In all three cases, one can be said "to destroy a reputation." But the three types of action destroy reputation in different senses.

7. The derivation of specific moral norms

Specific moral norms can be derived from modes of responsibility. That is plain from the work of many philosophers with the principle of universalizability and from the examples given above pertaining to other modes. I shall now try to clarify the process of derivation.

Its heart is a deduction which can be formulated in a categorical syllogism. In the simplest case, the normative premise is a mode of responsibility, which excludes a certain way of willing toward relevant goods. The factual premise is a description of a kind of action; it indicates what willing which bears on basic human goods would be involved in doing an action of that kind. The conclusion is that doing an act of that kind is morally wrong. Actions not excluded by any mode are morally permissible; those whose omission would violate some mode are morally required.

Many ways of describing actions, especially with a focus on results, do not reveal what is necessary to derive a moral norm. For example, if killing is defined as any behavior of one person which causes the death of another, the description is insufficient for moral evaluation. Descriptions of actions adequate for moral evaluation must say or imply how the agent's will bears on relevant goods. Such descriptions indicate which of the three sorts of doing, distinguished above, will be involved in an action.

Not all the modes of responsibility apply to all three sorts of doing.

Universalizability does. Parents who show affection for a favorite child but are cold toward another violate the Golden Rule in a doing which immediately instantiates the good of familial fellowship. Superiors who assign harder jobs to subordinates they dislike and easier jobs to subordinates they like violate universalizability in choosing means. Dormitory residents who party through the night while others try to sleep but complain when others make noise during daytime hours are unfair in accepting side effects.

Thus accepting side effects of one's choices can be wrong if one does it unfairly. Similarly, even without unfairness to anyone, someone excessively attached to some good can go wrong in accepting grave side effects--for example, the aging, champion boxer who ruins his health in trying to retain his title.

However, one cannot act at all without accepting some bad side effects. In any choice, one at least devotes a certain part of one's limited time and other resources to the pursuit of a limited good and leaves unserved other goods for which one might have acted. Hence, it is impossible to have a general moral principle entirely excluding the willing of every negative impact on a basic human good. One sometimes can accept bad side effects as inevitable concomitants of a fully rational response to the intelligible requirements of goods.

Thus, the principle that evil may not be done that good may come applies only to the choice of a means to an ulterior end, not to the acceptance of side effects. Sometimes the results of doing an evil and of accepting a bad side effect can be quite similar, yet the acceptance of the side effect, if not excluded by some other mode of responsibility, will be permissible. For example, a choice to kill a suffering person, whether by a positive performance or by a purposeful omission, is morally excluded, as a case of doing evil that good may come. But a choice to limit or terminate burdensome and costly treatment, with death accepted as a side effect, need not be wrong. The treatment of free choice in the next section will help explain why differences in willing have such great moral significance, even when the results are quite similar.

Actions can be described more or less fully. If a limited description of an action makes it clear that it involves a choice to destroy, damage, or impede some instance of a basic human good, then the wrongness of any action which meets that description is settled. Additional factors may affect the degree of wrongness, but further description of the act cannot reverse its basic moral quality. For this reason, moral norms derived from this mode of responsibility can be called "moral absolutes." For example, an absolute norm forbids killing one innocent person to prevent that person and several others from being killed by a mob.

Different modes work differently, so not all specific norms are absolute. Universalizability can exclude as unfair an action proposed under a limited description, yet allow as fair an action which includes all the elements of that description together with some other morally relevant features. For example, fairness demands promise keeping, whenever the only motive for breaking a promise is of the sort whose operation promises are meant to exclude. But someone who has another reason to break a promise--for example, that keeping it would have such grave consequences that even those to whom it was made would agree it should be broken--may break the promise without violating the Golden Rule.

In general, specific norms based on universalizability are nonabsolute. That may not appear to be so, since ordinary language sometimes builds the moral specification into the act description--e.g., by limiting "stealing" to the wrongful taking of another's property. However, instances of justifiable taking can include all the elements which are present in unjustifiable taking; the addition, not the subtraction, of relevant features makes the taking justifiable.

8. Free choice, personal identify, and character

Classical moral philosophers sought the wisdom to live good lives. By their standard, the ethical theory summarized thus far is inadequate. For being a good person is more than conforming each of one's acts to an appropriate moral norm.

One makes a choice when one faces practical alternatives, believes one can and must settle which to take, and deliberately takes one. The choice is free when choosing itself determines which alternative one takes. True, factors beyond one's control provided options and limited them. But, if free, only one's choice determined which option one would adopt.

The particular goal realized by a successful action is sensibly good and experienced as such, but the appealing goodness with respect to which one determines oneself in choosing to do that action is intelligible and transcends that experience. For example, recovery from a particular illness is sensibly good; health, to which one determines oneself in choosing to do what is necessary to get well, is intelligibly good. In many successful human actions, the goods concretely realized can also be realized by natural processes or spontaneous human acts without choice; by contrast, the sharing in and service to goods to which one determines oneself by choice can only occur in one's self-determining choice.

As self-creative, free choices transcend the material world. They are not events or processes or things in the world; they must be distinguished from the performances which execute them. The performances of particular acts come and go, but a choice, once made, determines the self unless and until one makes another, incompatible choice. Self-determination through choice means that the self is actualized and limited; one's orientation toward further possibilities is more or less settled. By choices, one not only brings about instantiations of goods, but participates in definite ways in the basic human goods.

There are large choices, which put one in the position of having to carry them out by many small choices. Examples of large choices are to become a philosopher, to get married, and to take up photography as a hobby. Some large choices can be called "commitments." To make a commitment is more than to adopt a long-range goal. Commitments bear directly upon goods such as religion, justice, friendship, authenticity, and so on. Since these are interrelated, any commitment will somehow bear on all of them. And since they include interpersonal harmony, every commitment joins one to a particular person or group.

The first moral principle requires willing in line with integral human fulfillment. Such willing must meet the conditions for effective and consistent participation in basic human goods. Without an integrated set of upright commitments, one cannot participate in goods effectively and consistently. Therefore, each of us must discern which commitments are personally appropriate, make and integrate them, and faithfully carry them out.

Some aspects of personal identity are given: One has a certain genetic make up, is brought up in a certain culture, and so forth. But the matrix of moral self-identity is one's free choices; mature people define themselves by their commitments. Still, a morally mature, good person is more than a set of upright commitments. For to faithfully carry out upright commitments, the whole personality must be developed and limited in line with them; they must shape feelings, beliefs, experiences, modes of behavior, skills, and so on. Thus, a good person is one whose whole self is formed by a comprehensive set of upright commitments.

Such a person has good character, whose facets are called "virtues." Since there are many ways of distinguishing facets of character, there are many classifications of virtues. But however classified, virtues are moral fruits, not moral principles. For virtues are only parts of a personality shaped by the carrying out of morally upright commitments, and such commitments are upright because they arise from and are shaped by propositional principles of practical reasoning and of morality.

9. The way of the Lord Jesus

Describing the good person is easy; living a good life often seems impossible. The good we achieve and enjoy is mutilated and threatened by ineptitude, failure, breakdown, ignorance, error, misunderstanding, pain, sickness, and death. We sometimes freely choose to violate known moral truths; we never perfectly fulfill our commitments. Perhaps we could live better private lives if we had the support of a good society, and we also need a good society because the human is naturally social. But there are many wicked people in the world, and powerful people seem especially likely to be wicked. Thus, every political society constitutionally compromises with systematic injustice and other sorts of immorality. All humankind lives in slavery, though some are always only slaves, while others sometimes also play the role of master.

Philosophical reflection seems unable to explain this situation and to show the way to freedom. Immorality, precisely insofar as it is rooted in truly free choices, is inexplicable and unpreventable. Apart from immorality, the most repugnant aspects of the human condition are epitomized by death, which seems natural and inevitable. Wrestling with the mystery of the human situation, ancient and non-Western philosophers ignore free choice, and modern and contemporary Western philosophers deny it. Almost all try to evade the reality of death by making some sort of rationally indefensible distinction between the morally significant human person and the human organism doomed to die.

The Christian gospel, I believe, offers a more adequate account of the situation. According to this account, God is a communion of three persons, who created human persons so that they might share in divine communion and live in human fellowship. In creating, God promised to forestall death, naturally inevitable for the human organism as such, if men and women cooperated with the divine plan. But from humankind's beginning, wrongful free choices blocked the formation and development of an inclusive human community, constitutionally uncompromised by evil. And so God permitted nature to take its course and humans to taste death, at least partly so that they might experience the wretchedness of their fallen condition, and be eager to escape it.

Human liberation, according to the gospel's proposal, can be gained in two stages by any who truly desire it. One of the divine persons became the man

Jesus, who lived a morally unblemished human life. In doing so, he not only provided a unique example of how to live uprightly in the broken human situation, but also made himself available as the head of the human community God had planned from the beginning. All are invited to make faith in Jesus and his cause the central commitment of their lives. In making such a commitment, the gospel teaches, Jesus' disciples enter not only into fellowship with one another but into the communion of the divine family.

The gospel teaches Christians that if they live their lives to implement their faith in Jesus, they will live the best human lives possible in this broken world. Following the way of the Lord Jesus, individual Christians can become good people, and on the basis of their common bond with Jesus they can work together to build up decent community in the Church and in their Christian families.

Yet this first stage of liberation is incomplete, since the upright must suffer at the hands of the wicked and all must suffer the human misery which culminates in death. The second, and final, stage of liberation requires a divine act of re-creation. This re-creation, according to the gospel, began with Jesus' resurrection from the dead, and will be completed by the raising up of all who die in faith, and their reunion in an unending divine-human fellowship, protected forever from the wicked.

If the Christian gospel is true, the normative ethical theory outlined in the previous sections remains adequate. The basic human goods remain, though they unfold in unexpected ways. The modes of responsibility remain, though they generate many specifically Christian norms, to govern actions people without faith either could not think of at all or would not think of as choiceworthy.

Most important, the Christian need not accept an Augustinian or Thomistic version of neo-Platonism, with its supposition that the human heart is naturally insatiable by human fulfillment, and naturally drawn to fulfillment in the Beatific Vision of God. For faith does not substitute a supreme instantiation of a supernatural good for integral human fulfillment.

Rather, it holds out the hope of an unending marriage feast. In this communion of divine and human persons, all the basic human goods will be instantiated without the defects imposed by the broken world and the limits imposed by death. And the more-than-human fulfillment which is naturally proper to God alone also will be enjoyed by his adopted sons and daughters.

ENDNOTES

[1]This paper has been previously published in a collection entitled Contemporary Ethical Thought and the History of Moral Philosophy (Marquette University Press, 1988).

SELECTED BIBLIOGRAPHY

Germain Grisez, <u>Contraception and the Natural Law</u> (Milwaukee: Bruce, 1964), xiii+245. Chapter three is an early version of the theory; for understanding its mature form, only the critique of "conventional" natural-law approaches remains helpful. The critique of consequentialism ("situationism") here, and up to "Choice and Consequentialism," mistakenly focuses on the noncommensurability <u>of the different categories</u> of basic human goods.

_____ , "The First Principle of Practical Reason: A Commentary on the <u>Summa Theologiae</u>, 1-2, Question 94, Article 2," <u>The Natural Law Forum</u>, 10 (1965), 168-201; abridged version: <u>Modern Studies in Philosophy: Aquinas: A Collection of Critical Essays</u>, ed. Anthony Kenny (Garden City, N.Y.: Doubleday & Co., 1969), 340-82. (Kenny did some significant, unauthorized editing, so it is best to use the original.) Of works listed in this bibliography, this article and the next are Grisez's only attempts at Thomistic exegesis. Elsewhere, he tries to do philosophy or theology, not history, and freely parts company with St. Thomas, often without saying so.

_____ , "Man, Natural End of" in <u>The New Catholic Encyclopedia,</u> 9:132-38. By examining the efforts of various groups of Thomists to make sense of St. Thomas's teaching on the natural end of human persons, and by pointing out many inconsistencies in which he says about the ultimate end, this article deliberately comes within a step of rejecting his position (and with it, the positions of both Aristotle and St. Augustine) on the ultimate end of human persons.

_____ , <u>Abortion: The Myths, the Realities, and the Arguments</u> (New York and Cleveland: Corpus Books, 1970), ix+559. Chapter six is a restatement of the theory, with its application to abortion and other killing, including capital punishment and war. Some find this presentation of the theory especially attractive, perhaps partly because it is easier to follow than later, more adequate versions. Certain critics, including Richard A. McCormick, S.J., still deal with this statement of the theory, and make objections whose answers they could find in later works.

_____ and Russell Shaw, <u>Beyond the New Morality: The Responsibilities of Freedom</u>, 3rd ed. (Notre Dame: University of Notre Dame Press, 1988), xi+ 256. Intended for use with beginning students as part of an introduction to ethics, this version of the theory is accessible, but somewhat simplified. Many important aspects of the theory and arguments for it are deliberately omitted, even from the 3rd edition.

Joseph M. Boyle, Jr., "Aquinas and Prescriptive Ethics," <u>Proceedings of the American Catholic Philosophical Association</u>, 49 (1975), 82-95. A clear account and critique of Hare's prescriptivism.

Germain Grisez, <u>Beyond the New Theism: A Philosophy of Religion</u> (Notre Dame and London: University of Notre Dame Press, 1975), xiii+418. The metaphysical foundations of the ethical theory are explained and defended in this book, which had the benefit of many years of work with Boyle and Tollefsen, especially on the book listed next. Chapters six through thirteen are an exposition and criticism of the modern and contemporary alternatives; chapter twenty-three deals with the irreducible complexity of the human person and community of persons.

74

Joseph M. Boyle, Jr., Germain Grisez, and Olaf Tollefsen, Free Choice: A Self-Referential Argument (Notre Dame and London: University of Notre Dame Press, 1976), xi+207. The most complete account of free choice and related elements of action theory, and a criticism of alternative views of these matters, which are so essential to ethical theory.

The Teaching of Christ: A Catholic Catechism for Adults, ed. Ronald Lawler, O.F.M., Cap., Donald W. Wuerl, and Thomas Comerford Lawler (Huntington, Ind.: Our Sunday Visitor, 1976), 640. Finnis and Grisez (Finnis more than Grisez) did the first draft of chapters eighteen through twenty-one, but their draft was revised considerably by the editors. Work on this project was the most important starting point of the subsequent development of the ethical theory in the context of moral theology.

Germain Grisez, "Choice and Consequentialism," Proceedings of the American Catholic Philosophical Association, 51 (1977), 144-52. The first presentation of the mature version (which corrects earlier ones) of the argument against consequentialism based on the noncommensurability of those goods and bads which are the intelligible grounds for the options between or among which a *free* choice must be made.

_____ , "Against Consequentialism," The American Journal of Jurisprudence and Legal Philosophy, 23 (1978), 21-72. The most thorough critique of consequentialism.

Joseph M. Boyle, Jr., "Praeter Intentionem in Aquinas, "The Thomist, 42 (1978), 649-65. A clarification of the notion of *side effect*.

Germain Grisez and Joseph M. Boyle, Jr., Life and Death with Liberty and Justice: A Contribution to the Euthanasia Debate (Notre Dame and London: University of Notre Dame Press, 1979), xiii+521. Chapters eleven and twelve benefit from Boyle's work in action theory; everything necessary to deal with life and death issues reaches nearly mature form here. The political philosophy in this book needs development and, perhaps, certain corrections. The authors now think it is usually wrong to withhold food and water from comatose patients.

John Finnis, Natural Law and Natural Rights (Oxford: Clarendon Press, 1980), xv+425. Chapters three through five deploy the ethical theory with originality, as a basis for Finnis's altogether independent philosophy of law. He gives special attention to epistemological issues raised by the empiricist tradition. There are some differences in ethical theory between Finnis, on the one hand, and Grisez and Boyle, on the other. But most differences are in formulation rather than in substance, and the more important substantive differences concern applications rather than the theory itself.

Joseph M. Boyle, Jr., "Toward Understanding the Principle of Double Effect," Ethics, 90 (1980), 527-38. A defense of the principle of double effect, with a clarification of the theory of agency it presupposes.

John Finnis and Germain Grisez, "The Basic Principles of Natural Law: A Reply to Ralph McInerny," The American Journal of Jurisprudence and Legal Philosophy, 26 (1981), 21-31. A defense against a Thomist of stricter observance.

John Finnis, <u>Fundamentals of Ethics</u> (Oxford: Oxford University Press; Washington, D.C.: Georgetown University Press, 1983), x+163. Finnis restates much of the theory, and engages in a rich dialectic both with the history of philosophy and with contemporary English-language work in ethical theory.

Germain Grisez, <u>The Way of the Lord Jesus,</u> vol. one, <u>Christian Moral Principles</u>, with the help of Joseph M. Boyle, Jr., Basil Cole, O.P., John M. Finnis, John A. Geinzer, Jeannette Grisez, Robert G. Kennedy, Patrick Lee, William E. May, and Russell Shaw (Chicago: Franciscan Herald Press, 1983), xxxiv+971. Chapters two through twelve are the most mature and complete statement of the theory thus far. Boyle contributed a total of more than six months of intense, *full-time* work to this volume. The rethinking in a theological context of the whole theory without reference to any particular issue (such as abortion or euthanasia) led to many important developments, and a considerable increase in the tightness of the system. Chapters nineteen and thirty-four provide a theological account of the ultimate end of human persons; chapters twenty-five and twenty-six explain the specificity of Christian ethics.

John Finnis, "Practical Reasoning, Human Goods, and the End of Man," <u>Proceedings of the American Catholic Philosophical Association</u>, 58 (1984), 23-36. A conciliatory comparison of the ideal of integral human fulfillment with the ultimate end as St. Thomas understands it. Finnis, whose view is closer than Grisez's to that of St. Thomas, here emphasizes points of agreement.

Joseph M. Boyle, Jr., "Aquinas, Kant, and Donagan on Moral Principles," <u>The New Scholasticism,</u> 58 (1984), 391-408. A criticism of Donagan's nonconsequentialist (Kantian) ethics.

John Finnis, Joseph M. Boyle, Jr., and Germain Grisez, <u>Nuclear Deterrence, Morality and Realism</u> (Oxford and New York: Oxford University Press, 1987), xv+429. A fresh, philosophical presentation of the theory, with a careful application to the morality of nuclear deterrence. The present paper is in part a considerably revised version of a first draft of chapter ten of this book.

Germain Grisez, Joseph Boyle, Jr., and John Finnis, "Practical Principles, Moral Truth, and Ultimate Ends," <u>The American Journal of Jurisprudence</u>, 32 (1987), 99-151. A restatement, clarification, and updating of many elements of the theory often criticized (and generally misunderstood) by philosophers in the (broadly speaking, Thomistic) natural-law tradition from which the theory was developed.

Catholic Teaching on the Laboratory Generation of Human Life

William May, Ph.D.

July 25, 1978 is a memorable date in history. It is, first of all, the birthday of Louise Brown, the "test tube" baby, the miracle child of modern technology. Although she was not the first baby to be conceived *in vitro,* she was the first child conceived in this way to be born. What is most significant about her birth is that it marks the first time in human history when new human life was born after having been conceived outside the body of a human person, that is, the mother. New human life can now come to be in the laboratory and not in the body of a woman.

Artificial insemination, whether by husband or vendor,[1] had already severed the generation of human life from the act of sexual union, and *in vitro* fertilization necessarily requires this separation, the significance of which will occupy us later. Artificial insemination, insofar as it requires biological technology and expertise and entails the severing of the bond between sexual intercourse and the generation of new human life, was the beginning of the shift from generating human life bodily through sexual union of man and woman to producing it in the laboratory. Accordingly, artificial insemination will be included as a mode of laboratory generation of human life. Nonetheless, with artificial insemination the life generated still comes to be in the body of a woman, and some mystery still shrouds its origin and early development. With the advent of *in vitro* fertilization, or the laboratory generation of human life in a more complete way, however, there has been, as it were, a "demystification" of the inception of human life. The contingencies beyond human control affecting its origin have been significantly reduced, and the origin and early development of new human life have now been brought, to considerable degree, under the control of human will and planning. We can now literally "make" babies, and our capacity to do so has become, within the decade since the birth of Louise Brown, much more sophisticated and "successful" than it was when Drs. Steptoe and Edwards managed the conception, gestation, and birth of Louise.[2]

July 25, 1978 is memorable, secondly, because it is the tenth anniversary of Pope Paul VI's encyclical on marriage and the generation of human life, *Humanae Vitae.* In his encyclical Pope Paul affirmed that there is "an inseparable connection, willed by God and unable to be broken by man on his own initiative, between the two meanings of the conjugal act: the unitive meaning and the procreative meaning".[3] The Pope appealed to this "inseparable connection" as the fundamental truth undergirding the Church's teaching on the intrinsic immorality of contraception, insofar as the choice to contracept severs the bond between these two meanings of the conjugal act. He had, it should be noted, given other reasons to show that contraception is intrinsically disordered; for example, he explicitly noted that contraception is immoral because it is directly opposed to the divine gift of fertility, something good in itself.[4] But his principal claim was this: the Church's teaching that "each and every marriage act must remain open to the transmission of human life" is "founded upon" the "inseparable connection" between the unitive and procreative meanings of the conjugal act.[5] In addition, Pope Paul emphasized that the conjugal act, by reason of its intimate structure as an act most closely uniting husband and wife, "capacitates them for the generation of new life *(eos idoneos etiam facit ad novam vitam gignendam),* according to laws inscribed in the very being of man and of woman".[6]

Pope Paul's concern in *Humanae Vitae* was with contraception and not with the laboratory generation of human life. Nonetheless, his teaching on the "inseparable connection" between the two meanings of the conjugal act plays a central role in the March 1987 *Instruction on Respect for Human Life in Its Origin and on the Dignity of Procreation,* in which the Congregation for the Doctrine of the Faith formally addressed the moral issues raised by various reproductive technologies. This document, drawing on the teaching about marriage and human procreation developed in the light of the Catholic tradition by Popes Pius XII, Paul VI, and John Paul II, insists that the generation of human life, if it is to respect the dignity of both parents and children, "must be the fruit and sign of the mutual self-giving of the spouses, of their love and fidelity".[7] In its treatment of heterologous fertilization, in which gametes, whether ova or sperm, from parties other than the spouses are used to generate new human life, the *Instruction,* not surprisingly, concludes that this way of generating human life is gravely immoral. It is so because heterologous fertilization is "contrary to the unity of marriage, to the dignity of the spouses, to the vocation proper to parents, and the child's right to be conceived and brought into the world in marriage and from marriage".[8]

Although some individuals find this judgment of the *Instruction* too limiting and restrictive of human freedom,[9] most people, whether Catholic or non-Catholic, can see its wisdom. In getting married a man and a woman "give" themselves exclusively to each other, and the "selves" they give are sexual and procreative in nature. Just as they violate their marital covenant by attempting, after marriage, to "give" themselves sexually, in coition, to another, so too they violate that covenant by choosing freely to exercise their sexual power of generating life with someone other than their spouse, the person to whom they have irrevocably given themselves, including their power to generate life. Moreover, a sperm or ovum "vendor," by freely choosing to bring new life into being by selling his sperm or her ovum for the purpose of generating human life, becomes a parent, a father or mother. Yet such a person refuses to accept the responsibilities of parenthood; and the child who comes to be as a result of their choice and who is, in truth, their own flesh and blood, will not even know them and will be deprived of their care, something to which it has a right. For all these reasons - briefly yet accurately set forth in the *Instruction* -- most people can see why it is morally bad to generate human life by laboratory methods that are heterologous in nature. For those who for some factor or another cannot grasp these reasons the tragic story of "Baby M" should be instructive.[10]

The "hard" case taken up by the *Instruction*, and the one in which Pope Paul's teaching on the "inseparable connection" plays such a key role, is that of homologous fertilization, when the gametes used to generate new human life are provided by the husband and wife. At times this entails artificial insemination of the wife by the husband; at other times it entails *in vitro* fertilization of the wife's ovum by sperm provided by her husband, with subsequent embryo transfer into her own womb. In this "hard" or, viewed somewhat differently, "simple" case there is no use of gametic materials from third parties; the child conceived is genetically the child of husband and wife, who are and will remain its parents. In this case there need be no deliberate creation of "excess" human lives that will be discarded (perhaps through a procedure that some term, euphemistically, "pregnancy reduction,"[11]) frozen, or made the objects of medical experimentations of no value to them. In this case there need be no intention of intrauterine monitoring with a view to abortion should the unborn child be found "defective." Nor need there be, in this case, the use of immoral means (masturbation) to obtain the father's sperm. In this case, apparently, there need be only the intent to help fulfill the legitimate desire of a couple, unable either by reason of the wife's blocked fallopian tubes or the husband's low sperm production or other causes, to have a child of their own and give it a home. Many people, both Catholic and non-Catholic, think that resort to the laboratory generation of human life is morally legitimate in this "simple case" of *in vitro* fertilization. They ask, quite reasonably, what could be morally offensive here? What wrong is being done? What evil is being willed?

Yet the *Instruction*, in company with Pope Pius XII and his successors, claims that even this type of homologous fertilization is morally wrong because it involves the deliberate willing of an evil. And to support this claim the *Instruction* appeals, first and foremost, to the teaching of Pope Paul VI on the "inseparable connection, willed by God and unable to be broken by man on his own initiative, between the two meanings of the conjugal act: the unitive meaning and the procreative meaning."[12] The evil willed in homologous fertilization is the "separation" of these meanings that, in God's plan, are inseparably connected. Applying this teaching to homologous fertilization, the *Instruction* appeals to the authority of Pope Pius XII, who had said that "it is never permitted to separate these different aspects to such a degree as positively to exclude either the procreative intention (as is done in contraceptive intercourse) or the conjugal relation".[13] The *Instruction* then concludes that

> *fertilization is licitly sought when it is the result of a "conjugal act which is per se suitable for the generation of children to which marriage is ordered by its nature and by which the spouses become one flesh." But from the moral*

point of view procreation is deprived of its proper perfection when it is not desired as the fruit of the conjugal act, that is to say, of the specific act of the spouses' union.[14]

In summary, a principal argument given in the Vatican *Instruction* to show that homologous fertilization, even in the "simple case" described previously, is morally bad employs as its major premise the teaching on the "inseparable connection" between the unitive and procreative meanings of the conjugal act. This document also uses two other lines of argument to support its conclusion, and these will be considered below, namely, the argument that generating human life in the laboratory is a form of "production" and hence an act that violates the dignity of the child produced, and the argument that generating human life in this way falsifies the "language of the body." But here our interest centers on the argument based on the "inseparable connection" of the two meanings of the conjugal act, a teaching central, as we have seen, to Pope Paul VI's encyclical, *Humanae Vitae*. The argument's conclusion, namely, that homologous fertilization is in itself immoral, follows *if* the premise on which it depends, namely, the inseparable connection between the unitive and procreative meanings of the conjugal act, is true. I hold that this premise is true. Yet it is not self-evidently so. People can reasonably question whether it is. The premise was used in *Humanae Vitae* to show that marital contraceptive intercourse is morally bad, and it was used in the *Instruction* to show that homologous fertilization is morally bad. But it is possible that the premise about the inseparability of the two meanings of the conjugal act is itself a conclusion, derived from the premises (1) that it is always wrong to contracept and (2) that it is always wrong to "make" or "produce" children. I shall consider this possibility below. But first I wish to offer some considerations, drawn from the Catholic understanding of marriage, that provide support for the truth of the proposition affirming the inseparable connection between the two meanings of the marital act, even if these considerations, derived in part from divine revelation, do not constitute, in themselves, demonstrative proof of the truth of this proposition.

MARITAL RIGHTS AND CAPABILITIES, THE MARITAL ACT, AND THE GENERATION OF HUMAN LIFE

When the teaching of Paul VI in *Humanae Vitae* and of the Congregation for the Doctrine of the Faith in its *Instruction* is examined from within the Catholic tradition, one can see, I believe, that these documents look upon the question of human procreation within the framework provided by the constant teaching of the Church on marriage and its relationship to the generation of human life, and that they regard this teaching as supporting the proposition about the inseparable connection between the unitive and procreative meanings of the conjugal act. An important point of departure is provided by what Pope Pius XII had to say in 1949, when he took up the question of homologous artificial insemination. In rejecting this way of generating human life, Pius XII spoke as follows:

We must never forget this: It is only the procreation of a new life according to the will and plan of the Creator which brings with it--to an astonishing degree of perfection--the realization of the desired ends. This is, at the same time, in harmony with the dignity of the marriage partners, with their bodily and spiritual natures, and with the normal and happy development of the child.[15]

Pius XII was evidently of the mind that God wills the generation of human life *only* in the marital act. Thus the choice to generate it outside the marital act is a choice that goes against the will of God. In 1951 he returned to this matter, saying,

To reduce the cohabitation of married persons and the conjugal act to a mere organic function for the transmission of the germs of life would be to convert the domestic hearth, sanctuary of the family, into nothing more than a biological laboratory ... The conjugal act in its natural structure is a personal action, a simultaneous natural self-giving which, in the words of Holy Scripture, effects the union "in one flesh." This is more than the mere union of two germs, which can be brought about artificially--i.e., without the natural action of the spouses. The conjugal act as it is planned and willed by nature implies a personal cooperation, the right to which parties have mutually conferred on each other in contracting marriage.[16]

The thought of Pius XII here is rooted in the Catholic understanding of marriage as a specific sort of human reality whose author is God Himself.[17] According to this understanding, married persons have capabilities, rights, and duties that nonmarried persons do not have. What are these?

By giving themselves to one another in marriage, husbands and wives not only acquire rights that nonmarried men and women do not have but they also give to themselves capabilities that nonmarried men and women do not have. Nonmarried men and women have the natural capacity, by virtue of their sexuality and their endowment with sexual organs, to engage in genital sex and to generate human life through such sexual activity. Yet they do not have the *right* either to engage in intimate genital acts or to generate human life. Although I cannot here show fully why they do not have the right to engage in genital sex,[18] I can briefly say why this is so. The reason is simply that they have not, by their own free choice, capacitated themselves to respect each other as irreplaceable and nonsubstitutable persons in their freely chosen genital acts. Such acts between nonmarried men and women do not *unite two irreplaceable and nonsubstitutable persons;* rather, they *join two individuals who are in principle replaceable and substitutable, disposable.* But human persons ought not to be treated as replaceable, substitutable, disposable things. Similarly, nonmarried men and women do not have the right to generate human life precisely because they have not, through their own free choice, capacitated themselves to receive such life lovingly, nourish it humanely, and educate it in the love and service of God.[19] Practically all civilized societies, it should be noted, rightly regard as irresponsible the generation of human life through the random copulation of unattached men and women. (It is a sign of a new barbarism that many in our society now assert the "right" of single men and women to have children, whether generated by heterosexual intercourse or by making use of the new "reproductive" technologies.)

Husbands and wives, on the contrary, have the right to the marital act, whose nature will be more fully investigated below. They have this right precisely because they have given themselves the capacity, through their irrevocable gift to themselves to one another in marriage,[20] to respect one another as irreplaceable and nonsubstitutable spouses. Likewise they have given to themselves the capacity to receive human life lovingly, nourish it humanely, and educate it in the love and service of God, for by marrying they have made themselves capable of receiving any new human life that should be given to them and of giving to it the home where it can take root and grow under the loving tutelage of its own father and mother, persons who are not strangers to one another but who are rather made one by *being* married.

An analogy may be helpful. I do not have the right to diagnose sick people and prescribe medicine for them. I do not have this right because I have not freely chosen to study medicine and to discipline myself so that I can equip myself with the knowledge and skills needed to do these tasks. But doctors, who have freely chosen to submit themselves to the discipline of studying medicine and acquiring medical skills, do have this right. They have this right because they have freely chosen to give themselves the capacity to do what doctors are supposed to do. Similarly, nonmarried men and women do not have the right to engage in intimate genital relations or to generate human life because they have not, through their free choice, given themselves the capacity needed to do these things. But husbands and wives have made the free choice to capacitate themselves to do these things because they have freely chosen to give themselves to each other in marriage and to do what married persons do, namely, give themselves to one another in the marital act and receive, through that act, the gift of new human life. The act proper to them is the "marital" act. Thus some comments on its nature are pertinent.

The marital act is not simply a genital act between a man and a woman who "happen" to be married. Husbands and wives have the capacity to engage in *genital* acts, as do nonmarried men and women, because of their sexuality and endowment with genitals. But they have the capacity (and the right) to engage in the *marital* act because they are married, i.e., because they are husbands and wives. The marital act, therefore, is more than a simple genital act between a man and a woman who happen to be married. It is an act that inwardly participates in their marital union, and it is one, furthermore, that respects the "goods" of marriage, i.e., the good of steadfast fidelity and of exclusive marital love and the good of children.[21] The *marital* act, therefore, as distinct from a *genital* act between a man and a woman who happen to be married, is one that is (1) open to the communication of spousal love and (2) open to the reception of new human life. A genital act forced upon a wife by a drunken husband seeking only to gratify his sexual urges and unconcerned with her legitimate desires is a genital act, but it cannot be regarded as a true marital act.[22] Similarly, a genital act between husbands and wives that is deliberately made hostile to the reception of human life, i.e., an act of *contra*ceptive intercourse, is also one that violates the marital act and is hence nonmarital precisely because it is an act deliberately made inimical to one of the goods of marriage.[23]

Thus the marital act is itself inwardly an act that is unitive or love-giving and procreative or receptive of the gift of life. It is so because it is *marital,* i.e., an act participating in marriage and its goods. The bond, therefore, that joins its two meanings, unitive and procreative, is the bond of marriage itself. "What God has joined together, let no man put asunder." There is an "inseparable connection, willed by God and unable to be broken by man on his own initiative, between the unitive and the procreative meanings of the marital act" because this act is the expression and sign of the marriage itself, a human reality inwardly open to the communication of conjugal love and to the reception of human life as a gift from God.

While husbands and wives have the right and capacity to engage in the marital act and, through it, receive from God the gift of life, they do not have a right to a child. They do not have this sort of right because a child is, like them, a person, not a thing that others can possess, nor is it an act to which others can have rights.

I believe that these considerations, drawn from the Catholic understanding of marriage--an understanding that in part derives from divine revelation--provide the context for the teaching on the "inseparable connection" of the unitive and procreative meanings of the conjugal act and help provide support for this teaching. Still, they do not demonstrate the truth of that proposition independently of Catholic faith, although they certainly make this proposition reasonable. A more demonstrative argument to establish the truth of the proposition about the "inseparable connection" will be advanced below. But before advancing it I want to examine a second line of reasoning advanced in the *Instruction* to show that all ways of generating human life other than by the marital act are morally wrong. This is the argument that the laboratory generation of human life regards the child as a "product" and is therefore a violation of the child's dignity.

"PROCREATING" HUMAN LIFE VS. "REPRODUCING" HUMAN LIFE

According to the *Instruction* of the Congregation for the Doctrine of the Faith, the child "cannot be desired or conceived as the product of an intervention of medical or biological techniques." Why? Because, it teaches, "that would be equivalent to reducing him to an object of scientific technology. No one may subject the coming of a child into the world to conditions of technical efficacy which are to be evaluated according to standards of control and dominion."[24] The *Instruction* then concludes:

Conception in vitro is the result of the technical action which presides over fertilization. Such fertilization is neither in fact achieved nor positively willed as the expression and fruit of a specific act of the conjugal union. In homologous IVF and ET, therefore, even if it is considered in the context of de facto existing sexual relations, the generation of the human person is objectively deprived of its proper perfection, namely, that of being the result and fruit of a conjugal act in which the spouses can become "cooperators with God for giving life to a new person."[25]

The *Instruction* is surely correct in judging that the generation of a
child through artificial homologous fertilization (including artificial insemination of an ovum within the body of the wife) is a technological procedure, an
instance of "making," and hence quite different in kind, as a human act, from the
generation of life in and through the marital act. When human life is given
through the marital act it comes, even when ardently desired, as a "gift" crowning
the act itself. The marital act is not an act of "making," either babies or
love. The marital act is something that husbands and wives "do;" it is not something that they "make." But what is the difference between "making" and "doing,"
and what is the human significance of this difference?

In "making" the action proceeds from an agent or agents to something produced
in the external world. Autoworkers, for instance, produce cars; cooks produce
meals; bakers produce cakes, etc. Such action is transitive in nature because it
passes from the acting subject(s) to an object fashioned by him or her (them). In
this kind of activity, which is governed by the rules of art, interest centers on
the object made (and ordinarily those that do not measure up to standards are
discarded--at any rate, they are little appreciated, and for this reason are frequently called "defective"). Those who produce the products made may be morally
good autoworkers or cooks or bakers or they may be morally bad, but interest in
"making" is in the product made, not the producers, and we would prefer to eat
good cakes made by morally bad bakers than indigestible ones baked by saints who
are incompetent bakers.

In "doing" the action abides in the acting subject(s). The action is immanent
and is governed by the requirements of prudence, not of art. If the action is
good, it perfects the agent(s); if bad, it degrades and dehumanizes them.[26]
I should note here that every act of making is also a doing insofar as it is
freely chosen, for the choice to make something is something that we "do," and
this choice, as self-determining, abides in us. But the important point here is
the difference between "making" and "doing".

As we have seen, the marital act is not an act of making. Rather, it is an
act freely chosen by the spouses to express their marital union, one open to the
reception of life and the communication of marital love. As such, the marital act
is an act inwardly perfective of them and of their life as spouses, the life of
which they are co-subjects; just as they are co-subjects of the marital act itself. Even when they choose this act with the ardent hope that, through it, new
human life will be given to them, the life begotten is not the product of their
act but is a "gift supervening on and giving permanent embodiment to" the marital
act itself.[27] When human life comes to be through the marital act, we say
quite properly that the spouses are "begetting" or "procreating." They are not
"making" anything. The life they receive is "begotten, not made."

But when human life comes to be as a result of various types of homologous
fertilization, it is the end product of a series of actions, transitive in nature,
undertaken by different persons. The spouses "produce" the gametic cells that
others use in order to make the end product, the child. In such a procedure the
child "comes in existence, not as a gift supervening on an act expressive of the

marital union . . . but rather in the manner of a product of a making (and, typically, as the end product of a process managed and carried out by persons other than his parents)".[28] The life generated is "made," not "begotten."

A human child, however, is not a product inferior to its producers. Rather, it is a person equal in dignity to its parents. A child, therefore, ought not to be treated as if it were a product.

To this the proponents of producing babies might argue: desire for the good, the coming to be of a new human person, leads to the choice, not wrong in itself, to bring the possible person into being. Granted, it would be preferable, if possible, to procreate the baby through the marital act. However, any disadvantages inherent in the generation of babies apart from the marital act are clearly outweighed by the great good of new human lives and the fulfillment of the desire for children of couples who otherwise cannot have them. They still wonder, what could be wrong with this?

This objection deserves an answer. The project of producing a baby precisely is to bring a possible baby into being to satisfy the desire to have a baby, and the choice precisely is *to produce a baby.* So, a choice to bring about conception in this fashion inevitably means willing the baby's initial status as a product. But this status is subpersonal, and so the choice to produce a baby is inevitably the choice to enter into a relationship with the baby, not as an equal, but as a product inferior to its producers. But this initial relationship of those who choose to produce babies with the babies they produce is inconsistent with and so impedes the communion of persons endowed with equal dignity which is appropriate to any interpersonal relationship.

Naturally, those who choose to produce a baby make that choice only as a means to an ulterior end. They may well intend that the baby be received into an authentic child-parent relationship, in which he or she will live in the communion which befits those who share personal dignity. If realized, this intended end for the sake of which the choice is made to produce the baby will be good for the baby as well as for the parents. But, even so, the baby's initial status as a product is subpersonal, and as a result the choice to produce the baby is a choice of a bad means to a good end. Moreover, in producing babies if the product is defective, a new person comes to be *as unwanted.* Thus, those who produce babies not only choose life for some, but--can anyone doubt it?--quietly dispose at least some of those who are not developing normally.[29]

I believe that the foregoing argument shows that it is wrong to "make" babies, and that homologous fertilization is a mode of making babies. I also believe, although I am not going to show why here, that contraception is immoral because it is a contra-life choice. Since producing babies is always wrong and since contraception is always wrong, the only morally acceptable way to engage either in love-giving or life-giving actions is by engaging in the kind of sexual act that is open to new life and to the communication of love. But this, as we have seen, is the marital act. It is for this reason that there is the inseparable connection between the unitive and procreative meanings of the conjugal act.

THE "LANGUAGE OF THE BODY"
AND LABORATORY GENERATION OF HUMAN LIFE

There is a third line of reasoning found in the *Instruction* to show that it is morally wrong to generate human life outside the marital act. This line of reasoning is based on the "language of the body." The *Instruction* observes that

> *spouses mutually express their personal love in the "language of the body," which clearly involves both "spousal meanings" and parental ones. The conjugal act by which the couple mutually express their self-gift at the same time expresses openness to the gift of life. It is an act that is inseparably corporal and spiritual. It is in their bodies and through their bodies that the spouses consummate their marriage and are able to become father and mother.*[30]

The *Instruction* then continues,

> *In order to respect the language of their bodies and of their natural generosity, the conjugal union must take place with respect for its openness to procreation, and the procreation of a person must be the fruit and result of married love. The origin of the human being thus follows from a procreation that is "linked to the union, not only biological but also spiritual, of the parents, made one by the bond of marriage." Fertilization achieved outside the bodies of the couple remains by this very fact deprived of the meanings and values which are expressed in the language of the body and in the union of human persons.*[31]

According to this argument, *in vitro* fertilization, which occurs outside of the bodies of husband and wife and outside of the bodily act by which their marital union is uniquely and properly expressed, is a way of generating human life that fails completely to respect the "language of the body." It is a way of generating human life that simply refuses to acknowledge the deep human significance of the personal gift, bodily and spiritual in nature, of husband and wife to one another that is aptly expressed in the marital act, a personal gift that is itself fittingly crowned by the gift of human life.

This argument, derived from the beautiful "theology of the body" developed extensively by Pope John Paul II,[32] is basically, so it seems to me, a variant of the argument based on the inseparable connection between the unitive and procreative meanings of the conjugal act. The truth central to it is that the marital act is a *bodily-spiritual* act wherein husband and wife "give themselves" to each other and truly become "one flesh". It is an act that "consummates," i.e., perfects and fulfills, their marriage by expressing in a bodily way their "gift" of themselves to one another as bodily, sexual, procreative persons who differ complementarily in their sexuality. In this act the husband gives himself to his wife in a receiving sort of way, and she in turn receives him in a giving sort of way. In this act the "nuptial significance" of the body, as a sign of the gift of the male-person to the female-person and vice versa, is revealed and displayed, and upon it the blessing of fertility can descend.

How different is this act, one immanent in nature and participating in the marriage of husband and wife and open to the gift of life, from the series of transitive actions involved in the laboratory generation of human life. The latter is in no way a bodily act of which the spouses are co-subjects, nor is it one in which they speak the language of marital love. Through the "language of the body" husband and wife open themselves to the gift of life and cooperate with God in its procreation. Through the laboratory generation of human life they merely provide materials, through distinct individual acts of their own and not through the act proper to them as spouses, that others will use to "make" life, to bring into being a "product" subject to technical control.

LTOT, GIFT, AND TOT

Before bringing this paper to conclusion, I want to discuss briefly the compatibility of some new reproductive technologies other than *in vitro* fertilization and embryo transfer with the teaching of the Church. My concern here is with the procedures known as LTOT (Low Tubal Ovum Transfer), GIFT (Gamete Intrafallopian Transfer), and TOT (Tubal Ovum Transfer).[33] Although the *Instruction* did not specifically address these procedures, it did, following the lead of Pope Pius XII,[34] articulate the basic principle to be used in determining whether or not these procedures are morally right and compatible with Catholic teaching. According to the *Instruction* a technical procedure "can be morally acceptable" "if (it) facilitates the conjugal act or helps it reach its natural objectives." But "if . . . the procedures were to replace the conjugal act, it is morally illicit."[35] Thus in what follows, my purpose will be to determine whether LTOT, GIFT, and TOT serve as *substitutes* for the marital act or serve to *facilitate* it and *help it reach its natural objectives*.

In LTOT an oocyte is removed from the wife's ovaries by laparoscopy and then, unfertilized, is reinserted in the mid or lower portion of the fallopian tube or in the uterus itself. Husband and wife then engage in the marital act and fertilization, should it occur, takes place as the natural result of this marital act.[36] In my judgment LTOT meets the criterion of a technical procedure that facilitates the conjugal act and helps it to achieve its natural objectives. As such, LTOT assists and does not replace the marital act. It is, therefore, in my judgment morally permissible and compatible with Church teaching.

GIFT is quite a different procedure. Developed originally by Ricardo Asch and his associates at the University of Texas in San Antonio, when first used it obtained the husband's semen by masturbation. Ova were removed from the wife's ovaries by laparoscopy. The semen and oocytes were then placed in a catheter separated by an air bubble to prevent fertilization outside the wife's body. The catheter tip was then inserted into the fimbriated end of the fallopian tube and the contents gently injected. Fertilization of the oocytes then took place within the wife's body.[37]

Since GIFT, as originally practiced, obtained sperm from the husband by masturbation, it was not in accord with Catholic teaching. The procedure was then modified to obtain the sperm in a morally acceptable way. In its modified form husband and wife engage in the marital act, using a perforated condom. Sperm collected in the condom are then placed into the catheter along with an ovum (or ova) removed from the wife's ovaries and separated by an air bubble to prevent fertilization from occurring outside the wife's body. The catheter is then introduced into the end of the wife's fallopian tube and its contents injected, with subsequent fertilization taking place within the wife's body.

Although some Catholic moralists have given their approval to the GIFT procedure,[38] claiming that it assists the marital act and does not substitute for it, I believe that it is not compatible with Catholic teaching. With Donald DeMarco and others,[39] I think it must be said that in the GIFT procedure the conjugal act is in truth incidental and not essential to the achievement of pregnancy. The bond between the marital act and the GIFT procedure is not essential. This is quite obvious from the fact that this procedure as such does not require the marital act. There is a complete dissociation between the marital act and the technical method which leads to conception. The *only* reason to engage in the marital act is to obtain the husband's sperm in a non-mastubatory way. But this is only incidental to the GIFT procedure as such. Conception does not take place as a result of the conjugal act, the personal, one flesh union of husband and wife. Rather, it takes place as a result of a technological procedure which, of itself, is not essentially related to the marital act. Gift, therefore, *substitutes* for the marital act so far as the conception of the child is con- cerned and does not facilitate it or help it to achieve its natural objectives.

Although the acronym "TOT" would make it seem that this procedure is similar to "LTOT," a close examination of this procedure shows that this is not the case. Developed by David S. McLaughlin, it differs from LTOT first in that the environment in which prospective fertilization is to take place is as high in the fallopian tube as possible (hence the elimination of the "L" in the acronym LTOT). But, secondly, it differs from LTOT in that fertilization does not take place as the result of a subsequent marital act. Rather, fertilization takes place after sperm (obtained from the husband either by masturbation or by the use of a perforated condom during a marital act) are introduced into the fallopian tube along with the wife's ovum after having been placed in a catheter, using air bubbles between sperm and ovum to prevent fertilization outside the body. In other words, TOT is more similar to GIFT than it is to LTOT. Its relationship to the conjugal act is, like that of GIFT, accidental and not essential insofar as the marital act is resorted to only in order to obtain the sperm used in a non- masturbatory way. Conception does not follow from the one flesh unity of husband and wife in the marital act; rather it follows from the technological introduction of sperm and ovum via a catheter into the distal region of the fallopian tube, and this technological intervention is *not* essentially related to the marital act. Thus in my judgment TOT, like GIFT, is in essence a way of generating human life that substitutes for the marital act and does not in truth facilitate that act's achieving its natural objectives. It is thus a procedure that is not compatible with Catholic teaching.

CONCLUSION

In this paper I have tried to show the reasons why it is morally wrong to choose to generate human life outside the marital act and to support the truth of Catholic teaching on this subject. I am convinced that, at the very deepest levels, a profound theological truth is at the heart of this teaching. According to Catholic faith, the Eternal Word of the Father was "begotten, not made." Catholic faith holds that human beings are the living images of God Himself, the "created words" that His uncreated Word became precisely to show us how deeply God loves us and wills to give us His very own life. It follows therefore, that His created words ought, like His Uncreated and Eternal Word, be "begotten, not made."

ENDNOTES

[1] I use the term "vendor" advisedly. On this see George Annas, "Artificial Insemination: Beyond the Best Interests of the Donor," Hastings Center Report 9.4 (August, 1979) 14-15, 43. Annas, a lawyer, noted that those "providing" sperm do so on the basis of a contract according to which they are paid. "The continued use of the term 'donor,'" he wrote, "gives the impression that the 'vendor' is doing some service for the good of humanity," which is not in fact true.

[2] The revealing, if inadvertent, remark of Dr. Robert Edwards after the birth of Louise Brown is worth noting. Edwards that: "The last time I saw *her*, *she* was just eight cells in a test tube. *She* was beautiful *then*, and she's still beautiful *now*" (Science Digest, October 1978, 9; emphasis added). Surely Edwards' statement is an eloquent testimony that human life begins at fertilization.

[3] Pope Paul VI, Humanae Vitae, n. 12: "Huiusmodi doctrina, quae ab Ecclesiae Magisterio saepe exposita est, in nexu indissolubili nititur, a Deo statuto, quam homini sua sponte infringere non licet, inter significationem unitatis et significationem procreationis, quae ambae in actu coniugali insunt."

[4] Ibid., n. 13: "Pariter, si rem considerent, fateantur oportet, actum amoris mutui, qui facultati vitam propagandi detrimento sit, quam Deus omnium Creator secundum peculiares leges in ea insculpsit, refragari tum divino consilio, ad cuius normam coniugium constitutum est, tum voluntati primi vitae humanae Auctoris. Quapropter cum quis dono Dei utitur, tollens, licet solum ex parte, significationem et finem doni ipsius, sive viri sive mulieris naturae repugnat eorumque intimae necessitudini, ac propterea etiam Dei consilio sanctaeque eius voluntati obnititur."

[5] Ibid., n. 12, text cited in note 3.

[6] Ibid., n. 12: "Etenim propter intiman suam rationem, coniugii actus dum maritum et uxorem arctissimo sociat vinculo, eos idoneos etiam facit ad novam vitam gignendam, secundum leges in ipsa viri et mulieris natura inscriptas."

[7] Congregation for the Doctrine of the Faith, Instruction on Respect for Human Life in Its Origin and the Dignity of Procreation, Part II, A, 1, with a reference to Vatican Council II, Gaudium et Spes, n. 50.

[8] Ibid., II, A, 2, with a reference to Pope Pius XII, Discourse to Those Taking Part in the Fourth International Congress of Catholic Doctors, 29 September 1949, AAS 41 (1949) 559.

[9] Many people, particularly in the affluent Western democracies, are quite favorably disposed to all the new reproductive technologies, even those involving use of gametic cells from third parties, the use of surrogate mothers, etc. One of the most extreme views, unfortunately not uncommon, is set forth in great detail by Joseph Fletcher, The Ethics of Genetic Control: Ending Reproductive Roulette (Garden City, NY: Doubleday Anchor Books, 1972).

[10] The "Baby M" case refers to the tragic story of a little girl, referred to as "Baby M," conceived by the artificial insemination of Mrs. Mary Beth Whitehead with sperm "provided" by Dr. Stern, whose wife did not wish to become pregnant because of a mild case of multiple sclerosis. Mrs. Whitehead, who had grown attached to the child, did not wish to give her over to the Sterns after her birth, and a lengthy, well-publicized trial took place, eventually giving custody of the child to the Sterns.

[11] "Pregnancy reduction" is the expression used by some doctors who deliberately kill within the womb "excess" children who have been conceived *in vitro* and implanted in their mother's womb to enhance the possibility of at least one child surviving pregnancy. In this type of case several babies are deliberately conceived *in vitro* and subsequently implanted in the mother's womb. But, since multiple pregnancies raise problems about the survival of all the unborn and since the parents are interested in having only one or possibly two children of their own, the "excess" number of unborn children is "reduced" by killing several.

[12] Instruction . . ., Part II, B, 4, a, citing Pope Paul VI, Humanae Vitae, n. 12 (text cited in note 3).

[13] Ibid., II, B, 4, a, citing Pope Pius XII, Discourse to Those Taking Part in the Second Naples World Congress on Fertility and Human Sterility, 19 May 1956, AAS 48 (1956) 470.

[14] Ibid., II, B, 4, a; emphasis omitted.

[15] Pope Pius XII, Discourse to Those Taking Part in the Fourth World Congress of Catholic Doctors, 29 September, 1949, AAS 41 (1949) 561.

[16] Pope Pius XII, Apostolate of the Midwives: An Address to the Italian Catholic Union of Midwives, 29 October 1951, text in The Catholic Mind, 50 (1952) 61.

[17] On the constant Catholic teaching that God is the author of marriage see the following: The Council of Trent, Session 24, 1563, in Enchiridion Symbolorum ed. Henricus Denzinger and Adolphus Schoenmetzer (ed. 33, Romae: Herder, 1984), nn. 1797-1812; Pope Leo XIII, Encyclical Arcanum Divinae Sapientiae, in Official Catholic Teachings: Love and Sexuality, ed. Odile M. Liebard (Wilmington, N.D.: McGrath, 1978), nn. 3, 5, 6; Pope Pius XI, Encyclical Casti Connubii, in Liebard, nn. 31, 64, 66; Vatican Council II, Gaudium et Spes, n. 48; Pope Paul VI, Humanae Vitae, nn. 8-9; Pope John Paul II, Familiaris Consortio, n. 11.

[18] For a fuller discussion of this point, see my Sex, Marriage, and Chastity: Reflections of a Catholic Layman, Spouse and Parent (Chicago Franciscan Herald Press, 1981), chapter 5. Also see my "Sexual Ethics and Human Dignity," in Persona, Verita e Morale: Atti del Congresso Internazionale di Teologia Morale (Roma, 7-12 aprile 1986) (Roma: Citta Nuova Editrice, 1988), pp. 477-495, especially pp. 488-489.

[19]Centuries ago St. Augustine rightly noted that one of the chief goods of marriage is children, who are to be received lovingly, nourished humanely, and educated religiously. See his De genesi ad literam, 9.7 (PL 34.397).

[20]On this see Vatican Council II, Gaudium et spes, n. 48.

[21]The Augustinian teaching on the threefold good of marriage (progeny, steadfast fidelity, and the "sacrament") was set forth by him in several places (see, for example, De Bono Conjugali, De Nuptiis et concupiscentia, passim). This teaching was accepted by later theologians and by the magisterium of the Church. The doctrine of the threefold good of marriage is central to Pope Pius XI's Encyclical, Casti Connubii, and the Fathers of Vatican II made it clear, in Gaudium et Spes, n. 48, with corresponding footnotes to sources in Augustine, St. Thomas, the Council of Trent, and Pius XI, that they made Augustine's teaching their own.

[22]Here the teaching set forth by Pope Paul VI in Humanae Vitae, n. 13, is pertinent. There he noted that a "conjugal act" (using this term in a purely descriptive sense) imposed by one of the spouses upon the other against the reasonable wishes of the other violates the requirements of the moral law.

[23]On the issue of contraception, which cannot be taken up here, see the essay by Germain Grisez, John Finnis, Joseph M. Boyle, Jr., and William E. May, "'Every Marital Act Ought to Be Open to New Life': Toward a Clearer Understanding," The Thomist (July, 1988); also printed in the book by the same authors, The Teaching of "Humanae Vitae": A Defense (San Francisco: Ignatius Press, 1988).

[24]Instruction . . ., II, B, 4, c.

[25]Ibid., II, B, 5, with an internal citation from Pope John Paul II, Familiaris Consortio, n. 14.

[26]Classic sources for the difference between transitive and immanent activity and the significance of this difference are: Aristotle, Metaphysics, Bk. 9, c. 8, 1050a23-1050b1; St. Thomas Aquinas, In IX Metaphysicorum, Lect. 8, n. 1865, Summa Theologiae, 1, 4, 2, ad 2; 1, 14, 5, ad 1; 1, 18, 1.

[27]Catholic Bishops Committee on Bioethical Issues, In Vitro Fertilization: Morality and Public Policy (London: Catholic Information Services, 1983), n. 23.

[28]Ibid., n. 24.

[29]The previous three paragraphs paraphrase material developed by Grisez, Finnis, Boyle, and May in the essay referred to in note 23.

[30]Instruction . . ., Part II, B, 4, b, with a reference to Pope John Paul II, General Audience on 16 Jan. 1980; Insegnamenti di Giovanni Paolo II III, 1 (1980) 148-152.

[31]Ibid., with a reference to Pope John Paul II, Discourse to Those Taking Part in the 35th General Assembly of the World Medical Association, 29 October 1983; AAS 76 (1984) 393.

[32]On this see Pope John Paul II, Original Unity of Man and Woman: Catechesis on Genesis (Boston: St. Paul Editions, 1981).

[33] The best treatment in English that I know of dealing with these procedures is Donald DeMarco, "Catholic Church Teaching and TOT/GIFT," in Reproductive Technologies, Marriage and the Church (Braintree, MA: The Pope John XXIII Center, 1988), pp. 122-139.

[34] Pope Pius XII, Discourse to Those Taking Part in the Fourth International Congress of Catholic Doctors, 29 September 1949, AAS 41 (1949) 560.

[35] Instruction . . ., Part II, B, 6.

[36] On this see Pope John XXIII Medical Moral Center, "Should Catholic Hospitals Encourage Low Tubal Ovum Transfer?" Hospital Progress, March 1984, 55-56.

[37] Ricardo Asch, et al., "Pregnancy after Translaparoscopic Intrafallopian Transfer," Lancet, Nov. 3, 1984, 1034-1035.

[38] E.g., Lloyd W. Hess, "Assisting the Infertile Couple," Ethics & Medics 11.2 (1986).

[39] See note 33.

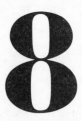

The Ethical and Legal Implications of Surrogate Motherhood

William J. Wagner, J.D.

The first instance of "motherhood for hire," often known as "surrogate motherhood," occurred in the United States at the end of the 1970's, that is, at about the time Louise Brown, the world's first "test-tube" baby, was born in England.[1] However, the new reproductive arrangement substantially touched public awareness only with an occurrence nearly a decade later. On May 5, 1986, five armed law-enforcement officers went to a blue-collar home in Brick Township, New Jersey, to take a five-week-old infant, by all necessary force, from the arms of its lactating natural mother.[2] This preliminary step in the enforcement of a motherhood-for-hire contract against Mary Beth Whitehead, together with her subsequent flight with her child, effectively introduced the arrangement to the public.

Under the circumstances, motherhood for hire could not be dismissed as one more private moral choice seeking social tolerance. In contrast to the "simple case" of *in vitro* fertilization, the case of motherhood for hire capturing the nation's attention had the form of a public conflict between adults hardly knowing each other, over who had the right to rear a child. The dispute was about the appropriate legal consequences of an impersonal business agreement. When viewed from this perspective, the arrangement's ethical implications appeared inseparable from its legal ones, even to some who would generally be inclined to treat morality as an exclusive private matter.

The dispute between Whitehead and the Sterns illustrates that parental status is, as the *Vatican Instruction on Respect for Human Life in Its Origin and on the Dignity of Procreation (Vatican Instruction)* teaches, "constitutive . . . of civil society and its order."[3] Decisions about who will have the right to rear a child are intrinsically of public significance. In every society, the civil law provides a pattern of sanctions giving force to a particular understanding of how such decisions ought to be approached. Even acquiescence by the law in an allegedly private choice to assign parental status is an event of public moment. In the pre-trial and trial stages of the Whitehead case, the apparatus of the civil law was used to enforce a private agreement conferring the right to rear a child.[4] The occurrence seemed a harbinger of some change in the law, that promised to transform the constitutive order of society in an unprecedented way.

In the natural mother's confrontation with law enforcement officers in Brick Township, a scene reminiscent of Eliza's flight across the ice in *Uncle Tom's Cabin*, the force of law was directed against the most primordial of human ties: a mother's bond with her nursing child.[5] On the moral level, this tie gives rise to emphatic rights and duties. Although the legal system cannot avoid being implicated, whether by enactment or acquiescence, in private arrangements that purport to confer parental status, the Whitehead case raises the question of the *moral* evaluation of the law's choice of response. A given legal answer may itself not be morally sound.

The question is not academic. Even as "Baby M" fades from memory, the lines are daily more sharply drawn in a contest that has taken shape, over the proper legislative response to motherhood for hire.[6] Options, now before legislatures, would appear to compromise the law's ethical basis, in the Catholic view, not less deeply than have the United States Supreme Court's abortion decisions. The outcome of the debate on motherhood for hire will emerge as a relatively fixed trend in the law in no more than ten years, and probably much sooner. Before us stands a precious opportunity to come to a morally sound policy position on the matter, and effectively to advocate that position before the country's legislatures.

This article seeks an ethically sound public policy position on the practice of motherhood for hire. It intends to address not the morality of motherhood for hire per se, but the morality of the law's chosen response to the practice. Still, an abstract evaluation of the ethics of personal choice in the matter is indispensible, as an inquiry preliminary to reaching the article's goal. If the practice is shown, as a matter of personal choice, to violate what may be termed public morality, for example, the civil law may validly restrict it. Methodologically, arguments about the morality of the legal response to the practice will also be easier to validate, if the morality of personal decision is clearly outlined, and distinguished. Finally, because the meaning of personal moral decision transcends social context, and the moral reality of social context transcends legal categories, it is important to acknowledge that the ethics of personal decision is an horizon fundamental to the quest for an ethically justifiable legal response to this or any societal problem.

In the present article, an abstract ethical analysis of motherhood for hire remains no more than an excursus, which sets the stage for an exploration of the further question of how the civil law should respond to the practice. In order to proceed at this second level, a statement is needed of generic goals that a sound ethics establishes for lawmaking in the area. Such a statement serves to mediate between abstract moral principles and the ethical demands peculiar to the requirements of lawmaking. This article includes such a statement, as an intermediate foundation of analysis. Upon that foundation, the article, in its final section, attempts to reach an evaluation of concrete legislative alternatives for responding to motherhood for hire now emerging in the United State.

The article describes these alternatives, which may be characterized as: 1) prohibition; 2) decommercialization; 3) approval with governmental validation; and 4) approval with "private ordering" validation; and it evaluates the soundness of each alternative, based on its statement of generic goals. The article, as a whole, seeks to provide a workable ethical framework for evaluating legal responses currently proposed to the practice of motherhood for hire in the United States.

I. THE ETHICAL IMPLICATIONS OF MOTHERHOOD FOR HIRE AS MATTERS OF PERSONAL DECISION

The *Vatican Instruction* judges that motherhood for hire is never ethically admissible. It justifies this conclusion in three separate, but complementary terms. The practice is said in the *Vatican Instruction* to be ethically inadmissible, because it violates: 1) certain basic goods; 2) certain essential personal duties; and 3) certain essential rights of others.[7] According to the *Vatican Instruction*, the goods implicated include the "unity of marriage" and the "dignity of the procreation of the human person;" the duties compromised are the mother's duty to her child ("maternal love"), her duty of fidelity to her spouse ("conjugal fidelity"), and her duty to herself to exercise her fertility responsibly, i.e. in a way furthering her own integral fulfillment ("responsible motherhood"); the rights violated include the child's "right . . . to be conceived, carried in the womb, brought in the world and brought up by his parents" and the family's right not to be divided "between the physical, psychological and moral elements which constitute [it]."[8]

The framework, that the *Vatican Instruction* applies in evaluating motherhood for hire, centers on the moral decision of the woman who chooses to alienate her maternity. Her decision is, in a sense, the pivotal one making the arrangement possible, so this focus is not inappropriate. Nothing is gained by romanticizing the plight of the gestational mother. At the same time, no framework for evaluating the ethics of personal decision regarding motherhood for hire is complete unless it allows an ethical evaluation of the choices of the genetic father who conceives a child in a motherhood for hire arrangement, and those of the commissioning party, who has no genetic relationship to the child, but who orchestrates the conception through the acquisition of gamete(s) from third-party donor(s).

The culpability of the commissioning party, whether the genetic father or someone else, may be compounded by an object that is not within the intention of the natural mother, at all, and, thus, not within the framework of moral analysis expressly contemplated by the *Vatican Instruction*. The commissioning party may intend to use and, perhaps, even to coerce the mother, in a manner violative of her dignity as a human person. I wish to adopt and develop the outlines of the reasoning of the *Vatican Instruction* as my starting point for evaluating the ethics of motherhood for hire. But, in so doing, I shall extend the analysis to cover this latter dimension of the commissioning party's action.

Motherhood for Hire Violates Basic Human Goods

A. The Unity of Marriage

Assuming the commissioning party is the genetic father and is married to another woman, the practice of motherhood for hire violates the unity of his marriage, since, in relation to the commissioning couple, the result is genetically asymmetrical reproduction. If the gestational mother is married to another man, then the arrangement violates the unity of her marriage for the same reason. Her action is worse in one sense, since she actualizes her procreative power to create a child benefiting a marriage other than her own; his action is worse in another action, since he diverts the resources of his household to raising the child whom he has chosen to conceive with another.

Proponents of motherhood for hire assert that there is no violation of the respective marriages of the two individuals who contribute genetically to the conception of the child, because they share no venereal pleasure. This argument misconstrues the opprobrium historically attached to adultery in nearly all cultures. If anything, illicit sharing in extramarital pleasure has only been the secondary ground for condemning adultery. The evil generally seen as primary has been illegitimate births whether within or outside the family unit, depriving the innocent spouse of the exclusive opportunity to procreate with his or her partner and, in the case of adultery by the wife, of certainty as to which offspring are his own.

Further, to the very real extent that adultery is a betrayal of the affective, as opposed to the procreative dimension of marital unity, motherhood for hire entails, in a certain sense, if not a pleasure bond, at least a bodily union between the gestational mother and the genetic father who has commissioned the pregnancy. Through the offices of a physician, his semen enters her body, and through it she shares, for instance, any venereal diseases from which he may suffer. Women have become infected with the HIV virus through artificial insemination by donor.[9] To the extent that she shares this communication and risk with a man not her husband, the gestational mother violates the unity of her marriage.

The purveyors of motherhood for hire attempt to answer these arguments, by alleging that the *consent* of the marriage partner is sufficient to remove any connotation of adultery from the arrangement. But, marriage, unlike simple friendship, is more than a "marriage of true minds." Marriage is an objective unity of "one flesh" that cannot be preserved through mere consensual dispensation by the marriage partner, after the manner of, say, a release from a prior commitment by a friend.[10]

One might suppose that motherhood for hire arrangements always involve a violation of at least one existing marriage, because the arrangements are promoted as a remedy for the infertility of married couples. Such is not the case. Unmarried individuals of both sexes have hired the maternity of unmarried women.[11] Such individuals may wish to raise a child alone. They may be

96

partners in a homosexual relationship. Paradoxically, in such cases, the absence of the concrete wrong of adultery serves to make the ethical objection stronger. The parties' actions, in such cases, violate the unity of marriage on another more profound level. They violate the unity of marriage as an available good and as a societal institution, since they pursue a part of what marriage offers, but in a manner that disengages the part from the available whole. In these cases, the actor does not feel constrained even to enter into a third-party marriage to provide for the child's upbringing.

Some argue that if the gestational mother does not contribute genetically to the child she carries but submits instead to the transfer of an embryo conceived by others, her action in carrying the child to term would not violate her own marriage, the marriage of the genetic parents, or the unity of marriage as a social institution. They assert, for this reason, that in the routine case motherhood for hire ought to utilize embryo transfer. Where the gestational mother accepts the transferred embryo for the sake of returning the chid to the genetic parents or to third-parties, this argument is unconvincing. The woman's gestational capacity would appear a no less integral aspect of marital unity than is her capacity to produce gametes.

Conversely, where the woman accepts the embryo intending permanently to adopt the resulting child, I would concede that her gestating of the child would seem not to violate the unity of her marriage, the child being adopted as much by her husband, as herself. Of course, such a case would more accurately be termed early adoption, than "surrogacy". Under most imaginable scenarios, the embryo available for such "adoption" would become so through other kinds of immoral acts implicating the "adopting" mother and her husband. Even if the couple is not so implicated (i.e. in the case of a genuine gestational emergency for the embryo conceived under normal circumstances), there are, for the time being, sufficient prudential reasons to oppose the development of such transfer techniques.[12]

Before leaving the issue of marital unity, it ought to be noted that the violations of the unity of marriage entailed by motherhood for hire have a novel feature: persons can commit them without contributing in any bodily way to the reproductive process. Parties commissioning a motherhood for hire conception without contributing genetically to the conception do just that. In such cases the unity of marriage is compromised in the more profound sense, because of the greater degree of disintegration reflected in the choice. It also bears stating that every kind of violation of marital unity that the practice of motherhood for hire makes possible is compounded, when money, either as means or end, induces the violation.

B. The Dignity of the Procreation of the Human Person

According to Roman Catholic moral doctrine, an approach to human reproduction must meet at least three requirements, if it is to be in accord with the dignity of the human person. The party who intends to reproduce must be willing to treat the person being procreated as an end in him or herself from the moment that the possibility of procreation comes into view.[13] The party reproducing must be willing to assume a relationship of unconditional parental loyalty to the person being procreated once that person comes into existence.[14] And, finally, he or she must act within a relationship with the one who provides the second gamete necessary for conception that adequately respects the dignity of the reproductive partner, that is to say, within the marriage relationship.[15] Motherhood for hire does not satisfy any one of these three requirements. Within a Roman Catholic perspective, the practice, therefore, is regarded as violative of the dignity of human procreation.

The requirement that *the child conceived always be viewed as an end in him or herself* is violated when the natural mother makes of the child an instrument to obtaining a medium of exchange not even itself a basic good: money. Reciprocally, where one views the transaction from the perspective of the commissioning couple whose end it is to obtain the child, the conclusion remains unavoidable that the child is "purchased" and a monetary value placed on a human person. From this aspect, the child conceived is treated also as an object rather than as an end in him or herself.

Some argue that the alienation of maternity in "surrogate motherhood" arrangements is not morally wrong, where the act is truly donative, because uncompensated beyond basic expenses, and the mother's motives are altruistic. This argument is not sound. Even on these terms, the mother assumes dominion over an incipient human person for the sake of the good of third persons (i.e. the commissioning couple). Again, the child is treated as a means rather than as the end that morality asserts that he or she must always remain. The fact that the end is, at least, the basic human good of friendship with a third party does not alter the intrinsic moral evil of reducing the child to a means.

Some answer the objection that motherhood for hire impermissably treats the child as a means to an end by arguing that, at the time the gestational mother disposes of the child by promise of custody to third-parties, whether out of altruism or for monetary gain, the child does not yet exist, rather only "pre-human" genetic material. The genetic package is said somehow to become a human person after the parties have arranged the transaction. According to this view, the mother is said to deliver no more than genetic material and a gestational service. However, ethically speaking, it would seem that as a somatic being the human person is entitled to personal respect from the moment the body is conceived, which, from a Catholic perspective, is also the presumed moment of ensoulment.[16] Even if the human person is not yet in existence at the time the arrangement is transacted, as is true when the motherhood for hire contract is signed prior to insemination, the dignity of a prospective human being is, in any case, offended in the transaction. An act may be morally wrong without violating the rights of another concrete individual. Examples can be taken from the criminal law concerned with recklessness.

The second requirement of respect for the dignity of the procreation of the human person, *unconditional loyalty,* is not compatible with an intent to terminate the parental relationship for any reason other than the best interest of the child. Some argue that the termination of parental rights by the gestational mother under motherhood for hire agreements is justified, because the termination of parental rights in cases of adoption are justified. However, the analogy is misplaced. The action of a natural mother yielding her child for adoption is morally justified because, through contingent events over which she has failed to exercise control, she cannot adequately care for the child. Relinquishment is justified solely on the ground of the child's best interest. By contrast, the termination of parental rights in motherhood for hire arrangements is, at best, for the sake of the third-party, rather than for that of the child. As such, it clearly violates the parent's fiduciary duty of loyalty to her offspring. Agreements to be bound in advance to deliver a child necessarily violate this principle, since the gestational mother cannot know, in advance, whether the commissioning couple will be fit to care for the child as of the future delivery date. The acceptance or conferral of money as an inducement to this breach of unconditional parental loyalty obviously aggravates the wrong.

The third element required by respect for the dignity of the procreation of the human person, *marriage between the child's genetic parents,* says that the violation of the unity of marriage represented by motherhood for hire is simultaneously a violation of the dignity of the person whose procreation is in prospect.

Motherhood for Hire Violates Essential Moral Duties

As the *Vatican Instruction* suggests, the wrongfulness of motherhood for hire can be further illumined by shifting the discussion from basic goods to essential duties. The wrong under discussion may, in fact, be substantially one and the same. Even so, the fuller scope and meaning of the wrong becomes clear when the matter is considered from this second aspect. From this vantage point, the *Vatican Instruction* specifies that motherhood for hire compromises three kinds of duties. They are: 1) duty to child; 2) duty to spouse; and 3) duty to self. Because I wish to expand the *Vatican Instruction's* framework for the sake of evaluating the ethics of the commissioning party, I shall also extend my consideration to a fourth kind of duty: 4) duty to neighbor.

A. Duty to Child

The offense against the good of the dignity of the procreation of the human person, which motherhood for hire represents, becomes concretely a violation of a duty to a child once the child comes into existence. The *Vatican Instruction* rightly indicates that this duty is the very opposite of the arm's length fairness characteristic of the market place; it is a duty of unconditional love. The execution of a promised performance to deliver over a child, under a contract signed before his or her conception, is a violation of a morally prior duty to the child. Mary Beth Whitehead's change of heart, in this respect, occurred within the *locus poenitentiae.* The gestational mother has a moral duty to resist the enforcement of the contract even after she has entered it. Such is not to say that she has a moral duty to refuse to relinquish custody of the child. The moral evaluation of a decision to relinquish custody would depend on her uncoerced judgment respecting the child's best interest at the time of its birth.

Some argue that the duty of the parent to the child can be fully satisfied by *delegation* to others. Witness the extensive use of nursemaids by upwardly mobile young professionals or the relinquishment of children to adoption. They, thus, conclude that a woman has a "right" to delegate to a "surrogate" the gestation of a child conceived from the woman's ovum or even to "delegate" ovum contribution to a "surrogate." This reasoning is specious, since such acts are not properly viewed as the delegation of a duty, but rather as the wrongful appropriation of an integral aspect of the personality of another.

Somewhat more plausibly, some argue that it is right for a gestational mother irrevocably to delegate the raising of her genetic and gestational child to the commissioning couple. Still, this argument is also defective. The duty of parental love is satisfied only where the parent assumes unconditional care on behalf of the child and relinquishes such care only when and to the extent that the child's best interest requires. Both relinquishing a child for adoption and hiring a nursemaid may themselves be wrong by this standard. Agreeing to terminate parental rights under a motherhood for hire contract must always be wrong, since such an agreement represents a fundamental refusal to assume unconditional care for the child, or at least a relinquishment of care assumed during gestation for a reason other than the child's best interest.

B. Duty to Spouse

The violation of the good of marital unity which motherhood for hire represents, when considered from the aspect of essential duties, is seen also to entail the violation of duties owed by the participating spouse to his or her marital partner. The unilateral disposal of one's bodily powers of procreation by extramarital procreation, sterilization, or abortion generally is to wrong one's spouse, who has a morally cognizable interest in one's fertility. Where the disposal of these powers results in asymmetrical procreation, either within or outside of the family unit, the spouse, who chooses to procreate unilaterally, simply wrongs his or her partner under this general principle, in this distinctive way. As I argued above, consent does not result in the defeasance of this duty. The duty in question is, more generally, that of marital exclusivity, or monogamy. Motherhood for hire is, in effect, a new form of polygyny or polyandry, the sort of arrangement which heretofore has been prohibited under laws against bigamy and polygamy.[17]

C. Duty to Self

Each person has a duty to attend to his or her own integral self-fulfillment.[18] The actualization of the procreative powers through motherhood for hire violates this duty. In this regard, the analogy, which has been made between motherhood for hire and prostitution is apt. The gestational mother, in such arrangements, makes a choice to realize her powers of procreation in a way which leaves the outcome disintegrated from either marriage or a relationship with her child. In her experience of pregnancy and childbirth in particular, the woman is alienated from her own bodily experience of union with the child developing within her, and, thus, necessarily is alienated even from an integral experience of her own body: her body says that the child is hers, but her intention says it is not. Her choice like prostitution, is objectively depersonalizing and degrading. The choice of the genetic father is likewise one to procreate in a manner disintegrated from marriage, although obviously not from relationship with the child. The fact that he may be in a marriage with another woman who is willing to assume the rearing role with him, does not change the fundamental disintegration implicit in the rejection of integral personal fulfillment entailed in his choice of extramarital generation.

D. Duty to Neighbor

The human person owes a duty to his or her neighbor not to actualize his or her sexual and procreative powers in a manner reducing the neighbor to a means rather than an end. This principle, of uncontested validity with respect to the ethics of unitive sexual pleasure, is, perhaps, less widely acknowledged as applying to the ethics of procreation. On this point, there is is a definite need to complete the framework explicitly provided within the *Vatican Instruction*. In motherhood for hire, a woman is not treated as an end in herself, as is a wife who becomes a mother through the unitive love of her husband. Rather, she is treated as a "vessel" and as a "source" of ova: that is as an instrument. Inducing her consent to this role merely means eliciting from her her own violation of her integral self-fulfillment in the sexual and procreative domain. This very serious wrong is the most public of the wrongs involved in motherhood for hire. It is a wrong to which the feminist critique of motherhood for hire is rightly sensitive.[19] The wrong is only aggravated when the commissioning party induces the mother to violate her integrity in this fashion, by means of monetary compensation. Such payment can be considered the moral equivalent of a bribe of an official to violate a nondefeasible duty.[20] The use of the coercive power of the civil law to compel the involuntary performance of an agreement to terminate parental rights, under a motherhood for hire arrangement, transform the act of merely inducing the mother to wrong herself, into what amounts to violence against the integrity of the mother's relationship with her child.

Where the commissioning party has no parental rights in relationship to the child based in genetics, the violation of the neighbor's personality, whether through his or her voluntary participation or through legal coercion would seem the more culpable. In such a case, the conflict of adult interests involved does not allow itself to be viewed as one natural parent combating the other, for the sake of the love of a natural child. Instead, it can be understood only as the quest for dominion over integral aspects of another's personality, for the sake of realizing an abstract personal project. On the facts of the Stern/Whitehead dispute, the wife of the sperm donor, among the adult participants, probably stood, for this reason, in what objectively is the most questionable ethical light.[21]

Motherhood for Hire Violates Essential RIghts

A. The Right of the Child

For the reasons given earlier, the practice of motherhood for hire violates parental *duty* to the child conceived. Focusing on the wrong which either natural parent alone does to the child in this kind of arrangement does not, however, exhaust the violation which the arrangement represents to the *rights* of the child, because the child has a right to more than one parent can give alone. The child has a right to a continuous relationship with a parental couple which is grounded in unconditional commitment and which issues forth in continuous personal-psychological love and nurturance. The child also has the right to experience a convergence in his or her social, genetic, and psychological identity. Motherhood for hire deprives the child of this wholistic unity of origin and rearing. The fragmentation of the modern world has given rise to what Robert Jay Lifton has identified as a severely crippling neurosis caused by discontinuity and unconnectedness from elements of identity, such as nature and past human generations.[22] As Leon Kass illustrates, motherhood for hire represents an extreme example of the modern fragmentation causing this painful psychic condition.[23] Deliberately to deny a child continuity and connectedness with a natural conception, gestation, and rearing within a unified family counts as the willing imposition of grave harm.

Proponents of the practice of motherhood for hire assert that the child does not have rights that can be violated by the arrangement, since he or she was not in existence when the arrangement was agreed upon, and, indeed, but for the arrangement would never have existed. In this view, the child is better off because of the arrangement, since the child exists only because the arrangement occurred. One flaw in this argument is that it presupposes that some net improvement in a person's general welfare can justify a deliberate violation of that person's human dignity. The argument would also serve to justify mercy killing. Another flaw in the argument is that the wrong, in the first instance, can be viewed as committed not against the child who comes to be, but against the hypothetical rights of prospective children whose procreation is in view at the outset.

B. Rights of the Family

The *Vatican Instruction* has been faulted for talking about the "rights of the family" on the ground that only individuals have rights. But, this opinion reflects an unduly individualistic and atomistic understanding of personal and social relationships. Individual identity is itself inconceivable without definition through familial and social relationship. Families and even voluntary associations, thus, must be viewed as having moral "rights" in an important sense. The *Vatican Instruction* claims that the practice of motherhood for hire violates at least one right of the family. This is the family's right to "physical, psychological and moral" unity and integrity.[24]

The claim is justified. Its importance and urgency become apparent when one notes that motherhood for hire severs the necessity of any link between marriage and procreative union, or between genetic and rearing parentage.[25] In this regard, it exacerbates the disconnectedness and discontinuity identified by Lifton as, perhaps, the single greatest threat in our own era to human wholeness and well being.[26] The harm threatened is not just for the children begotten through hire maternity, but for everyone. The practice shatters the organic meaning of "parent," "child," and "spouse," devalues the currency of the received language of courtship, love, commitment and relations between men and women, as well as those between adults and children. Were the practice generally adopted, it would make it more difficult to recognize a family, even when, by grace and the natural resiliency of human beings, one came into existence.

The relative value of "blended families" following divorce and remarriage, and of adoption are cited as authority for sanctioning the replacement of the traditional notion of family with a notion broad enough to include motherhood for hire. The precedents, in question, are both, at best, emergency responses to the de facto absence of family integrity not deliberately willed. It is mistaken to suggest that they provide any normative justification for broadening the definition of family to include motherhood for hire. If the definition of family were so extended, it would make room for a hierarchical caste system with two kinds of wives, social spouses and paid procreative concubines, and two kinds of children, companions and commodities. Such a stratification offends the American political tradition. For all reasons outlined here, motherhood for hire has unremittingly negative ethical implications. There is no reason to suppose it represents anything other than a significant regression in the developing moral awareness of humanity.

II. A STATEMENT OF THE GENERIC GOALS WHICH A SOUND ETHICS ESTABLISHES FOR LAWMAKING ON THE QUESTION OF MOTHERHOOD FOR HIRE

In the Catholic view, the full extent of moral obligation is, enforceable solely by God. The divine enforcement of moral norms is both omniscient and omnipotent. As such, it largely transcends the human ability to comprehend and, only by analogy, can it be considered to be comparable to the enforcement of human law. Within history, the tradition generally assumes that such divine enforcement is operative, as one aspect of natural law, in certain natural penalties that are the intrinsic outcome of disordered conduct. Ultimately, God is expected to execute a final eschatological judgment against all sinners. According to representative thinkers in the Catholic tradition such as John Courtney Murray, S.J. and Thomas Aquinas, one difference between the divine enforcement of moral norms and the enforcement of such norms under human law is the circumscribed scope of enforcement under human law.[27] Through its sanctions, human law does not and should not seek to enforce morality per se. It seeks only to effectuate the *common good,* by preserving, at a minimum, the elements of *public order, public morality,* and *justice.*[28]

If one is to arrive at a reliable statement of the generic goals for lawmaking that ethics establishes in the area of motherhood for hire, one must clarify, at the outset, that the eradication per se of the immoral personal choices of those engaged in the practice lies quite outside the role of civil law, as the Catholic tradition understands it. The practice of motherhood for hire should be outlawed for its immorality no more than should the old Protestant Comstock laws against contraceptives[29] be revived simply because the Church, I believe correctly, teaches that contraception is never morally admissible.

By contrast, where the bad moral choices in motherhood for hire have a notoriety interfering with the public moral health of society, the civil law may need to restrict individual freedom to make such choices for the sake of *public morality*. On this basis, for instance, restriction on the advertisement and brokerage of motherhood for hire arrangements would be justified.

Similarly, if it can be shown that the bad moral choices represented by motherhood for hire arrangements constitute an assault on society's *public order*, civil law may for this reason justifiably curtail them. In the Catholic view and, indeed, in the anglo-american legal tradition, the institution of marriage and the family are the basic "building blocks" of the social order, to which fundamental reference must be made in any just allocation of societal rights and duties.[30] Motherhood for hire impairs the order of these fundamental relationships. At a minimum, then, the state must withhold its enforcement mechanism from use as an instrument to effectuating such arrangements. This the law has traditionally done, by treating contracts impairing familial relationships as unenforceable and void as against public policy.[31] The law of marriage and the family must remain the exclusive legal matrix for enforcing a constitutive order of relationships in the domestic sphere.

The law of marriage and family establishes certain formal requisites, for recognizing de facto human sexual and procreative relationships as the basis of legally sanctioned rights and duties. De facto sexual and procreative relationships standing alone do not constitute legally cognizable marriage and family. Compliance with legal form is necessary before societal recognition through law is warranted. Yet, such legal requirements may not be arbitrary. They receive their normative direction from the natural givens of genetic and sexual relationship.

Even where the civil law strikes the correct balance in this regard, social practice will necessarily remain imperfect. Experience shows that some number of couples will become sexually involved outside of marriage and some number of children will be born out of wedlock. Such couples and children ought to be seen as having certain legally cognizable natural rights and duties, despite the absence of compliance with legal form necessary to create a cognizable marriage in a strict sense.[32] Conversely, even where there has been legal compliance so that a marriage exists, the state may, under its *parens patriae* power, need, in effect, to disregard the integrity of the family thereby formed, for the sake of protecting unemancipated or incompetent family members from abuse or neglect.[33]

An integral family remains always the ideal, but under the imperfect conditions of reality, a legal system may, depending on circumstances, need to give greater weight either to compliance with legal form or to the existence of the underlying de facto sexual and procreative relationship implicated, in deciding what recognition to give particular concrete claims. For example, it may give greater weight either to the presumption of legitimacy that arises from the spouses' legal marriage ceremony or to the natural rights of the genetic father, even though the mother is married to another.[34] While the law has a certain prudential latitude in deciding exactly how to balance these two factors, it should not detach the question of legal form from the underlying givens of de facto sexual and procreative relationship as the law's primary source of normative direction.

In the context of the new reproductive technologies, generally, and of motherhood for hire, in particular, alternative underlying matrices have, in fact, been suggested as sources of the basic normative direction in the area of domestic relations. They are: 1) the autonomous intention of the individual, under liberal individualism; and 2) positive conferral by the state, under theories giving overriding importance to the sovereign command of government. Each alternative is currently proposed as a substitute for the normative direction which traditionally has been provided for law and social order by the inherent moral structure of sexuality and procreative relationship.

In political terms, the law's response to motherhood for hire puts at stake the role of the natural family, as a meaningful subsidiary social unit capable of preventing the degeneration of social life into either complete individualism or collectivism. If the normativity of the structure of sex and procreation is sacrificed as the basis for formulating rules on legally cognizable marriage and domestic rights and duties, in favor of adopting a basis in one of these stated alternatives, either the market or the state can be expected to invade the sphere of intimate human relations, ultimately with devastating effect.

If it is to satisfy ethics, the law must accept, as a fundamental goal, the protection of the integrity of marriage and the family, as these basic institutions take shape within a normative matrix based on sex and procreation. To succeed, the law must seek to protect more than concrete families in being. It must, more fundamentally, seek to protect the common pool of intangible social terms, which make the formation and survival of such families possible. The law must seek to preserve the currency of genetic relatedness and covenantal committment, as societally meaningful terms, in order to make it possible for families to be formed and to flourish. On this ground, it may wish to rule out commercialized motherhood for hire contracts that tend, in general, to "poison the well" of social interaction between men and women and parents and children.

In addition to its role in protecting the family, the law has an equally fundamental role in protecting the moral dignity of the human person. Such recognition is a touchstone, according to most, of the moral legitimacy of any government. The law ought not, therefore, to give cognizance to the alienation of basic dimensions of personality, such as those involved in peonage, slavery, or indentured servitude.[35] Neither should the law allow the value of the human person directly to be assessed in dollars or otherwise quantified as expendable in a master calculus of social utility. On this basis, the law can prohibit money

105

passing hands or the enforcement of contracts either for custody of a child or termination of a natural parent's rights.

The challenge, in pursuing this objective, is to balance the inalienability of fundamental aspects of personality that is required to protect human dignity against the appropriate alienability of labor, that now allows women, for example, to function as full-fledged economic actors in society: a prerequisite to the meaningful exercise of individual political rights. Principles, in this area, should be capable of neutral application between men and women, adjusted only where masculine and feminine reproductive functions undeniably implicate basic goods in demonstrably different ways. Restrictions on the commercialized alienation of maternity should, for example, be matched by equivalent restrictions on sperm vending.

All of the considerations, which I have laid out with respect to the law's obligation to uphold the public order, could be recast in consideration of the law's obligation to uphold the value of *justice*. This would be done simply by shifting the focus of the discussion from societal goods to the claims of individuals and families that arise or tend to arise concretely as the public order is violated.

Respect for the family that properly balances the importance of formal legal requirements with that of the normativity of sex and procreation; respect for the dignity of the individual person; and public morality where relevant--such are the generic goals, which ethics proposes for the civil law as it responds to the practice of motherhood for hire. The evaluation of particular legislative proposals in the light of these generic goals requires the mediation of political prudence. According to St. Thomas, the rule of law must be based primarily on the free and reasonable appropriation of those governed, the force of coercion being available in the marginal case to bring the bad man into compliance with order.[36] Given the moral state of a particular society, the question for prudential judgment is how lines are best drawn to effectuate law that is properly grounded in the objective morality of justice and the public order, and, yet, that also is freely affirmed by the populace. The lawmaker must decide which evils can and must be tolerated in arriving at this balance. He or she must decide what indirect moral harms, perversely following from the pursuit of any one aspect of the good may outweigh the good to be achieved. Finally, he or she must ask how the generic goals prescribed by ethical considerations can be effectively communicated, within the categories of a particular legal system.

More concretely, the task of political prudence is to select the best *means* to the generic goals of lawmaking in a given area, under the conditions obtaining in a particular culture and legal system. In pursuit of the generic goals implicated by lawmaking on the matter of motherhood for hire, a number of concrete objectives present themselves as potentially appropriate means. Seven come to mind. They should be considered in the order of their descending importance in relation to two factors: the importance of the particular aspect of the societal good each seeks to secure, and the likelihood of its success in effectively serving its purpose. In the descending order I would give them in relation

106

to these two factors, such intermediate objectives include:

1. Nonenforcement of motherhood for hire contracts upon avoidance by the gestational mother;

2. The prohibition of fees for delivering custody of an infant;

3. The prohibition of fees in exchange for the termination of parental rights;

4. The *parens patriae* right of the state to intervene in custody allocations to safeguard the welfare of affected children;

5. The prohibition of advertising and brokerage that serves to induce participation in motherhood for hire arrangements;

6. The prohibition of procreation between partners who are not in a legally cognizable marriage, or at least a de facto monogamous heterosexual relationship;

7. The prohibition of procreating or gestating a child for the purpose of yielding custody to another.

A morally sound legislative proposal for responding to motherhood for hire will advance the generic goals set out above, through a prudent application of some or all of these means according to conditions obtaining in the culture and legal system.

III. THE CONCRETE LEGISLATIVE OPTIONS WHICH HAVE EMERGED FOR RESPONDING TO MOTHERHOOD FOR HIRE

Legal proposals, especially perhaps, when offered from the perspective of moral conviction, should be made, as far as possible, from starting points available within the existing system of law. Recommendations on the legal response that ethics mandates to motherhood for hire ought to begin inductively, by considering the foundation that the legal system may already provide for an ethically sound approach. In the present context, the point of departure for reform proposals should be the New Jersey Supreme Court's opinion in *In re Baby M.*[37] The New Jersey opinion represents both the most authoritative and best reasoned legal analysis that exists on how the *existing* law in a typical state jurisdiction should be read to govern the practice of motherhood for hire.

In Re Baby M

In its holding, the New Jersey high court ruled unenforceable the terms in the Whitehead-Stern contract that provided for allocation of custody rights and for termination of the natural mother's parental rights. The court concluded that the custody provision was unenforceable under a public policy against the exchange of money for the right to rear a child. The court found that the policy derived from the New Jersey anti-baby selling law enacted to end black market adoption.[38]

It also concluded that the contract provision terminating Whitehead's parental rights was unenforceable by reason of a second state policy, restricting the termination of parental rights to cases in which the state has made a *parens patriae* determination that termination is necessitated by present abandonment or unfitness on the natural parent's part.[39]

The Court considered and rejected a constitutional argument on the part of the Sterns that an abstract constitutional right of the individual to procreate free of the constraints of other natural familial rights and duties (an extension of the jurisprudence of *Roe v. Wade* and *Eisenstadt v. Baird*) preempted these public policies and mandated strict enforcement of both relevant contract provisions.[40]

It should be apparent that the New Jersey holding effectuates several of the intermediate objectives of a sound legal response to motherhood for hire, as these were developed above. Although not binding outside of New Jersey, the prestige of the New Jersey Court guarantees that the holding will be considered persuasive elsewhere. The New Jersey Supreme Court itself provides notice, however, that its holding is no ground for complacency. The policies on which its holding rests can be changed by new legislation. Constitutional arguments, essentially the inverse of those made by the Sterns, might well be found by the Courts to provide little brake in how far the legislature could go in this regard.[41]

At present, legislative proposals are being tested before courts and legislatures around the country which would affirm, strengthen, or reverse the policies on which the New Jersey Court based its decision. These proposals can be classed as falling into four types: 1) prohibition; 2) decommercialization; 3) approval with governmental validation; and 4) approval with "private ordering" validation.[42] The momentary legal stasis centering on *In re Baby M* can be expected to dissolve and re-form according to one of these four models, once the matter has been evaluated or adjudicated by state legislatures, Congress and the United States Supreme Court.

An Evaluation of the Four Legal Models for Responding to Motherhood for Hire

1. Prohibition

An outright prohibition of the alienation of maternity, whether on a commercial or altruistic basis, would fulfill all the concrete policy objectives I enumerated as applicable to lawmaking on motherhood for hire. In this sense, this option is preferable among those available. Arguably, it is the response called for in the final section of the *Vatican Instruction*.[43] This option would be analogous to the criminal provisions, still existing in many states, against bigamy, adultery, fornication, and sodomy.[44]

The Catholic view of civil law does not necessarily make this strong response mandatory. The civil law trend, moreover, is against such prohibitions, in other matters of sex-related conduct. Outright prohibition would tend to offend contemporary American sensibilities about personal freedom and privacy. Practically speaking, the ban would be virtually unenforceable. Such prohibition has been proposed and defeated in at least one state legislature.[44] This option stands little chance of being adopted in any American jurisdiction, and, even if it were, it might well be overturned by the United State Supreme Court.

2. Decommercialization

The option of decommercialization is best considered in two phases, according to the separate forms it takes depending on the specific legislative proposal. In its "weak" form, it gives what can be interpreted as guarded approval to the alienation of maternity, as long as the practice is transacted without legal coercion. In its "strong" form, this option not only rules out legal coercion of the gestational mother's performance, but excludes as well the exchange of fees for "surrogate" services and even imposes criminal sanctions for violating its restrictions. Both forms of decommercialization share the goal of substantially restricting the market for alienated maternity.

Decommercialization in its weak form

The weak form of the response is seen in statutes adopted by such jurisdictions as Louisiana and Nebraska.[46] Its effect is to make contracts alienating maternity void and unenforceable. In some cases, it varies its effect to make such contracts voidable at the instance of the gestational mother, rather than to make them simply void.[47] Commissioning parties are, in either case, denied certainty and predictability, since they are denied legal enforcement of the expectancy created by the gestational mother's promise to perform. There can be little question that such a measure would discourage the market for alienated maternity and would significantly reduce the incidence of the practice. Importantly, it would also withhold the symbolic approval inherent in state enforcement of the transaction.

Under this approach, however, some motherhood for hire transactions would continue to go forward, and money would regularly be exchanged for children and for the termination of parental rights. As long as there is no legal coercion, the approach may be seen as a guarded moral approval by the state of the practice. That guarded approval may be explicitly stated in the statutory scheme or it may merely be the signal implicit in the state's failure to move actively against the voluntary form of transaction.

The reduction in incidence, expected from this legislative response, would follow from uncertainty stemming from the gestational mother's right to change her mind and resist delivery of her child. There is reason, however, to doubt the desirability and efficacy of relying on the mother's right to change her mind as the sole restraint on the practice of commercial alienation of maternity. First, there is a real danger that unacceptable extralegal means, some illegal and even violent, would be found to substitute for legal enforcement.[48] In addition, even the voluntary present exchange of fees for termination of parental rights could evolve into a fairly significant market in maternity alienation. A statistically significant flow of transactions of this latter kind may make it inevitable that the society eventually would slide into approving and enforcing the practice on a commercial basis. Finally, the symbolism of allowing the de facto exchange of money for a child or the termination of parental rights, even on a voluntary basis, entails an unacceptable erosion of the society's commitment to human dignity and the welfare and rights of children. In the long run, decommercialization in its weak form is likely either to evolve further and to become decommercialization in its strong form, or to unravel and to become outright approval. The weak form of decommercialization probably does not present a stable option.

Decommercialization in its Strong Form

Like the typical version of decommercialization in its weak form, the option in its strong form makes motherhood-for-hire contracts void and unenforceable. But, unlike the weak form of decommercialization, the strong form of the option prohibits even the voluntary exchange of monetary compensation for the contemporaneous alienation of maternity, and it adds significant criminal penalties for attempts to enter such contracts or to facilitate their formation through brokerage and advertisement. Note that this legislative option does not prohibit the alienation of maternity on an "altruistic" basis, nor does it attempt to restrict human conception to the confines of marriage. On the other hand it does more than passively withhold state enforcement from private contract: it actively imposes negative sanctions for attempts to commercialize human reproduction. As such, this option finds what appears to be a workable middle ground, avoiding what could be perceived as undue conflict with personal privacy in the area of choice about marriage and procreation, but, at the same time, drawing a bright line that demarks the boundary between market transactions and the sphere of those intimate relationships necessary to the nurturance and moral dignity of human persons.

Michigan has enacted a statute which embodies this strong form of decommercialization.[49] In my opinion, Michigan's enactment represents the best possible legal response to motherhood for hire, as measured against the relevant generic goals of lawmaking developed above, that is feasible under present circumstances. It would seem to satisfy the legislative recommendation of the *Vatican Instruction*.[50] The extensive experience of lawmakers in Michigan with the high-volume motherhood-for-hire mill run by Noel Keane from out of Michigan may account for the soundness of the Michigan approach.[51] The American Civil Liberties Union has brought a suit for an injunction against the implementation of the Michigan Act, alleging that it violates the *Roe* right of individual freedom in procreative choice.[52] The outcome of the ACLU case will be the next significant landmark after *In re Baby M* for charting the American law response to motherhood for hire arrangements.

3. Approval with Governmental Validation

A prestigious national legal drafting committee, the National Conference of Commissioners on Uniform State Laws, has approved a uniform statute for suggested approval by all fifty states, that, in the first of its two alternate forms, has the effect of institutionalizing commercial motherhood for hire. The title of this uniform act is the Uniform Status of Children of Assisted Conception Act.[53] The alternate form in question is "Alternate A."[54] In contrast to any of the three particular approaches mentioned so far--prohibition, and weak or strong decommercialization--which all are arguably acceptable from the ethical perspective delineated in the earlier sections of this article, the National Conference of Commissioner's approach, despite its lucid drafting style, is morally unacceptable.

This uniform statute essentially adopts the statutory framework which has been developed in about half of the American states over the past thirty years to deal with Artificial Insemination by Donor.[55] Its fundamental principle is that parentage can be severed from genetic contribution and can be made to devolve from governmental conferral of status. Under the AID statutes, the husband of the child's genetic motherhood becomes not merely the "adoptive" father, but the father pure and simple. The actual genetic father is deemed, as a matter of law, to have no relationship with the child he has engendered. Conferral of parental status under these statutes is, it is true, triggered by private contractual transactions between the physician and each of the respective genetic parents or between the two genetic parents. But, the justification for the grant of status is freedom of contract, but positive conferral by the state. In many jurisdictions, such conferral is contingent on satisfying certain regulatory norms, such as that which requires that a licensed physician be used to accomplish the insemination.

The application of this framework to motherhood for hire by the National Conference of Commissioners implements the recommendation of the Report of the Ontario Law Reform Commission.[56] The transfer of the framework from the sphere of simple gamete contribution to that of gestation amplifies the role of governmental conferral as the fundamental basis of parental status. The Act requires judicial approval of the motherhood for hire contract in advance of conception.[57] Once the contract has been approved and conception occurs, and as long as the gestational mother does not exercise a limited right to terminate the agreement, the commissioning couple has irrevocable parental rights in the child conceived.[58] These rights extend to the wife of the genetic father, who has no genetic, gestational, or psychological relationship with the child, and they vest well in advance of childbirth, and, thus, suffice to override the wishes of the gestational mother even though she stands in a de facto relationship of nurturance with the child still within her womb.

Admittedly, concern for the welfare of the adult parties and the child in prospect is one ground that leads the Commissioners to require advance judicial approval of the motherhood for hire arrangement. Unfortunately, the consequence is to further accentuate the stress on governmental conferral as a basis of parental rights. The status being conferred extends not just to the positive status of "parent" but also to the collateral status of "surrogate", and to the negative status of "nonparent."[59] Some number of women are to be officially approved by the state as "surrogates" and their relationships with sperm donors or sperm owners are to be officially formalized. At the same time, these women are to be negatively defined as "nonparents". In effect, this legislation would modify American marriage law so that it would encompass not only marriage in a strict sense, but also a subordinate form of "marriage" with the content of reproductive concubinage. As such, the legislation represents a radical revision of the principles upon which American marriage and family law rests.

The solicitude that the Commissioners extend to the gestational mother not only requires advance approval of the contract as a requisite for enforcement, but also allows her a kind of "no-strings" termination of the contractual relationship up until roughly six months of gestation.[60] While the Commissioners intend this provision to mitigate the objectification or reification of the gestational mother that would be incurred by virtue of more unrestricted legal enforcement of the contract, the provision's effect is, again, to underscore arbitrary conferral by the state as the basis of parental rights. Ostensibly, the six month cutoff is inspired by the generally recognized right the gestational mother has, under *Roe v. Wade,* to abort a baby up until six months gestation notwithstanding contract terms to the contrary.[61] The Commissioners would seem to be balancing this right to end the pregnancy with an equal right to preserve a relationship with a living child.

If one focuses on the autonomy of decision making of the mother before 180 days gestation, this provision may count as working a significant amelioration of the harshness of simply enforcing the gestational mother's promised performance. But, if one focuses instead on the social meaning of the relationship between the mother and the child or on the substantive dignity, health, and wellbeing of the mother, the same cannot clearly be said. The Act sets the coercive force of law against the natural bond which the gestational mother may come to recognize as normative for her during the crucial third trimester of pregnancy, a period which includes the most vigorous physical interaction between mother and child prior to birth and which represents the most socially manifest part of pregnancy, since, at this stage, the expectant mother's condition is readily apparent to all those about her. Similarly, the maternal-infant relationship is denied normative significance prior to the mother's experience of childbirth, a potentially life threatening event that entails profoundly interpersonal, reciprocally traumatic if, on balance, gratifying interaction between mother and child generally conducive of bonding. Finally, the mother is deprived of the perspective of a return to postpartum hormonal and physical equilibrium from which to assess her own wishes regarding relationship with this particular child, whom she had yet to encounter *ex utero* at the time the contract was judicially approved, the child was conceived, or the termination of parental rights became irrevocable at roughly six months gestation.

One may ask why, once they decided to go as far as they did in accommodating the right of the gestational mother to change her mind, the Commissioners did not simply set the "date of no return" at a date *subsequent* to childbirth. On the most fundamental level, the answer must be that if the Commissioners aim, in fact, at replacing the natural order with positive governmental conferral, as the ground for recognizing parental status, they have to avoid linking maternal rights with a natural event such as either the completion of the mother's experience of gestation and parturition or the fact of the natural mother's abandonment of the child.

The choice of a date prior to childbirth as the point at which the woman's promised performance becomes enforceable has, moreover, the instrumental effect of establishing the possibility of an expanded, legally sanctioned commercial market, albeit a closely regulated one, in alienated maternity. The woman who is to gestate the child can trade future expectation against present profit, and the commissioning parties can acquire enforceable expectations in the right to decide the rearing fate of the child for present value. Because the woman's promise becomes irrevocable prior to the period of perhaps greatest likelihood that she will develop the motivation to withhold her performance, and because the commissioning party is guaranteed their expectation as of the symbolically critical moment of birth, the Act serves to encourage investment of money and emotion by commissioning parties in such arrangements, and to validate their expectations as worthy of special social recognition.

The comments to the penultimate draft of the Act stated that the drafters meant to withhold judgment on the morality of motherhood for hire arrangements.[62] The overriding justification they gave for their approach was concern for the predictability of the status of the children born in such arrangements, such predictability being of great importance to the law of intestate succession and class gifts.[63] In fact, such concern could be as easily accommodated by lodging the power to decide the status and custody of the child in the decision of the gestational mother at a time subsequent to childbirth. Inescapably, "Alternate A" of the Act represents a moral choice with respect to the status of motherhood for hire arrangements, since it chooses to treat the alienation of future powers of maternity as a good worthy of state enforcement, for the purpose of making such powers disposable in the course of advance planning by others. As such, the Act seeks to open distinctively feminine powers to economic exploitation by men. It responds to changing social and technological conditions by seeking to preserve and extend the possibilities of control through claims of property right.

In the scheme which the Act would introduce, however, markets and property interests are to be strictly limited and regulated by the government, for the sake of the state's *parens patriae* interest in maintaining a stable and societally beneficial order for generating new human beings. Both natural parent-child bonds and private market transactions alienating parental rights and relationships would seem to be subordinated as means for realizing this end.

The Act permits the payment of money for the right to rear a child and the receipt of money for the termination of parental rights.[64] The high degree of judicial control which the Act requires of such transactions may well constitute implicit recognition that such exchanges are a threat to the dignity and well being of children and others. But, the requirement of judicial scrutiny elevates the power and asserted authority of the state, without succeeding in securing the dignity of human persons. To the contrary, it implicitly rejects the inherent dignity of the human person and of basic human relationships, and replaces it with positive conferral by the state.

When informed international opinion is consulted, the Commissioners' approach would appear to have little chance of achieving enactment, for the present, anywhere other than in North America.[65] In Canada and in the United States, serious proposals for legislation of this kind have been advanced. If they are adopted in these countries, they might, in view of pervasive North American influence, also eventually be adopted elsewhere. In view of the prestige of the body which has promulgated it and the technical quality of its drafting style, the National Conference of Commissioners' Status of Children of Aided Conception Act represents perhaps the most serious occasion for a severely flawed legislative response to the practice of motherhood for hire.

4. Approval with Validation by "Private Ordering"

In its extreme form, this opinion, as recommended, each from his own theoretical perspective, by commentators like Judge Posner of the United States Seventh Circuit Court of Appeals[66] and the University of Texas' John Robertson,[67] calls for free alienation, by contract, of virtually all aspects of parental rights. Whether based on the model of abortion rights, as in the case of Robertson, or law and economics, as in the case of Judge Posner, this approach, in theory, fundamentally supplants the family with shifting, legally enforceable contractual relationships. Contract intention replaces nature as the source of rights and duties. Under this option the family dissolves into the marketplace of atomistic individuals. A necessary correllary of the approach is that persons are treated as property, whether as raw materials or finished product. In this extreme form, fortunately, this option does not appear likely to be enacted, at least in the near future.

The "private ordering" option, however, also exists in more moderate forms, which do not subject family ties to untrammeled market exchanges, but rather allow the market to operate, in this area, but only to a restricted degree. Such moderate forms of the "private ordering" option are still objectionable from an ethical perspective, and they stand in serious jeopardy of enactment. One example, in a sense, is the contract component of the National Conference of Commissioners proposal that was discussed in the previous section. In that example, however, the market is harnessed as an instrument of governmental policy and also restricted accordingly. In at least one other proposed legislative response to motherhood for hire, stipulated governmental regulation exists *without* displacing the freedom of contract or "private ordering," as the fundamental validating principle justifying the scheme. This proposal situates private ordering within a "consumer protection" framework. It has been promulgated by the American Bar Association Section on Family Law. The proposal is known as the Model Surrogacy Act (Model Act).[68]

The Model Act seems to make the value of freedom of contract, at least as this value operates with respect to possible reproductive projects, the justifying ground of validation within its scheme. In this respect, the approach of John Robertson of the University of Texas would seem to provide the most plausible theoretical basis for what the Model Act contains.[69] At the same time, the drafters of the Model Act restrict the scope of the freedom of contract, so-understood, with certain paternalistic goals in view. They wish to protect the child in prospect from being reared in an unfit family.[70] They wish to protect the "surrogate" from uninformed consent and to provide her with minimal employment conditions and benefits.[71] They wish to keep the price of surrogacy" services to an affordable minimum and to avoid the financial exploitation of the rearing parents.[72]

Resulting restrictions under the Model Act would prevent the family from being dissolved into purely atomistic market relationships. Yet, to the extent the market is restricted, the family preserves neither its traditional rationale nor profile. Rather, it would seem to be absorbed into a "new class" caste system. The Model Act yields significant roles and substantial power to various white collar social castes: lawyers, psychologists, and physicians.[73] Family status and relationships are given cognizance only insofar as these functionaries validate them by approval.[74]

The "private ordering" validation which the ABA Model Act provides is far from classic nineteenth century freedom of contract. Rather, it is freedom of contract within the limits of the "new feudalism" in which transactions are mass produced, the level of risk which the parties are permitted to assume is strictly allocated by the government, and entitlements are distributed according to a consumer-welfare model.[75]

Once the gestational mother has entered the "surrogacy" track, by being certified as "suited to be a surrogate," and once she has conceived a child, she cannot be prevented from aborting the baby to term. But, she has no right to change her mind about relinquishing custody and in this respect is subject to specific enforcement of the contract.[76] Although the model act requires that to be eligible for its protection commissioning parties must receive prior approval from a psychologist, the fact remains that, in this scheme, the baby is made a fit subject of mercantile exchange.[77] The effect of this Act is to commodify women and children.[78] The consumer-protection-style safeguards which the Act contains have a hollow ring within this framework which undermines the fundamental human dignity of persons.

History shows that the legally unrestrained operation of markets does not necessarily tend towards an egalitarian society. Unless regulated, it may tend towards the development of classes or castes which distribute economic power through nonmarket channels for the sake of private interests. Political action has usually been considered necessary for securing values, such as dignity and equality, which markets are not capable of sustaining. Under the Model Act, the operation of the market can be expected to have such a retrogressive effect, especially since the Act does not even posit equality as a goal. Rather, it is quite at home with empowering certain classes and subordinating others. It is cynical and poorly drafted legislation, estranged from the most basic understanding of basic human needs. If enacted, it would contribute to a grotesquely alienated society.

IV. CONCLUSION

From the ethical perspective that has been developed here, the practice of motherhood for hire is, like human slavery, always and everywhere morally objectionable. I have expressly identified this perspective as Roman Catholic and have adopted, as my point of departure, the *Vatican Instruction on Respect for Human Life in Its Origin and on the Dignity of Procreation*. Yet, the perspective is one grounded in reason and addressed to others in the political community, whether or not they are Catholics or even Christians. Ultimately, what the article advocates is not even its distinctive moral conclusion. It advocates only that the political community, from its diverse moral perspectives, join together in a legal response to motherhood for hire, that preserves the normative value of the family and the individual human person as fundamental to the public moral order of society, and that otherwise maintains the minimum conditions required by public morality.

This article's analysis leads to the conclusion that the best among legal proposals available on the question of motherhood for hire is the proposal I have termed decommercialization in its strong form. The Michigan statute on motherhood for hire exemplifies the approach. Such an approach does not forbid the alienation of maternity, as long as it is transacted without compensation, without legal enforcement, and without compromising the state's *parens patriae* power to intervene on behalf of the child. It does punish, with criminal sanctions, public actions designed to induce others to participate in motherhood for hire arrangements, as well as the exchange of monetary compensation for the custody of a child or the termination of parental rights. The article settles on this recommended legal response from out of a spectrum of responses which are, in theory, ethically acceptable. On this spectrum, outright prohibition was found to be too heavy, and decommercialization in its weak form too light a response. The alternatives, available in the Uniform Status of Children of Assisted Conception Act, "Alternate A," and the Model Surrogacy Act, are ethically unacceptable. The enactment of either proposal would compromise the moral legitimacy of the American system of law and significantly disrupt the public moral order of American life.

ENDNOTES

[1]Copyright 1989 William Wagner.

[2]*The Fierce War of Longing Over Baby M*, Wash. Post, Oct. 14, 1986, at E4, col. 4.

[3]Congregation for the Doctrine of the Faith, Instruction on Respect for Human Life in Its Origin and on the Dignity of Procreation: Replies to Certain Questions of the Day, reprinted in Pope John XXIII Medical-Moral Research and Education Center, Ethics and Medics 20 (Supp. April 1987) [hereinafter Vatican Instruction].

[4]In the pre-trial phase of litigation, the Superior Court issued an *ex parte* order calling for the forcible removal of the child from Mary Beth Whitehead, pending the outcome of the contract action. In the trial-level decision, the judge upheld the validity of the contract and ordered its enforcement against Whitehead. In re Baby M, 217 N.J. Super. Ct. 313, 525 A.2d 1128 (1987).

[5]H.B. Stowe, Uncle Tom's Cabin, *reprinted in* Harriet Beecher Stowe: Three Novels 78-80 (The Library of America ed. 1982).

[6]According to the National Committee for Adoption which monitors legislative activity on this question, as of June 17, 1988 fifty-nine bills or resolutions on motherhood for hire had been introduced in twenty-seven states. Twenty-seven would have, to one degree or another, prohibited the practice, and eighteen would essentially have permitted it. Fourteen would have created a committee to study the question. As of June 17, 1988, at least sixteen states had enacted some form of response to the problem. National Committee for Adoption, 1988 State Legislative Activity Regarding "Surrogate Parenting" (June 17, 1988).

[7]The Vatican Instruction's rather terse statement on motherhood for hire reads, in its entirety, as follows:

Is "Surrogate" Motherhood Morally Licit?--No, for the same reasons which lead one to reject heterologous artificial fertilization: for it is contrary to the unity of marriage and to the dignity of the procreation of the human person. Surrogate Motherhood represents an objective failure to meet the obligations of maternal love, of conjugal fidelity and of responsible motherhood; it offends the dignity and the right of the child to be conceived, carried in the womb, brought into the world and brought up by his own parents; it sets up, to the detriment of families, a division between the physical, psychological and moral elements which constitute those families.

Vatican Instruction, *supra* note 1, at 16.

[8]The conceptual division among goods, duties, and rights which this paper draws upon is, in the Vatican Instruction, implicit rather than explicit. The harm to the family which is last mentioned is explicitly referred to as a violation of familial "right" later in the document. Vatican Instruction, *supra* note 1, at 20.

[9]Under present modes of practicing artificial insemination by donor, infection by venereal disease is a distinct possibility. This danger becomes more menacing in view of the current epidemic of acquired immune deficiency syndrome. *Artificial Insemination and Aids*, Wash. Post, Health Mag., Jan. 5, 1988, at 17, col. 1 (Four Australian Women Infected with AIDS virus through AID). *See generally*, Mascola & Guinan, *Screening to Reduce Transmission of Sexually Transmitted Diseases in Semen Used for Artificial Insemination*, 314 New Eng. J. Med. 1354 (1986).

[10]The concept of marriage as being a union of "one flesh" derives from the *Genesis* account of creation, *Genesis* 2:24; and is appropriated by the New Testament. *Matthew* 19:4-6; *Mark* 10:5-8; *Ephesians* 5:31. The concept is a standard point of reference in magisterial teaching on Christian marriage. e.g. Vatican Instruction, *supra* note 1, at 18. The concept of matrimony currently operative in American law has, since the advent of no-fault divorce, departed considerably from the Christian ideal. *See* H. Clark, Jr., 1 The Law of Domestic Relations in the United States 68-81 (1987) [hereinafter The Law of Domestic Relations]. Nonetheless, the concept of marriage within the American legal system remains one founded on a morally distinctive, presumptively

exclusive community of interest, which has its roots in the Western and Christian traditions. Griswold v. Connecticut, 381 U.S. 479 (1965). It is with this broader civil law notion of marriage, along with the concomitant idea of family that goes with it, that motherhood for hire is in irreconcilable conflict.

[11]United States Office of Technology Assessment, Infertility: Medical and Social Choices 269 (1988) [hereinafter Office of Technology Assessment].

[12]Logic suggests that "surrogate embryo transfer" is only feasible prior to implantation. At this point, the gestational mother will not know that she is pregnant, much less that an emergency threatens the continuation of the pregnancy, unless she has, from the Catholic perspective impermissibly, planned the conception with the aim of such transfer. Even assuming that the delicate symbiosis of the post implantation placental relationship could be disrupted in one woman and re-established in another, without unduly injuring the fetus, the case of a woman who actually has the necessary advance warning of a threatened spontaneous abortion or miscarriage and is willing voluntarily to undergo the significant invasion and foreseeable emotional distress this operation would entail for the sake of permanently relinquishing her child to another might be exceptional.

It is possible, of course, that a reform of the abortion laws might give impetus to this kind of preparturient adoption. If induced abortion were otherwise prohibited, the incidence of *surrogate fetal transfer* might well expand to equal the number of women willing to receive the embryos and fetuses of other women. Clearly, the number of such willing recipients would be fewer than the number of present induced abortions. Even in the event that post-implantation transfer techniques were developed, which , at present, seems unlikely, prudence would, nevertheless, seem to dictate that the incidental evils attending their development would probably outweigh the good to be gained through saving lives currently lost to abortion. In terms of broader social impact, the techniques would be likely to tend generally to be used for purposes that would reduce women to objects of manipulation or violate parental rights and duties. Further, development of these techniques would require morally impermissible nontherapeutic and destructive experimentation on existing embryos and fetuses.

[13]The person's status as "end in him or herself" is expressed theologically as being made "in the image of God." Vatican Instruction, *supra* note 1, at 9. Respect to a human life, on this basis, is owed from the moment of conception. *Id.* at 10. It is owed, in an anticipatory way, from the moment the couple contemplates the marital act, since the procreation of another being is deemed to be an intrinsic aspect of the meaning of sexual intercourse. Pastoral Constitution on the Church in the Modern World (Gaudium et Spes) (1965), reprinted in *The Documents of Vatican II* 253 (W. Abbott & J. Gallagher eds. 1966) [hereinafter Pastoral Constitution] and Paul VI, Humanae Vitae, 60 Acta Apostolicae Sedis 481, 12 at 488-89 (1968).

[14]Procreation is understood in the Catholic tradition not merely transmitting life to children, but as both giving biological life to *and* rearing children to maturity. Having given life to the child, the parent has the duty and the right to rear it to maturity. Pastoral Constitution, *supra* note 12, at 254.

[15]Vatican Instruction, *supra* note 1, at 14-15. The spouses are required to treat each other as ends-in-themselves and with unconditional loyalty, which means that marriage is exclusive and indissoluble. Pastoral Constitution, *supra* note 12, at 250-51. Theologically, the Catholic understanding of these moral requirements is expressed in terms of sacramental union, which transcends the partners and is modeled on Christ's relationship with the Church. Pastoral Constitution, *supra* note 12, at 251.

[16]Sacred Congregation for the Doctrine of the Faith, Declaration on Procured Abortion, 66 Acta Apostolicae Sedis 730, 738 (1974).

[17]See generally The Law of Domestic Relations, *supra* note 9, at 127-35. The constitutionality of such laws was upheld in Reynolds v. United States, 98 U.S. (8 Otto) 145, 25 L. Ed. 244 (1878), but, under contemporary trends, it might be challenged.

[18]T. Aquinas, Summa Theologica, I.II. Q. 3 art. 1, 595-96 (Eng. Dominicans trans. reprinted by Christian Classics 1981) [hereinafter Summa Theologica].

[19]G. Corea, The Mother Machine: Reproductive Technologies from Artificial Insemination to Artificial Wombs (1986).

[20]J. Noonan, Bribes 683-706 (1984).

[21]The wife of the sperm donor was deliberately excluded as a party to the contract for the purpose of avoiding conflict of New Jersey's laws against child selling. However, it was her reluctance to accept the risks of pregnancy that led the couple to undertake a motherhood for hire arrangement with Mary Beth Whitehead. Whitehead's realization that she did not wish to go through with the arrangement was, in fact, triggered by the wife's attempts to control her behavior. She relates that she felt that "Elizabeth Stern was trying to take over her life. *Who Keeps "Baby M"?*", Newsweek, Jan. 19, 1987, at 49, col 1.

[22] R. Lifton, The Life of the Self (1976) [hereinafter The Life of the Self] Lifton's theory grows out of his work on the survivors of Hiroshima. *See* R. Lifton, Death in Life: Survivors of Hiroshima (1968). A well known application of his theory, that had legal ramifications, is described in K. Erikson, Everything in Its Path: Destruction of Community in the Buffalo Creek Flood (1976).

[23]L. Kass, Towards a More Natural Science 110-15 (1985).

[24]Vatican Instruction, *supra* note 1, at 16.

[25]Wagner, *The New Reproductive Technologies and the Law: A Roman Catholic Perspective*, 4 J. Contemp. Health L. & Pol'y 45 (1988).

[26]The Life of the Self, *supra* note 21.

[27]Summa Theologica I, II, Q. 96, art. 2., *supra* note 17, at 1081; J.C. Murray, We Hold These Truths 155-174 (1960) [hereinafter We Hold These Truths].

[28]Declaration on Religious Freedom (Dignitatis Humanae) 7 *reprinted in* The Documents of Vatican II 687 (W. Abbot and J. Gallagher eds. 1966).

[29]The original Connecticut Comstock law against contraception, which was overturned, as amended, in Griswold v. Connecticut, 381 U.S. 479 (1965), was originally Chapter 78, Public Acts of Connecticut (1879), and later Section 8568 of the General Statutes, Revision of 1949. Comstock also successfully lobbied the federal government for a law restricting contraception. This was 18 U.S.C. 1461 and 1462. For a general discussion, see 1 The Law of Domestic Relations in the United States, *supra* note 9, at 362. For a discussion from the Catholic perspective, see We Hold These Truths, *supra* note 17, at 157.

[30]From the perspective of the Catholic Church, see Pastoral Constitution, *supra* note 12, at 257-8. For the principle in American law, see Meyer v. Nebraska, 262 U.S. 390 (1923) and Pierce v. Society of Sisters, 268 U.S. 510 (1925).

[31]E. Allan Farnsworth, Contracts 341-47 (1982).

[32]For instance, under American constitutional law it is recognized that the illegitimate child has a right to support from his or her natural parent. Levy v. Louisiana, 391 U.S. 68 (1968).

[33]Under American law, natural parents rights may be terminated involuntarily because of unfitness or abandonment, as long as certain due process safeguards are met. Santosky v. Kramer, 455 U.S. 745, 763 (1982).

[34]The Law of Domestic Relations in the United States, *supra* note 9, at 341-44.

[35]As reflected, for example, in the thirteenth amendment to the U.S. Constitution: "Neither slavery nor involuntary servitude, except as a punishment for crime whereof the party shall have been duly convicted, shall exist within the United States, or any place subject to their jurisdiction."

[36]Summa Theologica, I.II. Q.96, art. 4 and 5, *supra* note 17, at 1019-1021.

[37]*In re Baby M*, 109 N.J. 396 (1988).

[38]*Id*. at 423-25 and 434-44.

[39]*Id*. at 425-44.

[40]*Id*. at 447-52; Roe v. Wade, 410 U.S. 113 (1973) and Eisenstadt v. Baird, 405 U.S. 438 (1972).

[41]*In re Baby M*, 109 N.J. at 452 n.16. This text is important and worthy of complete citation here:

> If the legislature were to enact a statute providing for enforcement of surrogacy agreements, the validity of such a statute might depend on this strength of the state interest in making it more likely that infertile couples will be able to adopt children. As a value, it is obvious that the interest is strong; but if, as plaintiffs assert, ten to fifteen percent of all couples are infertile, the interest is of enormous strength. This figure is given both by counsel by the Sterns and by the trial court [citation deleted]. We have been unable to find reliable confirmation of this statistic, however, and we are not confident of its accuracy. We note that at least one source asserts that in 1982, the rate of married couples who were both childless an infertile was only 5.8% [citation deleted].

> On such quantitative differences, constitutional validity can depend, where the statute in question is justified as serving a compelling state interest. The quality of the interference with the parents' right of companionship bears on these issues: if a statute, like the surrogacy contract before us, made the consent given prior to conception irrevocable, it might be regarded as a greater interference with the fundamental right than a statute that gave effect only to a consent executed, for instance, more than 6 months after the child's birth. There is an entire spectrum of circumstances that strengthen or weaken

the fundamental right involved and a similar spectrum of state interests that justifies or does not justify particular restrictions on that right. We do not believe it would be wise for this court to attempt to identify various combinations of circumstances and interests and attempt to indicate which combinations might and which might not constitutionally permit termination of parental rights. We will say this much, however: a parent's fundamental right to the companionship of one's child can be significantly eroded by that parent's consent to the surrender of that child. That surrender, if voluntary and knowingly made, may reduce the strength of that fundamental right to the point where a statute awarding custody and all parental rights to adoptive couple, would be valid.

Further, the threshold of constitutional protection might not be reached if the court held that enforcement of the contract was not even state action under Shelley v. Kraemer, 334 U.S. 151 n.15.

[42]Commentary on developments in reproductive technology and the law has sought to distinguish the various models available for a legislative response. Generally, such attempts have not succeeded in identifying the truly salient differences among approaches. The report of the United States Office of Technology Assessment identifies them as "static, private ordering, inducement, regulatory, and punitive." Office Of Technology Assessment, *supra* note 10, at 261. The Ontario Law Reform Commission identifies alternatives as "private ordering," "state regulation," and "hybrid" or "flexible." Ontario Law Reform Commission, Report on Human Artificial Reproduction And Related Matters 130 (1985) [hereinafter Ontario Law Reform Commission]. The University of Virginia's Walter Wadlington suggests the following division: 1) static; 2) private ordering; or 3) state regulation. Wadlington, *Artificial Conception: The Challenge for Family Law*, 69 U.Va.L.Rev. 465, 496-97(1983). These schematizations revolve around supposedly germane distinctions between status quo and progress and between government intervention and private choice. There is not space here to develop why these distinctions are less than satisfactory. For the purposes of the present article, suffice it to say, with respect to the first distinction, that the balance between permanence and change which is always necessary in law is a purely formal dichotomy, which has nothing to offer by way of substantive direction, and, with respect to the second, that the distinction between state regulation and private choice does not go deep enough, since both approaches entail the use of governmental coercion against individual claims.

[43]"Legislation must also prohibit, by virtue of the support which is due to the family . . . 'surrogate motherhood'." Vatican Instruction, *supra* note 1, at 20.

[44]See Model Penal Code and Commentaries, Part II, 430 (1980). The constitutionality of such laws was upheld in Bowers v. Hardwick, 106 S. Ct. 281 (1986) over arguments that they were invalid, in view of the procreative liberty espoused in Roe v. Wade, 410 U.S 113.

[45]In Maryland, for instance, S. 795 (sponsored by State Senator Stone prior to June 1988) and S.613 (sponsored by State Senator Mitchell prior to June 1987) were apparently general prohibitions that died without legislative enactment. National Committee for Adoption: 1988 State Legislative Activity Regarding "Surrogate Parenting" (June 1988); National Committee for Adoption, 1987 State Legislative Activity Regarding "Surrogate Parenting" (June 1987).

[46]Nebraska Legislative Bill No. 674 (July 8, 1988); Louisiana Act No. 583 (R.S. 2713) (Sept. 1, 1987).

[47]This approach is reflected, for example, in the judicial holding of Surrogate Parenting Associates, Inc. v. Commonwealth of Kentucky *ex rel*. Armstrong, 704 S.W. 2nd 209, 213 (1986).

[48]The case of Alejandra Munoz is illustrative. This Mexican woman was kept involuntarily confined in the home of the sperm donor during the duration of her pregnancy. *Surrogacy Arrangements Act of 1987: Hearings on H.R. 2433 Before the Subcommittee on Transportation, Tourism, and Hazardous Materials of the House Comm. on Energy and Commerce*, 100th Cong. Sess. (1987) (Statement of Alejandra Munoz).

[49]Sections 1-13 of P.A. 199 of Michigan Public Acts of 1988. The same approach is seen in the report of the New York State Cuomo Commission. See Proposed Surrogate Parenting Act, in The New York State Task Force on Life And The Law, Surrogate Parenting: Analysis and Recommendations for Public Policy A-1 (1988). It is also evident in the federal legislation sponsored in 1987 by Rep. Thomas Luken. H.R. 2433, 100th Cong., 1st Sess. (May 14, 1987).

[50]Whether my recommendation fulfills the directive of the Vatican Instruction depends, in part, on what the drafters meant by "prohibit." The Vatican Instruction does concede that "[the civil law] must sometimes tolerate, for the sake of public order, things which it cannot forbid without a greater evil resulting." Vatican Instruction, *supra* note 1, at 20. This would seem to be a basis for moderating the measure of prohibition for the good of the public order. The limited degree of prohibition recommended here is intended to accomplish this end. Whether my recommendation fulfills the directive also depends on the definition of "surrogate motherhood," a term the Vatican Instruction uses but never defines. If the Vatican Instruction, in using this term, means "commercial surrogacy" or "motherhood for hire," then my recommendation fully accords with the directive.

[51]Noel Keane, who considers himself the "father" of commercial "surrogacy," has written and spoken extensively as an advocate of motherhood for hire. e.g. Keane, *Legal Problems of Surrogate Motherhood*, 1980 S. Ill. U.L.J. 147. Keane challenged the state's application, pending a specific legislative response to motherhood for hire, of its adoption-law prohibition of the exchange of fees for the severance of parental rights to motherhood for hire arrangements. Keane lost the case. Doe v. Kelley, 307 N.W. 2d 438 (1981), *cert. denied*, 459 U.S. 1183 (1983).

[52]Jane Doe v. Attorney-General of Michigan, Civil Action No. 88-89032CZ (filed in Wayne County Superior Court 1988). The ACLU challenge is directed against the Michigan Act's prohibition of commercial exchanges of money for parental rights. It admits that the state has an interest in not enforcing a motherhood for hire contract, in the "extremely rare situation where the surrogate mother changes her mind and wants legal custody of the child." Plaintiff's Brief in Support of Plaintiff's Motion of Preliminary Injunction filed by American Civil Liberties Union Fund 14-15.

[53]National Conference of Commissioners on Uniform State Laws, Uniform Status of Children of Assisted Conception Act (typescript and without prefatory note and comments) (approved and Recommended for Enactment in all the states, Aug. 1988) [hereinafter Uniform Status of Children Act].

[54]*Id.* at 3-9.

[55]Unif. Parentage Act 5, 9A U.L.A. 592-93 (1979). For suggested relevance of this AID approach to other reproductive technologies, see Krause, *Artificial Conception: Legislative Approaches*, 19 Fam. Law Q. 185, 194 (1985). For a critique of the approach, see Annas, *Fathers Anonymous: Beyond the Best Interests of the Sperm Donor*, 14 Fam. Law Q. 1 (1980).

[56]Ontario Law Reform Commission, *supra* note 41, at 239-245.

[57]Uniform Status of Children Act, *supra* note 52, at 3-4.

[58]*Id.* at 7-8.

[59]The Uniform Act provides that "a donor is not the parent of a child conceived through assisted conception," Id. at 2, "a person who dies before a conception using his sperm or her egg is not a parent of any resulting child born of the conception," Id., and "the surrogate and her husband, if any, are not parents . . . " Id. at 8.

[60]"A surrogate who has provided the egg for the assisted conception pursuant to an approved agreement may terminate the agreement by filing written notice with the court within 180 days after the last insemination pursuant to the agreement. Upon finding . . . that the surrogate has voluntarily terminated the . . . agreement . . . the court shall vacate the order . . . The surrogate incurs no liability to the intended parents for exercising her right of termination. If the court vacates the order . . . the surrogate is the mother of the resulting child, and her husband, if a party to the agreement is the father." Id. at 7-8.

[61]In the draft originally considered by the National Conference of Commissioners, the draft Comment to the sections on motherhood for hire noted that "the six-month period was selected to track, as closely as possible, the Supreme Court's decision in Roe v. Wade. Just as a pregnant woman can choose to abort during the first two terms of pregnancy, the statute permits the surrogate to choose to keep the child she is bearing during the first six months." National Conference of Commissioners on Uniform State Laws, Status of Children of the New Biology 10 (draft for approval) (July 1988). Presumably, the same Comment will also appear in the final version of the Uniform Act as it was eventually approved.

[62]"The Committee offers this provision while remaining neutral on the question of whether surrogacy is desirable." Id.

[63]The Comment goes on to talk about the importance of certitude for the children and their parents involved in motherhood for hire arrangements. The key external reference in charting the meaning of this certitude, however, is found in Section 11, "Succession and Gift Rights." Id. at 10. The same section appears in the Act, as approved. Uniform Status of Children Act, *supra* note 52, at 10-11.

[64]The Act provides that "adequate provision must be made" under the contract for "all reasonable health care costs associated with the surrogacy" and that "unless otherwise provided in the surrogacy agreement, all court costs, counsel fees, and other costs and expenses associated with the hearing shall be assessed against the intended parents." Uniform Status of Children Act, *supra* note 52, at 5-6. The act is silent about what the contract may dictate regarding additional fees, and would appear to permit them.

[65]Department Of Health & Social Security (U.K.), Report Of The Committee Of Inquiry Into Human Fertilization And Embryology (M. Warnock Chair) 47 (1984).

[66]Posner, *The Ethics and Economics of Enforcing Contracts of Surrogate Motherhood*, originally given as the Brendan Brown Lecture delivered at the School of Law of the Catholic University of America on November 17, 1988, 5 J. Contemp. Health Law & Pol'y 21-31 (1989); Posner, The Regulation of the Market in Adoptions, 67 BOSTON U. L.R. 59 (1987); Landes & Posner, The Economics of the Baby Shortage, 7 J. LEGAL STUD. 323 (1978).

[67]Robertson, Embryos, Families, and Procreative Liberty: The Legal Structure of the New Reproduction, 59 S. CAL. L. REV. 942 (1986); Robertson, Procreative Liberty and the Control of Conception, Pregnancy, and Childbirth, 69 VA. L. REV. 405 (1983).

[68]Section of Family Law Adoption Committee and Ad Hoc Surrogacy Committee, Draft ABA Model Surrogacy Act, 22 FAM. LAW Q. 123 (1988) [hereinafter Model Act]. The Model Act was approved by the Council of the American Bar Association's Section of Family Law, at its January 1988 meeting. It was considered and rejected by the ABA House of Delegates in February 1989. Where not approved by the House of Delegates, a section proposal does not constitute the policy of the American Bar Association.

[69]Section 1 of the Model Act states that its purposes include, among others, to "facilitate private reproductive choices by effectuating the parties intentions while minimizing the risks to the parties." Id. at 125.

[70]The Model Act provides that "[b]efore the insemination and not more than one year before the insemination, the intended parents shall be examined by a certified or registered social worker who shall obtain a complete social history of the intended parents and determine *whether the intended parents appear to be suited to* going through the process of having a child through surrogacy and *raising a child born of a surrogacy agreement.* (emphasis added)". *Id.* at 129.

[71]The Model Act stipulates that "[b]efore the insemination and not more than 18 months before the insemination, the surrogate shall be examined by a licensed or registered mental health practitioner . . . The licensed or registered mental health practitioner shall examine the surrogate to determine whether, to a reasonable degree of psychiatric or psychological certainty the surrogate . . . is mentally and emotionally capable of entering into a surrogacy agreement." *Id.* at 128-29. The Act also requires that "before the insemination and not more than one year before the insemination, the surrogate shall be examined by a certified or registered social worker who shall obtain a complete social history of the prospective surrogate and determine whether the prospective surrogate appears to be suited to being a surrogate." *Id.* at 129.

[72]The Model Act specifies that "the minimum and maximum fee to be paid to the surrogate shall be determined by an administrative body of three persons, called the . . . Surrogacy Fee Agency. The . . . Surrogacy Fee Agency shall not set the minimum fee at less than $7,500. The maximum fee shall not be more than $12,500 . . . The surrogacy agreement may, however, waive the payment of a fee . . . if the surrogate is related to the intended parents or if [they] have known each other for a period of more than three years . . . " *Id.* at 125.

[73]The legal validity of the arrangement does not hinge on court approval, as under the National Conference of Commissioners' proposal, considered above, but rather on its being channelled by a "qualified facility," which would be a private facility licensed by the state. Such facilities, like present day surrogacy service businesses, would view themselves as delivering some combination of brokerage and medical services. *Id.* at 140 and 141. The Model Act makes it legally mandatory that such licensed facilities bring physicians, psychologists, psychiatrists, lawyers, and social workers into the process. *Id.* at 127-130.

[74]Various forms of approvals by physicians, social works, and mental health professions are required before the agreement will be recognized as valid under the Model Act. *Id.* at 127-130.

[75]See generally M. Glendon, The Family and the New Property (1981).

[76]If she aborts when not "medically necessary," however, she will be liable to the "intended parents" for money damages. *Id.* at 133. The Model Act provides that "[a]fter the child is born, either of the parties shall have the right to specific performance, that is, the right to have the court order and enforce the delivery of the child to the intended parent or parents." *Id.* at 133.

[77]The legislative scheme contained in the Model Act has the form which one would expect to cover a commercial joint venture in any other regulated area.

[78]For a discussion of the concept of commodification, see Radin, *Market-Inalienability*, 100 Harv. L. Rev. 1849 (1987).

Acknowledgments: I would like to thank my student research assistants, Patricia Jehle and Christine Bianchine, for their invaluable research assistance in the preparation of the present article.

9

Recent Advances in Infertility Evaluation and Treatment

Thomas W. Hilgers, M.D.

The problem of infertility is immense! It clearly is on the increase and, in 1982, the National Survey for Family Growth in the United States, estimated that fecundity was impaired in 22.2 percent of potentially fertile married couples.

The couple with fertility problems should be viewed as having serious difficulties. Unfortunately, all too often, the medical community responds superficially. The community, in general, responds in the same fashion. Historically, reproductive problems have been viewed as simply "all in your head" and the solution to them has been to "go home and relax". Such responses should be considered archaic and the time has come for us to move beyond them.

Church members with these problems often feel that the Church is insensitive to their needs. Documents such as *Donum vitae* are viewed by many as negative. The Church is once again "saying no" to potential solutions to very difficult problems. In such complex situations, "saying no" is indeed an obvious oversimplification. First of all, while the moral decisions to the questions involved often do say "no", they also provide a resounding yes! They say no to certain technologies which are not morally licit and *cannot* be condoned under any circumstances. On the other hand, they give a resounding yes to *the supreme gift of life* and to the new testament commandments which Christ gave to all of us. *Taken in context,* the entire teaching of the Church is *a resounding affirmation* of the *dignity of the human person.* Unfortunately, that, alone, does not assist the infertile couple with the resolution of their infertility problem.

Where the Church's statement of "no" seems to so deafeningly drowned out the affirmation which the Church is providing, is in *the utter lack of a Catholic medical response* to these couples whose needs are enormous. When *the Church preaches without actions to back it up, there will always be a dichotomy* between what one wants to believe and what actions are undertaken. In other words, while many Catholic couples would like to believe *Donum vitae,* many may not choose that course because there simply is no apparent answers available to them or no apparent interest in finding an answer.

The Pope Paul VI Institute for the Study of Human Reproduction is a response to the challenges presented in an attempt to provide a Catholic answer. Others have attempted to do the same. However, they have focused their attentions on providing a Catholic alternative in the technological realm so that there would be *a Catholic competitor* to such technologies as *in vitro* fertilization. Gamete intrafallopian transfer (GIFT) is such an program. In my opinion, and as you will see from this presentation, I believe that such pursuits hold little hope of reaching out to large numbers of couples with infertility problems.

The Pope Paul VI Institute is clearly technological in its orientation. We use laser and microsurgical techniques, advanced ultrasound technologies and hormonal evaluation. However, we also use more simple techniques that, by being simple, are often ignored by other investigators. The simplest technique we have is the Creighton Model Natural Family Planning System which, in my opinion, has given us a *whole new insight* into the problems of human fertility.[2] It has provided a research opportunity which I am going to share with you today.

Donum vitae recognizes the need for research. The document states that "scientists therefore are to be encouraged to continue their research with the aim of preventing the causes of sterility and of being able to remedy them so that sterile couples will be able to procreate in full respect for their own personal dignity and that of the child to be born."[1]

CREIGHTON MODEL NATURAL FAMILY PLANNING

The Ovulation Method of Natural Family Planning was first described by Drs. John and Lyn Billings in Melbourne, Australia. It was introduced into the United States in 1971 and I had the personal privilege of meeting with Dr. John Billings on his first tour of this country in 1972. My interest in the method began immediately and an intensive investigation of the method started, under our auspices, in 1976. As a result of the research that we have done with this method, we have developed a new standardized model of the Ovulation Method often referred to as *the Creighton Model*.[2]

The Creighton Model is a means of teaching the Ovulation Method in which the method *is fully standardized* with duplication or replication of results from one couple to the next. *The versatility of the method* is thus increased in the hands of our teachers, who are trained to manage fertility patterns at the most advanced level. This standardization of the method has produced a significant impact on our ability to look at the human menstrual cycle and human fertility in a fashion which has not been done previously. One of the astonishing realizations in reproductive medicine is that, in spite of all the technological advances, there has been no orderly study of the fertility events of the menstrual cycle (with the exception of the work of Vollman[3] who's emphasis was mostly on the statistical parameters of the menstrual cycle and the basal body temperature events).

128

While I am a gynecologist and have been trained to be an "expert" in vaginal discharges, it has become more and more amazing to me that *no systematic study of vaginal discharges has ever been done.* Our work, which began in 1976, was an opportunity for us to begin a lifelong study of these events. As these events have unfolded, a number of exciting findings have come forward.

In Figure 3, one sees the charting of the Ovulation Method in a way which is recognizable by most.[4] The first cycle shows five days of menstruation, followed by four dry days and then the beginning of the mucus discharge. The mucus discharge usually begins as a sticky, cloudy or tacky, cloudy discharge and progresses to become clear, stretchy or lubricative. *The last day* in which the mucus is *clear, stretchy or lubricative* is referred to as *the Peak Day. Following the Peak Day, there is an abrupt change in the mucus discharge to either a sticky or tacky, cloudy discharge or a dry observation.*

The Peak Day has been studied extensively and shows a very close correlation to the timing of ovulation.[5] The beginning of the mucus discharge correlates with the rising levels of estrogen as the follicle approaches ovulation (Figure 6). The cervical mucus is vital to sperm survival and the penetration of the sperm through the cervix at the time of fertility. The menstrual flow is the result of the sloughing of the lining of the uterus (endometrium) secondary to the decline in the progesterone and estrogen hormones which are produced in the previous cycle.

The dry days prior to the beginning of the mucus discharge are infertile because the ovary is not yet preparing for ovulation and the mucus is absent. From the fourth day following the Peak Day until the beginning of the next menstrual period is also infertile. The *fertile time* is from the first day of the beginning of the mucus discharge until three full days past the Peak Day.[6]

The length of the post-Peak phase averages about 12 days in duration and is a good indicator of the length of the luteal phase of the menstrual cycle.[7] This phase of the menstrual cycle is critical to the support of pregnancy and, if inadequate, can lead to a variety of different reproductive problems.

The Ovulation Method can be used as a means to avoid pregnancy and is extremely effective in doing so. Extensive studies have been done on the effectiveness of the method to avoid pregnancy and it is equivalent to the method and use-effectiveness of oral contraceptives if it is properly taught by well trained teachers.[8-9]

This method can also be used to achieve pregnancy and is *not a method of contraception.* In Figure 4, one observes the use of the method to achieve pregnancy. The acts of intercourse are occurring during the time of fertility and subsequent pregnancy occurs. This figure also demonstrates the use of the Vaginal Discharge Recording System (VDRS) (Figure 2). This system is a scientifically unique contribution of the Creighton Model to natural family planning.

WHAT IS NORMAL FERTILITY?

In order to understand reproductive abnormalities, *it is essential* to have an understanding of what normal fertility is. One of the major drawbacks to most research currently occurring in the field of infertility is the lack of an appropriate understanding of what is normal. Not long ago, I attended a conference at Johns Hopkins University where Drs. Georgeanna and Howard Jones (the founders of the Norfolk In Vitro Fertilization Clinic) spoke. Dr. Georgeanna Jones admitted that they had not studied couples of normal fertility. From a scientific point of view, this was astonishing. It is clearly difficult for one to understand what is abnormal when one does not understand what is normal. As a result of this void in understanding, a number of misstatements have been made with regard to the effectiveness of the technological means for achieving pregnancy. For example, it is frequently heard on the national media that *in vitro* fertilization approaches the natural conception rate. However, nothing could be further from the truth.

The *Ovulation Method* is the most *precise* means of identifying the true time of fertility in a given menstrual cycle. We have studied the effectiveness of the method as a means of achieving pregnancy in couples of normal fertility and found that 76.0 percent of them became pregnant in the very first cycle that they used the days of fertility.[10] By three cycles, 90.0 percent had achieved pregnancy and by six cycles 98.0 percent. This study corroborates a collaborative study previously conducted by the World Health Organization.[11] Unfortunately, data from such studies is rarely referred to and the *in vitro* programs still look to studies done many years ago which show only a 20 to 30 percent success rate in any given cycle.[12,13]

With a better understanding of what is normal, one can better define what is abnormal. For example, the current medically accepted definition of infertility requires *one year* in which no pregnancy occurs in a couple using *random* acts of intercourse. However, with the Ovulation Method, when intercourse is *fertility-focused,* one can make the identification of infertility within *six months* of use of the method. This is *important* because the quicker one is able to recognize the problem, the quicker one is able to work on correcting it. Also, it is my opinion that the longer the infertility problem is in existence, the more difficult it is to treat.

THE CREIGHTON MODEL IN INFERTILITY

The *Creighton Model* allows us to study the patterns of mucus discharge as they occur during the course of the menstrual cycle and as they relate to the times of fertility and infertility. This system is different from previous natural methods of family planning because it focuses on the identification of the true phases of fertility and the true phases of infertility in a standardized fashion. Previous methods, especially basal body temperature systems, focus predominantly on the post-ovulatory phase of the cycle and, when the temperature increases, it identifies *a time of naturally occurring infertility*. Thus, such systems are not helpful in making a positive identification of the time of fertility. Indeed, the long term emphasis on the use of basal body temperatures, which is still the prevalent practice, has actually given us erroneous information with regard to our understanding of human ovulation. The biphasic temperature patterns, used almost universally to diagnose human ovulation, may actually be in error as often as 70 percent of the time.

As one begins to look at the patterns of the mucus discharge using the Creighton Model standardized version of the Ovulation Method, one then begins to see certain patterns which relate more to infertility than to normal fertility. The information obtained in this fashion can *only* be observed with those women who are charting the mucus symptom in this fashion. If such charting is not occurring, it cannot be identified! Thus, as you will see, the system becomes not only one which assists in the treatment of the infertile couple (by identifying the best time of fertility), but it also becomes *a system of further evaluation* of the infertility problem itself.

In Figure 5, five different menstrual cycles are charted according to the Creighton Model. Cycles A through D are ones typically seen in women with reproductive problems. Cycle E is a more normal cycle.

In Cycle A, we see the mucus discharge present on only one day in the cycle and observed in very small quantities. We refer to this as a *limited mucus cycle*. In Cycle B, we see that the mucus is present for the normal length of time, five days, but on each day the amount of mucus is reduced. We refer to this type of cycle as an *intermediate limited mucus cycle*. In the third cycle, Cycle C, there is no mucus discharge observed. This type of cycle is called a *dry cycle*.

These three patterns are much more commonly observed in women with infertility. In our study of normal fertility populations, these three types of cycles were observed in only 21.7 percent of the population and none of those patients had dry cycles. However, in the infertility population (regardless of cause), these types of cycles were observed in 65.7 percent of cases with 11.4 percent being dry cycles. The difference between these two populations of patients is statistically, highly significant!

In an expansion of our studies of patients with endometriosis, we studied 152 patients who had surgical correction of their condition. In that group of patients, 77.6 percent had limited mucus cycles or dry cycles. These are significant deviations from the patterns observed in women of normal fertility.

In Cycle D, the post-Peak phase is five days in duration. As you will see later, this correlates very well with a short luteal phase, a condition associated with repetitive miscarriages.

131

Cycle E could be considered a regular mucus cycle and, if observed in a woman with infertility might suggest that there is a male factor problem as a primary cause of the infertility. However, I would caution against making that automatic presumption since there may be other possible related causes.

After having begun to realize that abnormal patterns of the mucus discharge can be identified in women with infertility and that these abnormal patterns are far more common in this group of patients, we then moved to see whether or not there might be some underlying physiologic abnormality which could be identified as a potential cause. At first, we thought that the inability to achieve pregnancy was related to the limited amounts of mucus present or perhaps the absence of mucus. However, as we have studied this further, *now over twelve years*, we recognize that what we first saw in the charts was really *the tip of an abnormal physiologic iceberg* and that, over these past several years, we have been able to "chip away" at the foundations of that iceberg.

In Figure 6, we have a menstrual cycle charted with the estrogen and progesterone levels present. The estrogen levels rise preovulatory as shown in the diagram with the black bars. The progesterone levels rise after ovulation as indicated by the grey bars. This particular cycle represents the estrogen and progesterone profiles of a normal menstrual cycle in a woman of proven, normal fertility.

In Figure 7, we see a woman with *a dry cycle* where the hormone profiles are also present. There are several features which are striking when looking at these profiles. First of all, the preovulatory rise in estrogen is significantly lower than the preovulatory rise in the previous cycle (Figure 6). In addition, the postovulatory elevation of both progesterone and estrogen is also *significantly lower*. The *inadequate rise in estrogen* during the preovulatory phase of the cycle suggests that the follicle, which is the source of the preovulatory estrogen, *is not developing or functioning normally* as it progresses toward ovulation. Whether this is truly an ovulatory cycle or not cannot be determined from the data available from either the Ovulation Method chart or the hormone studies. That issue will be discussed later. None the less, as we began to see this type of hormone profile, we began to recognize that *the absence of the mucus* may be the result of inadequate stimulation of the cervix by the preovulatory estrogen. At the same time, however, the low levels of preovulatory estrogen could also represent the abnormal functioning of the developing follicle and thus a deeper cause of infertility than simply the absence of the mucus discharge.

In Figure 8, we see another *dry cycle* presented with its hormone profile. In this case, the preovulatory estrogen levels are somewhat higher than in the previous example but the same overall pattern exists. In this particular cycle you will note that, on days 24, 25 and 26 of the cycle, the woman also had premenstrual spotting as indicated by the B on the chart which indicates brown bleeding. This premenstrual bleeding is the result of inadequate support of the lining of the uterus (endometrium) by progesterone. The hormone profile supports that contention.

In Figure 9, the chart shows a *limited mucus cycle*. Again, the hormone profile is also presented. Once again, the estradiol levels are low and the progesterone levels are suboptimal. What is also pertinent in this particular cycle is *the length of the post-Peak phase*. In this particular case, the woman's post-Peak phase was 19 days in duration. At the time we studied this cycle, we didn't know why this would be the case. However, subsequent study has shown that women who have the *luteinized unruptured follicle syndrome (LUF Syndrome)* will exhibit, on occasion, a prolonged post-Peak phase. Thus, the Creighton Model record allows us to obtain a high level of suspicion for the presence of the unruptured follicle syndrome, one of *the more common ovulation disorders* which will be discussed later. The important observation, however, seems to be, that the limited amounts of mucus is representative of *abnormal follicular growth and development,* probably *abnormal function of the follicle* and subsequently *abnormal functioning of the corpus luteum.*

As we can begin to appreciate, the Ovulation Method is *critical* to the *refined evaluation* of the infertility problem. By understanding the Peak Day and its association with ovulation, hormones can be measured during the post-Peak phase of the menstrual cycle in such a fashion as to give a clear picture of the pattern of the hormone production during that phase of the cycle. It is common practice for physicians to measure progesterone levels *based upon a given day* of the cycle as opposed to the day's relationship in the cycle relative to the timing of ovulation. This often gives erroneous information.

In Figure 11, we see a different type of hormonal defect, referred to as a *late luteal defect.* In this case, the preovulatory estrogen levels are within normal limits and the postovulatory production of progesterone is progressing very nicely over the first six or seven days of its production. However, on day 21 of the cycle, six days after the Peak Day, there is *an abrupt fall* in both the progesterone and estrogen levels (see arrow). This abrupt decrease in the production of these hormones, which then lasts for six days prior to the onset of menstruation, is an abrupt fall-off in the hormonal support provided to the lining of the uterus (endometrium). Most probably, this also has an effect on the feedback mechanisms to the pituitary gland which produce the important hormones necessary for the overall control of the menstrual cycle (FSH and LH). This type of hormonal defect is not uncommon in women with infertlity problems but the diagnosis is often missed (as are all of the mucus abnormalities in women not charting their cycles). *Only with the properly timed assessment of these hormones,* in a way which allows for a profile of their production to be studied, can this subtle change be identified.

In Figure 10, a 24 day cycle is shown in which the post-Peak phase is only five days in duration. This is a *short post-Peak phase* (the normal length post-Peak phase is approximately twelve days in duration) and it is corroborated with the hormone profile which shows a seven day luteal phase (identified by the presence of the short luteal phase production of progesterone). Patients with such inadequate luteal phases are prone to miscarry when they achieve pregnancy. This is a long and well recognized condition, although not common. It has previously been a difficult condition to identify, but the Ovulation Method makes it quite easy.

Premenstrual spotting is also common in women with fertility problems. In our studies, we found that 14.9 percent of 114 patients with infertility problems had premenstrual spotting as opposed to none in the normal controls. Premenstrual spotting, is defined in the Creighton Model as three or more days of light, very light or brown bleeding prior to the onset of the menstrual period. In Figure 12, we see the chart of a woman who had had four miscarriages prior to our seeing her for the first time. On days 22 and 23 and days 26, 27 and 28, bleeding is present during the premenstrual phase of the cycle. If one looks at the hormone profile, one sees that the amount of *progesterone* produced during the post-Peak or luteal phase of the cycle *is clearly sub-optimal*. It is because of the low amount of progesterone that this premenstrual spotting is present. It is also because of the low amount of progesterone that this woman has had repetitive miscarriages. Treatment aimed at supporting the production of progesterone can clearly be expected to be of assistance to this couple.

In Figure 13, we see a cycle in which the post-Peak phase is 17 days in duration. This particular cycle was followed throughout its course with *advanced ultrasound* evaluation. Indeed, this woman had the luteinized unruptured follicle syndrome as identified in Figure 14. This ultrasound photograph was taken on Peak + 17. Over the last ten years, we have observed a number of women with prolonged post-Peak phases and infertility. *All of them* had the unruptured follicle syndrome. Thus, the Ovulation Method becomes an essential tool in our ability to identify potential causes of infertility. The unruptured follicle syndrome is a form of anovulatory cycle and so long as the follicle does not rupture and the egg is not released, then pregnancy cannot occur.

Finally, one might wonder about male infertility. Many physicians, when considering women with infertility problems, recommend artificial insemination as one of the first steps in the management of their difficulties. We have seen, over the years, a number of pregnancies that have occured in patients where the sperm count has been documented to be extremely low. In Figure 15, we see a patient who achieved a pregnancy at a time when her husband's sperm count was 771,000 per cc. In addition, the motility of his sperm was markedly reduced to 30 percent and there was an increased number of white blood cells in the seminal fluid. This particular case is significant because the seminal fluid analysis was performed only 16 days prior to the estimated time of conception. The patient subsequently delivered a normal, full-term, healthy baby. We now have a patient pregnant in which her husband's effective sperm count was only 30,000 per cc. Thus, because the sperm count is low, all hope for pregnancy is not removed. In these two cases most medical specialists would consider pregnancy impossible. But with fertility-focused intercourse, pregnancy occurred.

POTENTIAL CAUSES

As we have studied our patients with infertility over the last several years, we have been able to identify a number of potential causes for the problems that have been observed. Extensive hormone evaluation of these cycles consistently reveals abnormalities. We find that the progesterone and estrogen levels during the postovulatory phase of the cycle are frequently low. We find that the pre-ovulatory estrogen levels, representing abnormal follicular function are often low. We find that the follicle stimulating hormone (FSH) levels are often low and we are now intensively investigating the role of *Beta-endorphins* in this entire process. To go into greater detail on the hormonal aspects of this goes beyond the scope of this paper, but it does integrate with other advanced observations we have made.

For over ten years we have studied the menstrual cycle with *advanced ultrasound technology.* With this technology, we can evaluate ovarian function in a way in which we have never been able to in the past. By looking at the ovarian follicle as it grows and develops toward ovulation, we can identify several different types of *ovulation disorders.* Over these past ten years, we have studied over one thousand menstrual cycles. This is one of the largest clinical experiences in the advanced ultrasound study of the menstrual cycle that has ever been accumulated.

The ovulation disorders observed by ultrasound can now be divided into several different categories. They include the situations where the dominant follicle is *too small,* where the dominant follicle is *too large,* where the follicle *does not rupture,* where the follicle is *empty,* and where the follicle ruptures but it *is poorly timed* with the occurrence of the Peak Day. Our preliminary data suggests that 13.5 percent of patients have follicles that are *too small.* This is significant because if the follicle is too small, it lends to an increased spontaneous abortion rate in patients who become pregnant in such cycles. An additional 10.8 percent will have follicles that are *too large.* When the follicle is too large, the pregnancy rate is very low.[15]

The unruptured follicle syndrome occurs in about 15.0 percent of our patient population.[15] In this group of patients, the follicle grows and develops but does not rupture and release the ovum. Thus, the cycle is anovulatory.

We have just completed the largest study of the menstrual cycle in which the *Empty Follicle Syndrome* has been sonographically defined. This syndrome, newly described, effects a large proportion of women with infertility problems. In our study, 50.0 percent of the women had follicles which were empty as ovulation approached. We can define this by ultrasound through the identification of *the presence or absence of the cumulus oophorus* (a mass of cells that surrounds the ovum and measures about 5.5 millimeters in diameter) (Figure 16).[16]

Our success rates in the treatment of these conditions are as good as any center in the United States if not better than most without using the artificial reproductive technologies. And, in fact, I would predict that with further investigation, our success rates will be greatly in excess of those currently reported when we understand further the pathophysiology of these underlying disorders.

We recently completed another study in women who have had *miscarriages* and found that their mucus cycles *were markedly limited* when compared to a group of control patients. This is very significant! It lends credibility to the notion that *ovulation disorders* are underlying many of the difficulties that are observed in reproductive abnormalities. It also holds hope for *the eventual cure of miscarriage,* a better understanding of some high risk pregnancies and even the potential of identifying some currently unknown causes of fetal defects.

In our research we have identified abnormal mucus cycles, abnormal luteal phase hormone production, an increased incidence of premenstrual spotting, variability in the length of the post-Peak phase, abnormal tail-end bleeding during menstruation, and a variety of ovulation disorders as identified by ultrasound which seems to underlie a number of these cycle patterns.

We believe if research continues in this area that the etiology of these conditions will become known and their treatment, eventually, will become much more successful. We have already found that the follicle stimulating hormone production by the pituitary gland is significantly lower in the women who exhibit these abnormalities. We believe that there is a cause and effect relationship between this sub-optimal production of FSH and the presence of these disorders. In addition, recent work performed by other investigators suggests that these patients also have end organ receptor disorders in both the ovary[18] and the cervix.[19] This could explain the abnormal mucus production patterns in these patients and also some of the ovulation disorders that we are observing.

However, when one looks at the question of FSH, one gets into a very complex arena of *neuroendocrinology.* The driving force behind FSH production is the pulsatile secretion of GnRH (Gonadatropin Releasing Hormone). The GnRH is produced in the hypothalamus in a pulsatile fashion and is responsible for the release of FSH and LH, also in pulses, from the anterior pituitary gland. The GnRH pulses are similar, then, to a *fertility pacemaker.* However, the pacemaker varies throughout the course of the menstrual cycle. In the early follicular phase, the pulses are about sixty minutes apart. As ovulation approaches the pulses are about 90 minutes apart. During the week after ovulation they are about two hours apart and late in the cycle about three hours apart. All of this is under the control of progesterone, estradiol, Beta-endorphins and other neuroendocrine substances which may not yet be known. Those that might play a role are such hormones as prolactin, testosterone, androstenedione and DHEAs.

It will take further, very extensive evaluation in order for us to further identify the causes of the abnormal ovarian function which clearly exists in this group of patients. We are already looking at the pulses of the GnRH production. We were one of the first groups to look at Beta-endorphins and the role they play in the regulation of the menstrual cycle.[20]

In addition, we have an extensive beginning experience with new and quite novel approaches to treatment; all consistent with Church teaching. A good deal of our research effort goes into the further evaluation of *treatment modalities* which reach to the underlying causes of these infertility problems.

There has been a lot said about the artificial reproductive technologies over the last several years. There are many couples with infertility who have been badly misled by their potential effectiveness. Even more so, they have been misled as to what the potential for improvement in these techniques allows. *One of the problems that underlies all of this is that investigators have failed to look at the underlying causes of infertility and other reproductive disorders.* They have failed to look carefully at the underlying disorders. They have failed to try to study what normal fertility is and thus, they have been working under a misunderstanding of the overall efficiency of the human reproductive system. Many preliminary presumptions were erroneous and, thus, we have been led down an artificial technological path which does not present a potential for assisting large numbers of women with infertility problems.

The Catholic Church stands as the one institution in our world which fosters the dignity and respect for the individual integrity of the human person. It is a principle which we cannot and should not abolish. The Church recognizes, in its compassion, the difficulties of infertile couples. But the Church asks for those couples not to abandon their own God-given integrity. The Church also asks that we continue to do research. This is what we are about, this is what we are attempting to do. Instead of saying no, we want to say yes!

REFERENCES

[1] Instruction on Respect for Human Life in its Origin and on the Dignity of Procreation: Replies to Certain Questions of the Day. Congregation for the Doctrine of the Faith. _Origins_, March 19, 1987.

[2] Hilgers, T.W., Prebil, A.M., Daly, K.D. and Hilgers, S.K.: The Creighton Model for the Development of Natural Family Planning Education and Service Programs. Creighton University Natural Family Planning Education and Research Center , Omaha, NE, 1980.

[3] Vollman, R.: _The Menstrual Cycle_. W.B. Saunders Co., Philadelphia, 1977.

[4] Hilgers, T.W., Daly, K.D., Hilgers, S.K. and Prebil, A.M.: The Ovulation Method of Natural Family Planning: A Standardized, Case Management Approach to Teaching - Book I. Creighton University Natural Family Planning Education and Research Center, Omaha, NE 1982.

[5] Hilgers, T.W., Abraham, G.E., Cavanagh, D.: Natural Family Planning I. - The Peak Symptom and Estimated Time of Ovulation. Obstet. Gynec. 52:575, 1978.

[6] Hilgers, T.W. and Prebil, A.M.: The Ovulation Method - Vulvar Observations as an Index of Fertility/Infertility. Obstet. Gynec. 53:12-22, 1979.

[7] Garcia, C. and Hilgers, T.W.: Clinical Estimates of the Luteal Phase (In press).

[8] Hilgers, T.W., Prebil, A.M. and Daly, K.D.: The Effectiveness of the Ovulation Method as a Means of Achieving and Avoiding Pregnancy. Paper presented at the Continuing Education Conference for Natural Family Planning Practitioners, Omaha, Nebraska, July, 1980.

[9] Doud, J.: Use Effectiveness of the Creighton Model of Natural Family Planning. Int. Rev. Nat. Fam. Plan. 9:54-72, 1985.

[10] Unpublished data.

[11] A Prospective Multicentre Study of the Ovulation Method of NFP, III: Characteristics of the Menstrual Cycle and of the Fertile Phase. World Health Organization. Int. Rev. Nat. Fam. Plan. 1:1-19, 1984.

[12] Barrett, J.C. and Marshall, J.: The Risk of Conception on Different Days of the Menstrual Cycle. Population Studies. 23:455-461, 1969.

[13] Vollman, R.: Assessment of the Fertile and Sterile Phases of the Menstrual Cycle. Int. Rev. Nat. Fam. Plan. 1:40, 1977.

[14] Hilgers, T.W.: Cervical Mucus Anomalies in Patients with Endometriosis. Presented at the Second International Conference on Endometriosis, American Fertility Society, Houston, Texas, May 1-3, 1989 (Abstract).

[15] Unpublished data.

[16]Hilgers, T.W., Dvorak, A.D., Tamisiea, D., et al: Sonographic Definition of the Empty Follicle Syndrome. J. Med. Ultrasound. 8:411-416, August 1989.

[17]Unpublished data.

[18]Ronnberg L., Kaupilla, A. and Rajaniomi, H: Luteinizing Hormone Receptor Disorder in Endometriosis. Fertil. Steril. 42:64-68, 1984.

[19]Abuzeid, M.I., Wiebe, R.H., Aksel, S., et al: Evidence for a Possible Cytosol Estrogen Receptor Deficiency in Endocervical Glands of Infertile Women with Poor Cervical Mucus. Fertil. Steril. 47:101, 1987.

[20]Vrbicky, K.W., Wells, I.C., Baumstark, J.S., Hilgers, T.W., Kable, W.T., and Elias, C.J.: Evidence for the Involvement of Beta-Endorphin in the Human Menstrual Cycle. Fertil. Steril. 38:701-704, 1982.

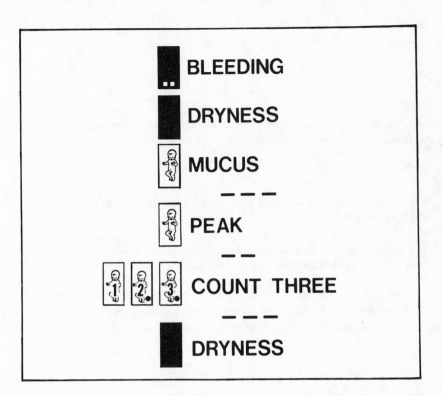

BLEEDING

DRYNESS

MUCUS

- - - -

PEAK

- - -

COUNT THREE

- - - -

DRYNESS

Figure 1: The stamps used with the ovulation method are generally red, green, yellow and white. In this black and white book the upper stamp is red, the second is green and the third is white. In the 5th line, the days marked "2" and "3" are green. The markings at the bottom of the stamps are the key to its color.

YELLOW STAMPS
USED ONLY UPON INDICATION
AND WITH TEACHER'S ASSISTANCE

Vaginal Discharge Recording System

H = Heavy Flow	**O** = Dry	**B** = Brown Bleeding
M = Moderate Flow	**2** = Damp Without Lubrication	**C** = Cloudy (white)
L = Light Flow	**2W** = Wet Without Lubrication	**C/K** = Cloudy/Clear
VL = Very Light Flow (spotting)	**4** = Shiny Without Lubrication	**G** = Gummy (gluey)
	6 = Sticky (¼ inch)	**K** = Clear
	8 = Tacky (½-¾ inch)	**L** = Lubricative
Always record the presence or absence of mucus during the light and very light days of the menstrual flow.	**10** = Stretchy (1 inch or more)	**P** = Pasty (creamy)
	10DL = Damp WITH Lubrication	**Y** = Yellow (even pale yellow)
	10SL = Shiny WITH Lubrication	
	10WL = Wet WITH Lubrication	

In addition, record how often during the day that you see the most fertile sign of the day and record it in the following fashion:

X1 = Seen only once that day   **X3** = Seen three times that day
X2 = Seen twice that day   **AD** = Seen All Day

Figure 2:

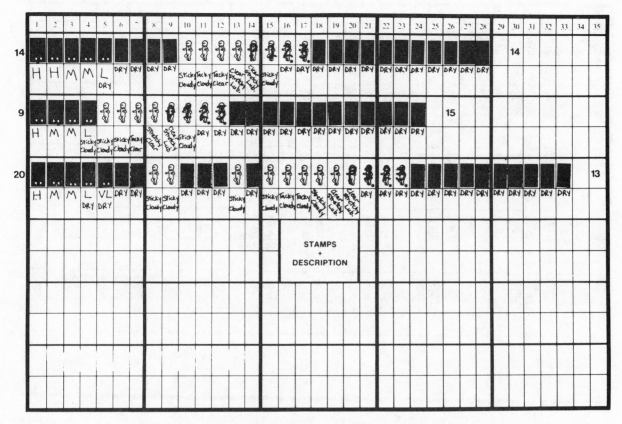

Figure 3: Three typical cycles charted - stamps plus descriptions.

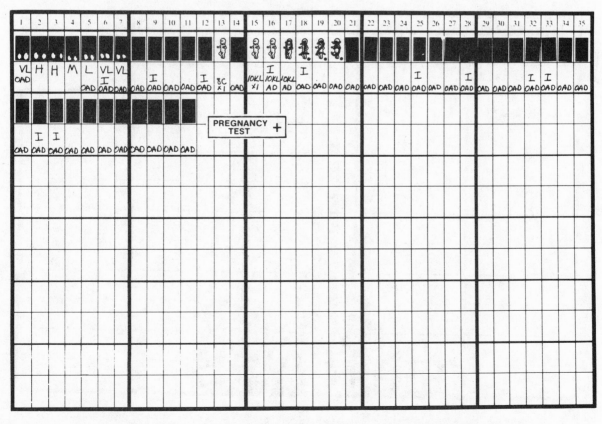

Figure 4: The use of Creighton Model Natural Family Planning to achieve pregnancy.

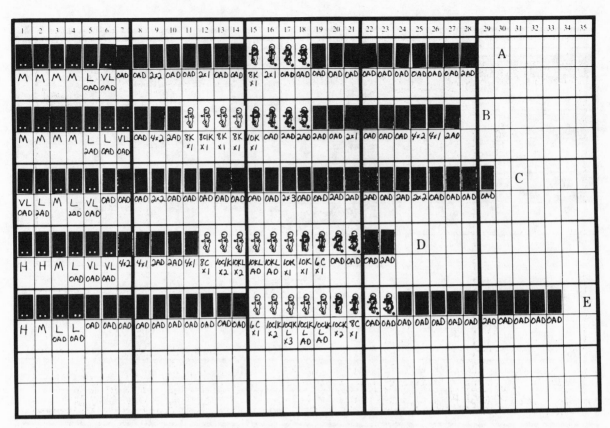

Figure 5: Charting examples observed in infertility.

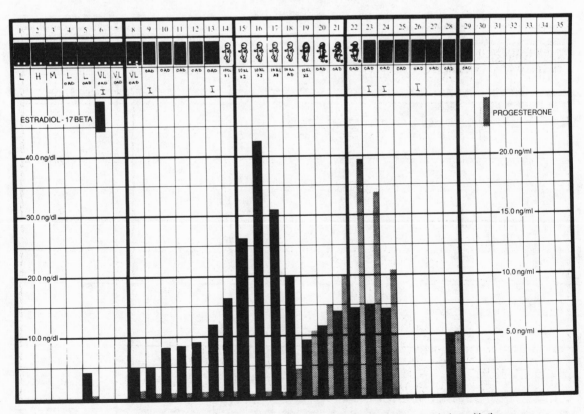

Figure 6: Daily serum levels of estradiol - 17 beta and progesterone shown in correlation with the mucus discharge as charted for the Creighton Model in a woman of normal fertility.

142

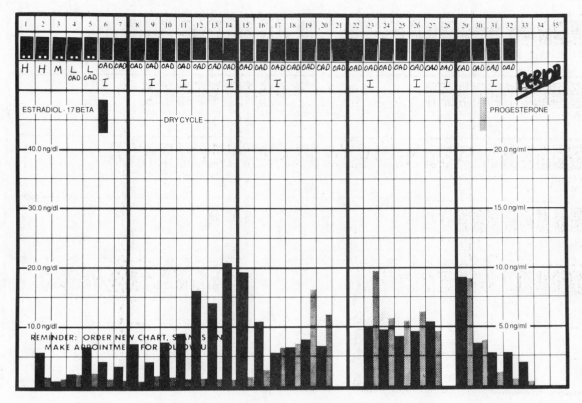

Figure 7: Hormone profile observed in a woman with a dry cycle.

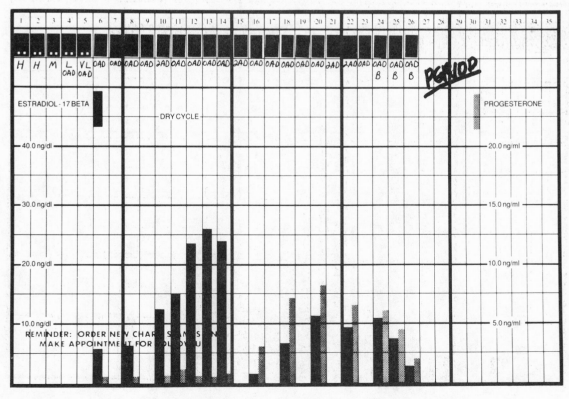

Figure 8: Hormone profile observed in a woman with a dry cycle.

143

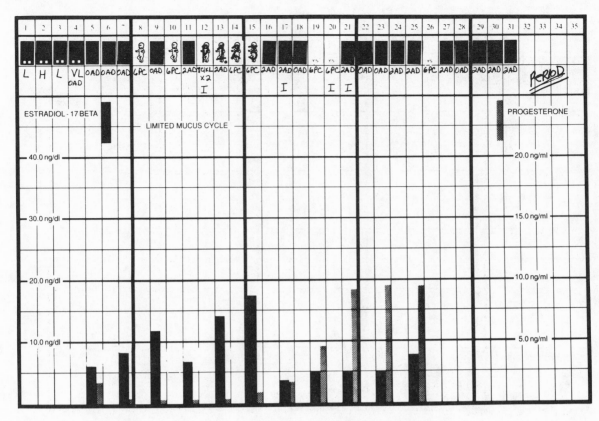

Figure 9: Hormone profile observed in a woman with a limited mucus cycle.

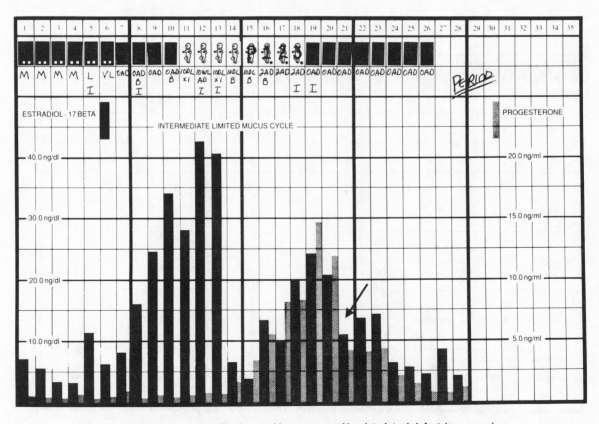

Figure 10: Hormone profile observed in a woman with a late luteal defect (see arrow).

144

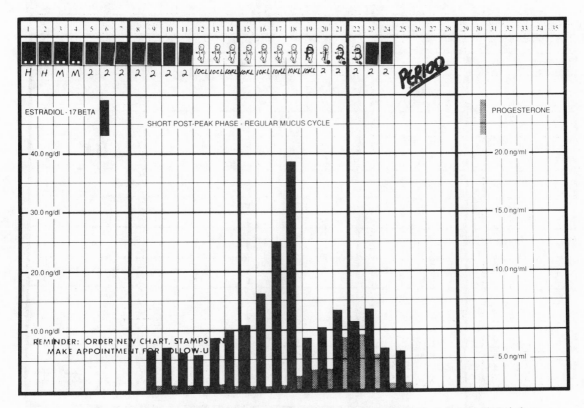

Figure 11: Hormone profile observed in a woman with a short post-peak phase confirming a short luteal phase.

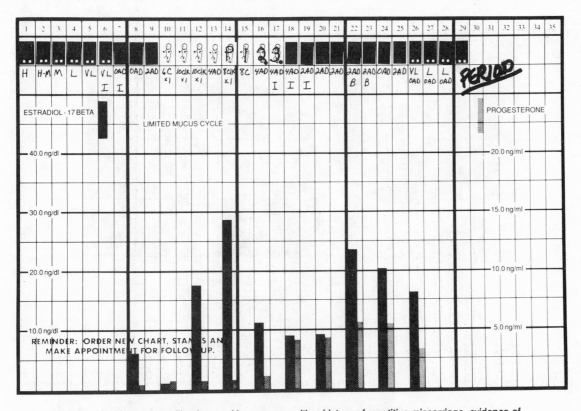

Figure 12: Hormone profile observed in a woman with a history of repetitive miscarriage, evidence of premenstrual spotting and suboptimal progesterone production.

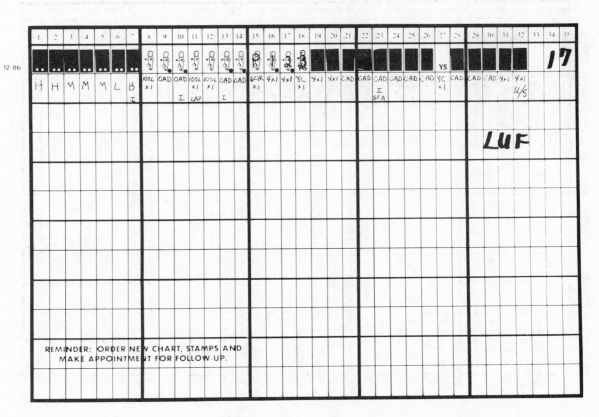

Figure 13: Woman with a prolonged post-peak phase (17 days) and the LUF syndrome.

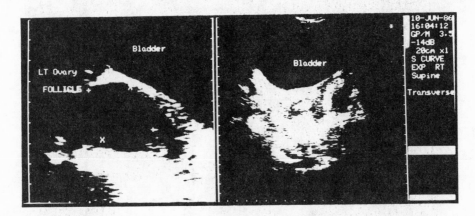

Figure 14: Ovarian Ultrasound done on P+17 of cycle in Figure 13. The luteinized unruptured follicle (LUF) is seen on the left. Secretory, premenstrual endometrium is seen on the right.

146

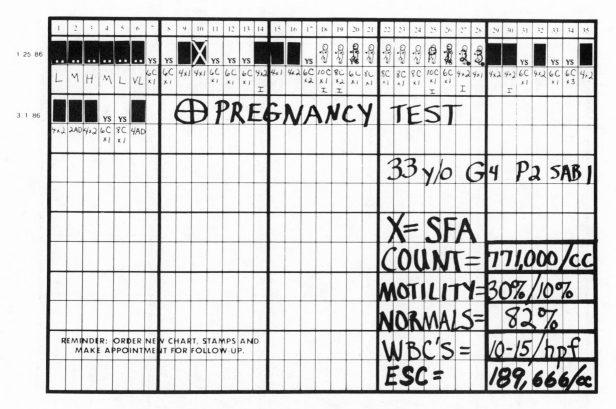

Figure 15: Achievement of pregnancy with natural insemination and a very low sperm count.

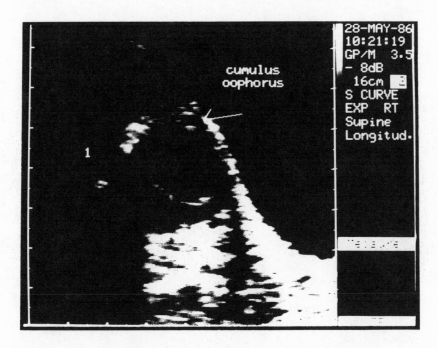

Figure 16: The ovarian follicle with the cumulus oopherus just before ovulation.
Ultrasound photograph.

10

The Christian Imperative to Follow the Teachings of the Church: The Testimony of Couples

Pope Paul VI Institute Patient - Couples

INTRODUCTORY REMARKS

DR. HILGERS: One can talk about these issues from a highly technical point of view, from a medical perspective as we just have; or from a theological or a legal perspective--all of the different perspectives that you have seen. As you can probably tell by now, it is my feeling that unless we can bring this down to reality, we are going to have a difficult time understanding the real significance of these various perspectives. Our work and our commitment, at the Pope Paul VI Institute deals with just such work. I am especially excited about this next hour because three couples will represent three different kinds of situations and problems relative to reproductive disorders. Thus these couples have generously responded to a request I made of them to share their own experiences with you.

KEITH AND ANNETTE

First are Keith and Annette who came to the Institute some time ago with an infertility problem. They had been charting their cycles for probably one to three years. We have them involved in the process of their infertility evaluation and treatment. Annette had endometriosis for which she's had major surgery. They are in a difficult position: still in the process of attempting to achieve pregnancy. They have not yet achieved that pregnancy however, and they are going to share with you where they are right now and hopefully where they are headed in the future. Their concerns, as well as their feelings, are very real for them.

KEITH: We want to thank you; Dr. Hilgers; (at least we think we do.) When we heard of your work several years ago we thought that it would be very good if we could come and work with you. We had it in mind that we wanted to stuff envelopes, however. We did not think we would be talking about our infertility in front of a group such as this!

149

As Dr. Hilgers said we've been diagnosed as being infertile, or having unexplained infertility. What that means to us is that we both can feel guilty about why we cannot have children. And we feel guilty all too often, unfortunately. Every month we think that perhaps today there will be another solution as a result of the surgery or as a result of some procedure we will go through; but we still have not yet become a family with a child. It is difficult.

Dr. Janet Smith yesterday said that people need to hear that NFP couples are happy with the Church's teaching. Well, Annette and I are one such couple. We have a personal acceptance of the Church's teachings on the pro-life issues raised in *Humanae Vitae* and *Donum vitae*. We've come to this acceptance based upon some experiences we had a number of years ago. In my particular case, I was fortunate to have a high school teacher who took the time to explain what was in *Humanae Vitae* as well as the Sacrament of Marriage itself. From that class and from the discussions we had, it was explained to me what the Church's teaching was so that I could incorporate it into my own moral life. I had explained to me the difference between the procreative and unitive aspects of marriage and how important they are to the Sacrament of Marriage.

ANNETTE: My upbringing has been a very strong Catholic one and all of the children in my family went to Catholic grade school and high school and I attended Creighton University. I think just being around Catholic teachings and values all of my life has really helped form what I feel to be true as far as the Church teaches it as far as the truth. I've been very lucky to go to a class where Fr. Val Peter, talked about Christian marriage and how we can make that real and good in our own lives.

Another thing that really effected me was that Roe vs. Wade was passed in 1973 when I was twelve years old. My mom was a former nurse and was really saddened by that decision. She became actively pro-life and got the kids in our family involved. We wore the little metal bracelets that commemorated the unborn children that were being killed. Also, we worked at State Fairs or festivals that had pro-life booths giving out information about abortion to anybody who was interested. I think that also was important in my upbringing.

KEITH: From those diverse backgrounds we met at Creighton University when we were students and started dating and went to dinner and movies like all the other people do, but we also did a lot of talking. We talked about the things that we had in common and one of the things that we realized pretty quickly was that we did have a common moral framework to work from. As a result of this and a number of other things, we decided to get married. As part of our engagement, we continued to look at the Sacrament of Marriage through the Engaged Encounter Program. In addition, we took natural family planning classes. The NFP program also helped emphasize for us the importance of marriage and the importance of our relationship. From that background and from our experiences, I can honestly say that we have a cerebrocentric relationship today.

ANNETTE: Having the background and faith commitment which God has given us, these other methods which have been discussed this weekend (artificial insemination, *in vitro* fertilization, and surrogate motherhood) really aren't a temptation to us because we see how they reduce the humanity of everyone involved: the technicians, the spouses, the babies, and also how they divorce the procreative from the unitive aspects of the marital act. So even though we are in this bad situation of infertility, we feel that getting involved with these reproductive technologies would be much worse. And we are not tempted in this regard. Our pressure comes from a general feeling that there are babies everywhere and we don't have one; seeing other people with children and realizing we may never have our own is the hardest part for us.

KEITH: I'm not sure how much you as an audience realize that every month there is a very up and down cycle as the result of going through infertility. As time comes toward Annette's period, we go from a sense of great joy, hope and faith, to "Unfortunately, things didn't work again this month for us." We go from a very high, high to a pretty low, low, when we despair or feel very badly about it. Luckily, in my case, I don't also have to go through the physical symptoms of that; I'm sure that Annette has a worse time in this sense than I do.

In addition, there are unfortunately some insensitive things that happen to us. Everybody is well meaning and well intentioned, but to ask us to--just relax, not worry about it, and things will go away--when we know better, is difficult for us to hear. In fact, we even had a case where one of our friends called and asked Annette for support because she was gaining too much weight during her pregnancy. This was very difficult to hear when Annette didn't have a pregnancy to worry about.

There are other things--like having to go to coffee break with your friends at work while they share all their children's stories. I don't have a child to walk in the park. The other strollers in the neighborhood are filled while ours is empty.

ANNETTE: We just want to give some examples of how going through this difficult experience of infertility has bonded us closer together as a couple. One of the things we had to go through was soon after we started trying to achieve a pregnancy we went through a miscarriage. Just having to go through that death-- the shock of it, the denial, no, it's not really happening to us, the grief over the loss, the guilt that maybe we caused it, and even the resolution which probably is still going on today--is something that I'm sure has brought us to a deeper understanding of each other and of ourselves.

After the miscarriage, we wanted to believe, (and everyone kept telling us), it will be okay, this was just nature's way of getting rid of a deformed fetus or something like that. We did keep trying for months; we didn't want to come to Dr. Hilgers and say we had a problem, and just deciding to be evaluated in the first place was a big step for us to get over that denial.

Once we got over that there were other procedures that had to be gone through: seminal fluid analysis, blood tests, ultrasound, laparoscopy. While those procedures were not pleasant, they have brought us closer together, made us feel like a team. We were working on the problem *together*. That seminal fluid analysis, where you have to use a perforated condom, was not something we wanted to experience. It was rather interesting since neither one of us had any experience using a condom. It was pretty awkward. Dr. Hilgers warned us--"You just have to have a sense of humor about it." We did, and it worked much better that way. It brought us closer together and although difficult, we got through it.

Then after all the evaluation, it was decided that I had to have surgery for the endometriosis and other problems. This was a very frightening thing for me to undergo. I had never really had major surgery before and just the thought of going under general anesthetic, really scared me. I was afraid I would never wake up. I was appalled at the thought of having someone cut my abdomen open to fix everything. It was very difficult for me. Keith had to help me although he himself felt worried. Would I come out of this okay? He had to face an empty house every night. I had to stay in the hospital for five days. It was a difficult time for us and we were glad when it was all over.

After the surgery, other things went wrong. My hormone levels weren't good. I had to take some pills and some shots, four HCG shots every month. To cut down on the expense and trouble of coming into the office every time, Dr. Hilgers' staff teaches the couple how to give the shots themselves at home. This required a lot of trust. First on the part of Dr. Hilgers and his staff that we could do it, but also Keith had to trust that he could do something that usually only medical people do; and for my part I had to trust that he could give the shots correctly. Your husband wields a lot of power over you when he comes after you from the rear with an inch and a half dart. It's not a pleasant thought. All the things we have undergone together have been challenges which we have faced as a team.

Infertility problems have not ruined our marriage. In fact, it's strengthened it. We've learned to deal with or communicate about this problem on many different levels. For this we drew on our initial instruction in NFP. For instance the spiritual level: we pray to God together that he will bless us with a child, or at least give us the grace to accept whatever his will for us is, even if it's not to have our own children. The physical aspect: we hug each other a lot to affirm each other, especially around the menstruation time. It's really kind of a sad thing. We usually go out to eat, just so we can feel that it's okay; there's still hope, we still have each other, and that is very important to us. The intellectual aspect: we like to go on long drives in the country. We get away from the TV, from the phone, from everything at home and talk about what we've been through or what lies ahead of us. Those types of things. Then we know where each of us is in our thoughts. The creative aspect: I've been able to volunteer at our parish school. That really helps me. Even though we can't have our own children right now, at least I have contact with other children and can get joy and can give them joy in helping them with their studies. When I come home Keith asks me what funny things did the children do today. That's a positive outlet for us.

The emotional aspect; we try to share too. We've gone through lots of procedures that evoke strong emotions in us: fear, doubt, anxiety, despair, hope. Just sharing that together. Talking about how we feel has really given us a deeper understanding of each other. Earlier, Dr. Hilgers said that intimacy of the mind and the heart is the best part of love and the best part of sexual fulfillment. We have definitely found that to be true in our marriage. And this has really helped us to deal with this difficult problem of infertility.

KEITH: So you might ask what's ahead for us. Well, IVF, GIFT, artificial insemination, surrogate motherhood, those procedures are not an option to us, for the reasons that we talked about earlier. We just don't believe that they are right. Adoption is a possibility but we are not yet willing to say that it's our only possibility. We are hoping and praying that things will still work out. We feel fortunate that we had the Church's instructions described to us so we could think and pray about them.

If we could leave you with one thought, it would be this. You have a *munus* to spread the Church's instruction; we all do. Religious, doctors, lawyers, teachers, everyone. As Fr. Lawler pointed out, someone has to hear the truth before they can believe it. Or put another way, we have to be taught the faith before we can think in the light of faith. We have to get the instructions of *Humanae Vitae* and *Donum vitae* out to others. If we let God work through us we can spread His word about the wonderful gift of human life.

KATHLEEN AND BILL

DR. HILGERS: Prenatal diagnosis is something that we deal with day in and day out. Every time that we have a woman who is pregnant and has an ultrasound examination that's a form of prenatal diagnosis. The question of prenatal diagnosis has been raised at this conference. As obstetricians we use and have used prenatal diagnosis for many years in evaluation of the unborn for the purposes of that child. It's only been in the last 15 years or so that prenatal diagnosis has been turned into a search and destroy mission; trying to identify the child that's abnormal and then abort it. We do prenatal diagnosis on a regular basis in the areas of ultrasound, for example, and in women who may need an assessment for their child for lung maturity, prior to Cesarean Section. We do amniocentesis for that. These procedures are always done to help the child. The properly ordained function of such procedures or tests are for the child, they are not to be done to help destroy the child.

Katheen and Bill came to me about 13 months ago on referral from a Catholic priest in a rural community here in Nebraska. Kathleen was pregnant with her fourth child. They had one child born that was a perfectly healthy baby. They had two other children born with a very rare form of muscular dystrophy, leukodystrophy. One of those children died at 10 months, the other at 15 months. They also have one adopted child as well. When they came to me they wanted to know about this fourth pregnancy. We sat down and we had a long talk about this whole question of prenatal diagnosis and in this case amniocentesis, looking for a genetic abnormality. I rarely do these and the reason I rarely do them is because they usually do not have a great significance or importance.

The risks are significant enough to not want to do them, and for the most part they are done only for the ultimate destruction of the child. I sat down and talked with Bill and Kathleen and I explained this to them. I said it was quite clear their anxiety was high and it was very understandable. I said, if the results come back abnormal we will not abort this child. They gave me every assurance that they too would not abort the child.

As the story turned out, we did the prenatal diagnosis and the procedure went well. The child did well and today they have a beautiful, beautiful daughter who is perfectly normal and healthy. The story they have to tell is the commitment to life that they gave to me and will now give to you.

BILL: First of all, if we would take you back through our history, we wouldn't have enough time to cover everything that has happened to us. If you will allow us, we are going to start our narration when we came to Dr. Hilgers.

KATHLEEN: Last fall when we found out that God had decided to change our "comfortable" life and that we were going to have to take on a big change, it was very difficult. We've been married 21 years, we have two teen-age sons; we've been working on building up a family business. The last thing we had planned was to have a baby. We had been told 15 years ago, after the birth of our third child, whom we lost at 15 months, that we were never to attempt a pregnancy again. The odds were too much against us.

At that time, we had no idea why our two babies had died. The doctors were puzzled. They couldn't give us any answer; they just knew we had a problem. Our daughter, on as high a medication as she could be on, still would have up to 75 seizures a day, and there was nothing the doctors could do to help her. So we watched her suffer through this for ten months; and when we did lose her I was four and a half months pregnant with our second child, Mark. He turns 18 in two weeks. He is healthy and we thank God for that. Then two years later we had Aaron, and the same thing happened again. The doctors didn't know what was wrong; they just knew we were going to lose him.

So needless to say, when we found out we were expecting, we went through all kinds of emotions, all kinds of questions. We were frightened. "How would we handle watching another baby die? How would our sons be able to watch their little sister or brother die?" We just knew that is what it was going to be. Then of coure we had all the other realities we had to face. "Would I be able to withstand another pregnancy?" I was having a lot of problems early on with this pregnancy. I had had difficulties with one of my previous pregnancies. We had our age factor; and of course, at our age, we'd been told of all the problems this would cause the baby because of our age--Down's Syndrome, etc. We just had so many doubts. "Did we even have insurance coverage?" This seems minimal, but we did not have insurance with our first baby that we had lost. She spent six and a half months in the hospital, so to us insurance was a real concern.

We really did not know which way to go. I went to a doctor and all I was given was a phone number for an abortion clinic. We weren't given any support. We were sent to a geneticist, for genetic counseling. All we were told was that this baby had these chances: 25% of being healthy, 50% that it will be a carrier, and 25% that we would lose this baby too. Well that 25% figure didn't mean anything to us because we'd already lost two out of three babies.

So then we were fortunate in talking to our parish priest. He said, "Wait a minute, slow down, you're in shock. You don't have to solve this problem today. Let me get you in touch with Dr. Hilgers." So that's how we came here to Omaha to Dr. Hilgers. And we thank God for that. Dr. Hilgers listened to our fears; he understood our fears; he treated them as real fears, for the first time. From the beginning of this last pregnancy, everybody looked at us as if: "What's your problem? Why are you so afraid?". They hadn't been through what we had been through with our previous children; watching them die day by day--which is exactly what it was. But Dr. Hilgers understood this and we were able to look at everything from a new perspective. We took it step by step, day by day and just went from there.

We did also have some further genetic counseling here in Omaha and we learned that there was a doctor on the East Coast that still had some autopsy cells that he had frozen from the last baby we lost 15 years ago. We found out, as a result of his testings, what pathology our two babies had. We also found out that if the baby I was carrying now would have this affliction, we would lose her within two years just as we did the others. There was no cure. All we would know would be that the baby was afflicted. There would be nothing more we could do for her, if she should be so afflicted.

So, we talked to Dr. Hilgers at length and we finally agreed that we were taking the right course in having an amniocentesis done. We did assure him that the last thing we wanted (or even had in our minds), was an abortion. We just wanted to know if the baby was afflicted or not. Then, if it was, we could plan. If the baby's going to be healthy, we could plan. Knowing what we were dealing with was the only way, at that point, we could cope. We just were so emotionally distraught. We knew from the past that the hardest part is not knowing. At least, we felt if we knew, we could go on from there.

BILL: From the start of this last pregnancy, we both knew we were suffering from shock and despair. The good Lord was talking to us all the time, but it took us a couple of months to start listening--past our fears. By coming to Dr. Hilgers, in the back of our mind we thought, "No, we are not pregnant; the good Lord is not going to send us another child that we will have to watch die. It can't be possible."

One test that we did enjoy was the ultrasound. It was our first step to reality. Yes, there is a child there. It looks as if it is doing pretty well. It was enough to uplift us to a certain degree.

However we are still not sure, if this were presented to us again, if we would have an amniocentesis. During the pregnancy, Kathy did go through some difficulties after the amnio was done. It could have been the amnio that brought on labor. If we would have had to suffer through premature birth and ultimately lost Nicole, I don't know if we could have lived with that decision. So, if we were to go through this again I don't know whether we would want aminocentesis.

It struck us how much danger we could have been in and how much danger Nicole could have been in, not only physically but spiritually. We could have been sent someplace that would have said, "Let's get rid of the child, let's save the mother". We were concerned with Kathy's health also. She went from a lady who was out helping me in an active lawn service, to a lady who couldn't even climb the stairs. So we had fears for her health also. But if we had gotten different counseling instead of changing our fears into something positive, it could have led us down a path of destruction. The first thing many medical practices might say is "Okay, we don't want to watch the child suffer; you don't want to watch the child suffer: abortion is the answer." In our case, I don't know how we could live with those kinds of thoughts. In our minds we knew that we were either going to have a healthy child or another angel. The angel would have been a lot harder to see through to the ultimate, but instead we have a six month old baby who is robust. And the thought of having somebody pressure us or, through concern for our sake, agree with us in our despair, and not turn us around is very frightening to us today.

We don't bring you this story today to make you feel sorry, because it is a tragic thing. We had a lot of beauty in our children that we lost. We saw so many miracles, so many, many miracles in their life and in their death. (And to encourage somebody to say, "Okay, we've diagnosed your child as being in a condition where it cannot live beyond two years.) Why put the child through, why put yourself through it? Let's just go ahead and terminate the pregnancy." You can't believe how many blessings that you deny yourself by taking this route. So many people don't realize what joy these children bring; they have so many blessings to offer us. If we had had genetic study done previously, would we have had the courage to go on and try to have more pregnancies? We wouldn't have Mark; we wouldn't have had Aaron; would Nathan be in our life if we had had less competent and compassionate medical care?

We told Dr. Hilgers, when Nicole was born it was like 1,000 pounds of weight immediately lifted off of our shoulders. Both of us experienced the same high. We are still high. We are settling down a little bit and when she starts pulling hair, and getting into waste paper baskets and spilling everything we may not think she's quite so cute. But to do anything other than what the good Lord planned for us is, I don't know how to express it, not enough. Please have the courage to tell others that the Church's teachings are right. There is no doubt about that in our minds. Because we stayed firm with the Church and its teachings, we have got a little girl, six months old that we adore and her brothers and sisters adore. Had she turned out any different, we would have loved her in a different way. It would be a struggle, but we would have coped because we have the good Lord on our side.

The main thought that we really want to leave with you is: when we have Dr. Hilgers and Pope Paul VI Institute to help us develop new ways to help our Christianity and our self respect, we have a tool that is a gift of God.

RON AND KATHY

DR. HILGERS: Ron and Kathy have been my patients for eight years and they have also had fertility problems. They represent a couple who has been down the path a few more years. In 1980 we began their evaluation process. Kathy also had endometriosis and underwent surgery. There were other problems; significant hormonal disorders which were treated. Subsequently, they have had two pregnancies which have resulted in healthy live-born children. As I think they'll testify to, they were not easy pregnancies. They are currently using natural family planning. They have been using it successfully to avoid pregnancy for the time being. Kathy also has some other problems related to premenstrual tension, which is another area that we work in. She is being treated very successfully because she's charting her cycles. I'd like to introduce Ron and Kathy.

RON: We begin by thanking our God for bringing us here to be with you and to share our lives with you. We hope that by our sharing we can, in some small way, benefit you. God has poured out His gift of life upon Kathy and me through the miracles of our two daughters, Sarah and Laura. Our joy in them is increased one hundred-fold by the pain and effort of our infertility process. We appreciate them immensely and our bond of love is stronger because of that suffering. Our marriage and our friendship are rooted in God and we know Him in the sacraments.

KATHY: My journey into adulthood was all too typical. It began without any sexual guidance. Premarital sex, although it seemed wrong, fulfilled my need to be loved and wanted. Pregnancy and the terror of an abortion are what followed. I was twenty years old. I was ignorant of sexuality, of chastity and how to cope with being pregnant. The father of the child rejected me. My parents rejected me. My friends panicked and ran away from me. Co-workers and priests at a Catholic hospital did not offer me any support and guidance. Everyone was confused, including myself, and we operated in that panic of fear. Instead of reaching out, everyone pulled away. I was never so alone. My parents took me to the abortion clinic and there I experienced the horror of death; yet also the presence of Christ, who always loves us. Forgetting the abortion and the child that I allowed to be murdered is never possible. But learning from that experience and growing in Christ's love and forgiveness to help others is the path that I now choose to take.

Ron and I were married two years later. Shortly after we started dating, I sat down one night with him and I told him the story of my abortion and I said, "If you can't handle this, leave now, because I can't handle the pain anymore of people deserting me when they hear about it." And he just sat there quietly on the couch and it seemed like hours and I said, "Well?" And he said, "Well, have I left?" And that was the beginning of a good communication between us. We began to talk about our deep feelings. He brought a lot of joy into my life. He brought my family back together, and he still brings joy into my life.

We naturally just expected children to be part of our union; but society's pressures to wait, and our desire to experience life as just a couple, led us to the use of artificial birth control methods. Emotionally, they were very unpleasing. Sexually they were very depriving and spiritually, they did not seem appropriate. My health ultimately caused us to reject them. God's life-giving grace then led us to the experience of Marriage Encounter. Our life as a couple took on new meaning beyond all comprehension.

RON: The Marriage Encounter experience led to a new communication and understanding between us. We came to know the love and commitment of other people who were focused on their relationship, on their relationship with God, and on their relationship with the Church. It was then that natural family planning came into our lives as taught by the Couple to Couple League. Tom and Ann Pogge brought to us a new view of our sexuality, of the most wonderful gift we have to give to our spouse, and how this method could help us to achieve pregnancy which we were now expecting to occur. Infertility and its darkness were creeping into our lives but we did not yet fully realize it. Guilt about the past had settled in. We were unsure and we were searching. Tom and Ann, our friends, led us to Dr. Hilgers. We have come to know that he is a man about God's own work and we love him dearly.

The Ovulation Method, or the Creighton Model, was better for us and was easy when both of us participated. The awareness and added dimension of NFP caused us to grow in our sexual love and our spiritual love.

KATHY: Dr. Hilgers and his staff were gentle and kind. Their approach to our infertility was careful and very well planned and reassuring. My own emotional upheaval and guilt, however, caused Ron and me many months of pain. I felt I was being punished. But forgiveness from God and others was not the question. It was my own guilt and pain. It took me twelve years to forgive myself for the abortion in spite of the fact that I had experienced God's forgiveness earlier. Our sexuality seemed to turn into a lab experiment, however. Everybody knew when we were together. As we looked around at what was being promoted elsewhere (that is artificial insemination, *in vitro* fertilization and so on), we were confused and questioned if the path we were following was all right. Then I went to my dear friend, a priest, and talked to him about it. I said "Is this right? Are we even doing the right thing to have the surgery for the endometriosis repair?" And he looked at me honestly and he said, "Kathy, if your sink was leaking you'd call a plumber." He said, "Get your plumbing fixed." I felt so much better then. So my plumbing got fixed.

When I was diagnosed with endometriosis I could shed much of the guilt and know that it was not just in my head, as I'd been told many times. I now had a medical infertility problem I could label.

We stayed with Dr. Hilgers and are still with him today. We believe in our Church's teaching. We find the support we need among some family and friends, and especially in each other. There were well meaning remarks of people; "just relax, you're trying too hard," or, "Here hold my baby, maybe it will help," or those who would ask, "Don't you have any children yet?" There were so many crushing blows to my womanhood. I felt worthless as a wife.

The healing that followed the surgery came not only to my body but to my spirit as well. I was able to look forward and to love my husband. It was a time when we truly enjoyed each other. Our new home was finished and we were together in the quiet of the country in the winter. Our desire was not to violate God's laws, but to gain life through them; to be co-authors of life, if it be His will. He did will it to be so and we were ecstatic and thankful. We found out the morning of Ron's back surgery that I was pregnant; and he walked that day.

However, my pregnancy with Sarah, became an everyday struggle. Progesterone injections, extra examinations, extreme care became the norm. The effort, however, was totally insignificant and completely melted away when Sarah was in our arms at last. Our joy overflowed.

We used NFP to avoid pregnancy for the first time after her birth and with success. We found that showing our love through the fertile time was only limited by our creativity. We learned even more about each other and the gift of our sexuality.

Our second pregnancy, we thought, would be smoother, but the opposite occurred. My Progesterone levels never got out of the cellar. Ron tenderly gave me Progesterone injections four times a week from 17 days post-Peak to the day before she was born. They became very painful at the last.

We almost lost Laura many times for many different complications. I had to have an emergency cerclage in the fifth month and I spent approximately six months of that pregnancy on my back in Ron's chair. It was very trying but most of all very, very humbling. I learned so much about life and love; about giving and receiving and about patience. These struggles and pain were wrenching; however, the reward was immeasurable when I looked into the loving eyes and experienced the gift of life in our two daughters. We have been so very blessed with them.

RON: Where we have come and where we are going, we place in our Lord's hands. We are still an infertile couple. Changes in employment and insurance carriers have excluded infertility testing from our insurance coverage. Four years have passed during which time we have tried to achieve pregnancy and failed. Because of extreme premenstrual symptoms, Kathy is now receiving Progesterone suppositories on prescribed days of her cycle.

KATHY: With the Progesterone suppositories that I take, I remember at first I felt so wonderful. The first month after I took them, I thought "Now this is in my head. There's no way I can go from feeling so rotten with headaches, shakes, all the symptoms." And then one month it was very hectic and I forgot to take my Progesterone, I forgot that I forgot to take it, and a few days into the time that I should have been taking it, Ron said to me, "Kathy, are you taking your Progesterone?" And I said "Oh my gosh, no." And I was so relieved because it wasn't in my head. It really was a medical problem, and the medicine really did help and it's something that I need.

RON: We will never give up hope. Life is given by God in so many ways. If our sharing with you can help bring the gift of life to anyone, anywhere, then our effort has been worth it and we will be blessed and thankful. If we leave you with nothing else, Kathy and I urge you to love as God loves. Love enough to teach young people about the sacredness of their bodies. Love enough to teach about the horror of abortion. Love enough to teach about the bond of marriage and the joy of human sexuality and the freedom of natural family planning. Our Church, we firmly believe, is right in its teaching. For within its boundaries, love flourishes. The forks in the road are many. The proper path is narrow. Please teach along the narrow path.

CONCLUDING REMARKS

DR. HILGERS: I do appreciate the kind comments. You know, as I was listening to these three, (and I know them all pretty well,) Ron said something about their loving me and I thought, "Wow, that's neat, because I love them too!" I love all of them and that may sound strange for a doctor to say in regard to a patient. But it all connects with those concepts of human sexuality that I was talking about yesterday. You can, in fact, love in a very real, and a very good and a very healthy and a very sexual way, a very free and a very liberating and a very exciting way, and that's the kind of love I have for them. They have been through a lot, but if there's anybody in this room who does not think they are better for what they have been through, then I think they need to look again.

Life has its difficulties. We live in a society that wants to push a button to solve all of its problems. I call it the "band-aid society". Everything we want to correct has a band-aid solution. Band-aids are fine and they have their place but some things don't lend themselves to a band-aid. With some things you have to get to the core, to the foundation. You have to be willing to be at the foundations, if you expect the kind of human, personal, spiritual, physical, emotional growth that we have the capability as human beings with God-given integrity and dignity to pursue.

As I sat here and listened to these three couples, I saw three very bonded relationships that have grown out of all the difficulty. And I have been moved not only by these three stories but over all the years of my own medical practice by people such as these. And I hope today that you have been moved by them as well. I know that they've been scared to do this! We met earlier this week. It's kind of tough to get up in front of a group like this and share these kinds of experiences. On behalf of all of us, I want to convey our gratitude and our thanks to all of you for presenting your stories to us today.

ADDENDUM: On November 2, 1989, Keith and Annette gave birth to a beautiful daughter, the reward for their commitment to the _Gift of Life._

11

The Meaning of Virtue in the Christian Moral Life and Its Significance to Bioethical Issues

Rev. Romanus Cessario, O.P.

First of all, I would like to express my appreciation to the Pope Paul VI Institute. It remains a real and felt privilege for me to address the 1988 National Conference on "The Gift of Life." Of course, this interdisciplinary conference affords me the opportunity to become better acquainted with recent advances in reproductive technology. Thus, I owe Dr. Thomas Hilgers and Sr. Marilyn Wallace, R.S.M. a double measure of gratitude since they have provided me the opportunity both to learn as well as to speak.

Before I begin my contribution to the theological aspect of our discussion, I would like to recall a principle which Paul VI, however obliquely, enunciated in the course of *Humanae Vitae*.[1] As you will see, this principle will become axiomatic for me. At the beginning of section three entitled "Pastoral Directives," we find a statement of theological purpose which should guide all Catholic moral practice. So I would like to read this text as a way of introducing us into the meaning of virtue in the Christian moral life.

> *The Church, in fact, cannot have a different conduct toward men (and women) than that of the Redeemer: she knows their weaknesses, has compassion on the crowd, receives sinners; but she cannot renounce the teaching of the law which is, in reality, that law proper to a human life restored to its original truth and conducted by the Spirit of God.*[2]

I am especially struck by the phrase "that law proper to a human life restored to its original truth," for I believe it actually describes the kind of life which develops in those who practice the virtues. Yet, before speaking about the implications of a virtue-centered morality for the difficult issues of bioethics, I would like to remark briefly on the way certain contemporary theologians misinterpret what Paul VI calls the "law proper to a human life restored to its original truth." In order to do so I have divided this paper into three parts. Thus, the first section of the paper examines several themes in contemporary moral methodology. The second section provides a general statement about the relationship between moral theology and the *sacra doctrina*. Finally, the third section briefly considers why the life of virtue remains the only legitimate means

for fulfilling the "law proper to a human life restored to its original truth."
First, then, to contemporary themes.

PROPORTIONATE REASON AND THE ETHICS
OF PERSONAL RESPONSIBILITY

During an earlier draft of this paper, I titled this section "St. Ignatius,
St. Alphonsus, and St. Elsewhere." Then, I had considered actually outlining the
moral methodologies of two Roman theologians, the German Jesuit Josef Fuchs[3]
and the Redemptorist Bernard Haring.[4] These authors, as you know, have influenced most leading revisionist moral theologians in America, especially Charles
Curran.[5] One could argue, therefore, that they figure among the principals
in the current debate over bioethical norms. Upon reflection, however, it seemed
preferable simply to signal two or three basic themes which appear in most
revisionist moral theology, especially as it has been developed in the United
States. In brief, these themes focus principally on (1) the freedom of the individual and (2) the consequences or end results of an action.

As you know, revisionist moral theologians receive their name from the fact
that their announced purpose includes a radical revision of pre-Conciliar casuistry.[6] Nevertheless, the revisionist project, as it has developed up to
this point, actually exhibits some marked similarities to the casuist model of
moral theology. As a result, we can signal at least two features of casuist
morals which hold a central place in the revisionist project. First, casuists
placed a great deal of emphasis on the function of conscience in the moral life.
Secondly, they developed a quite complex principle of double effect as a means
for resolving difficult moral cases. Traditionally, then, moral theologians have
recognized the importance of a person's freedom and an action's consequences in
moral discourse.

As you know, the revisionists treat these same issues. But revisionist moral
theology employs these elements which would form an integral part of any moral
theory in an altogether different way. In particular, revisionists of the "free
and responsible" school focus on the immanent act of choice or decision, whereas
revisionists of the "consequentialist" school focus onto the results of a transient action. Thus, we frequently hear theologians argue as if human freedom or
an act's consequences themselves constituted self-contained and free-standing
arguments to determine an action's moral value. Curran's theology of compromise,
for example, simply asserts that the conscientious exercise of personal liberty
frequently requires that one not conform to the moral norms which embody the
original truth of human life.[7] And, as you know, *Donum vitae* refutes
the common claim that certain actions are morally justified simply because the
conception of a child results. Revisionist moral theology, in short, confuses
immanent and transient actions.

First of all, then, let us consider the ethics of personal responsibility.
One of the most common appeals made against observing moral norms, including those set forth in *Donum vitae*, rests on the supposition that the principal moral good for any human individual always remains the freedom to choose.
To cite an obvious example, consider the fact that abortion advocates describe

themselves as "Pro-Choice." To be sure, freedom, as St. Thomas Aquinas reminds us, remains one of the promised effects of Christ's redemptive death. Nonetheless, New Testament freedom always orders the human person towards choosing the infinite Goodness of God.[8] Indeed, the political concerns of the free world and liberal democracy do not always help us remember this essential truth. Notwithstanding this cultural obstacle, the Christian tradition offers no support of the view that the ability to choose among the largest number of alternative options constitutes a normative value for directing the moral life. Only when moralists separate human life from the truths of revelation do we find human *praxis*, shaped by the virtue of prudence, degenerating into *techne*.

Of course, Christian theology does consider the role of intentionality in the life of the individual. The Church, moreover, as numerous doctrinal controversies witness, rightly upholds the authentic role of the human person's created freedom in pursuing the goals of the moral life. Still, the Christian theologian values free choice not as an end in itself, but as a means whereby the human person engages in the prudential process of attaining God. Since Christian freedom never means simply self-determination or self-realization, the Church sets forth moral teaching to ensure that the exercise of free choice always includes the basic choice for "human life restored to its original truth" and Beatitude. As the Fathers of the Second Vatican Council have declared, man is the only creature that God has desired for himself.[9]

Thus, even in the face of ubiquitous criticism, the Church remains faithful to her own identity and mission. As a sign of salvation and an instrument of the divine will, the Church remains Emmanuel for all of us. Consequently, the Church sees no alternative to providing specific directions on what concretely constitutes the economy of God's love. In doing so, the Church is essentially following the norms given by Thomas Aquinas. He, in fact, gives us three arguments why the Church must take her teaching authority seriously. He tells us, first of all, that everybody and not just a few have a right to know the truth about moral matters. Secondly, since morals pertain to personal salvation, they have to be learned quickly. And finally, dependent upon the wisdom contained in revelation, the Church can present sacred doctrine "without admixture of error." Needless to say, his arguments presuppose the divine assistance that we call grace; for, in the last analysis, we are measured not by human norms but by those proper to God alone.

As you know, certain revisionist theologians take sharp exception to this view of personal freedom and responsibility within the Church. Indeed, many argue that "the law proper to human life restored to its original truth"--especially in matters of reproductive technology--constitutes an infringement on the exercise of personal freedom.[10] Consequently, we are not surprised to discover that today the People of God remain inclined to accept, at least, specific moral instruction as the hard price one pays for being Catholic. To tell the truth, many Catholics prefer to minimize any understanding of Church teaching, rather than choose to recognize it as authentic means whereby the human person can discover union with God. Thus, the moral law, rather than serving freedom, becomes its enemy.

Accordingly, in order both to favor human initiative and to promote personal responsibility, the revisionists have sought ways to provide flexible interpretation of the New Law's normative character. In so doing, they have set aside the proposal of *Donum vitae* to speak about the "purposes, rights, and duties which are based upon the bodily and spiritual nature of the human person."[11] They have also set aside the place of virtue in the moral life. Rather, the ethics of personal responsibility so emphasizes the exercise of freedom that respect for the God-given finalities of human nature--what Paul VI calls the "law proper to a human life"--receives scant, if any, notice in the formulation of moral argument. In effect, the revisionists frequently prescind from our supernatural call to holiness.

In addition, the revisionists' project to make the exercise of personal responsibility an ultimate moral norm requires the theoretical construction called pre-moral/non-moral/ontic evil as an essential component of its scheme. As Louis Janssens puts it, "Ontic evil and moral evil are not the same."[12] In brief, this theory supposes that every action, even one adequately defined and constitutive of a complete moral species, still maintains a sort of independent and morally neutral status until subjective factors, such as the personal motive or intention of the agent, definitively determine its moral character. In other words, it denies any moral status to a given act such as blasphemy, lying, suicide.

Obviously, those who would make human autonomy the principle criterion of the moral life find this division between evil as a moral category and evil as a kind of quasi-ontological existent helpful for explaining their point of view. Why? Because the category of pre-moral/non-moral/ontic evil provides the theoretician with an excuse for ignoring the nature of an action in itself. By this phrase, "the nature of the action in itself," I intend the particular shape of moral being which a properly defined action necessarily embodies. All in all, there exist general statements in morals, founded on the nature of human activity, that have meaning which can be verified without being bound up with an example. And, of course, only in this context can one begin to defend absolute moral norms.[13]

Consider, for instance, a case which should interest the membership of this Conference. The distinction between the kind of homologous artificial insemination which substitutes for the conjugal act and the kind which serves to facilitate it clearly means little to many revisionist theologians.[14] The distinction, moreover, also provides one of the most difficult challenges for those who must explain the Church's position on AIH. In addition, the Church agrees that general statements about these two kinds of actions can serve the purposes of moral instruction. So we can expect that moral theology will defend the validity of this practice. Of course, since most people assume that any form of AIH simply assists nature accomplish its purpose,[15] it should come as no surprise at all that few recognize the validity of these general statements or the moral truths which they embody.

Of course, the ability to formulate general statements in morals which are not bound up with a particular example of an action implies the existence of what realist moral theologians call moral objectives. In other words, the act of artificial insemination, for example, embodies a specific moral nature or moral objective. Therefore, forms of AIH which substitute for the conjugal act actually constitute a specific kind of action--what the theologians sometimes call a moral "object" (or objective)--different from the "object" of those forms which simply facilitate sexual congress. As a result, in the former case, because the technique constitutes a complete separation of procreation from the conjugal act, one can measure to what extent the action in itself falls short from fulfilling "that law proper to a human life." In this instance, of course, the law appropriate to matrimony or wedded love applies.

Admittedly, which techniques actually constitute a complete separation remains a matter of dispute. But, since this issue forms part of another discussion, the question need not detain us here. In addition, why "human life restored to its original truth" requires the unity of procreation and the conjugal act also belongs to another area of theological investigation. Actually, Christian anthropologists should set forth the theological implications of the conjugal union between man and woman. On the other hand, the moral theologian may affirm that a given action (for example AIH) can be defined in such a way that any realization of the action already possesses a moral nature as real as the nature of any other created thing. For the realist moral theologian, then, moral being belongs to the whole order of creation. To take a simple example, auto-erotic behavior already brings about deleterious effects on personal development and virtue before one considers the motives of the unchaste person or the consequences of the unchaste act. Masturbation and prurience, for instance, have a way of dehumanizing the Christian condition, even if revisionists dismiss them in the interests of some kind of technical nominalism.[16]

By this I mean that revisionist moral theologians advance the view that actions, such as the standard non-facilitating techniques of AIH, masturbation, and so forth, simply considered in themselves, as actions, amount to nothing more than "physical" reality. For instance, one could purport to describe AIH as the morally-neutral removal of semen from the husband and its insertion in the womb of the wife. Of course, even revisionists must recognize that this particular form of begetting a child does not conform to the measure of natural intercourse. Thus, to account for the fact that artificial insemination entails something defective, they propose the philosophical fiction of pre-moral, non-moral, or ontic evil. I call it a fiction because, in fact, evil can only result from the absence of some perfection which ought to exist in a created thing. To consider evil a positive reality actually amounts to an illusion. To put it differently, the revisionist construal of AIH ignores the rupture of the "one flesh" of man and woman in marriage inherent in the very action itself. Obviously, such a position clears the way for a moral analysis focused on the creative dispositions, such as the good purposes, of the individual. Nevertheless we see once again their preference for *technē* over virtue-shaped *praxis*.

Besides, the Christian tradition acknowledges only two ways of looking at evil. These include the *malum poenae*, or the punishment suffered as a result of sin, and the *malum culpae*, or the actual fault itself which constitutes the defect of sin.[17] According to Catholic teaching, both varieties of evil, if you will, remain metaphysically related to the existential state of original sin. As you know, the Church holds that the sin of Adam is communicated to every person born into the world. To be sure, certain of these "punishments" result from personal moral agency only in a derived way, for example, earthquakes, famines, or other natural disasters. Nevertheless, all natural disorders remain clearly connected to the sinful and broken condition of the human race which results from the sin of Adam and find restoration only in the New Adam. As a result, only theological faith which invites the human person to share in the redemptive suffering of Christ provides whatever rational apology one can give for such evils. As you know, *Donum vitae* recalls this truth in the case of infertility.[18] On the other hand, there exists nothing within the theological tradition which speaks about pre-moral/non-moral/ontic evil in the way that the revisionists have employed these categories. Although one author does speak about "creative regret" when personal initiative or circumstances requires the performance of an "ontic" evil. Still we perceive the unnecessary distancing in this regard from the Christian tradition.

It is interesting to note that this is not the first time in the history of moral theology that theologians have sought to carve out large areas of moral neutrality by recourse to mental constructs and hypotheses. For instance, Blaise Pascal's *Fourth Provincial Letter* provides a good example of how something similar occurred in the Church during the 17th century. Then, French Catholicism, tortured by conflicts between Jansenist and orthodox Catholics, witnessed a curious attempt on the part of, yes, Jesuits, to ease the rigorist moral standards presumably promoted by those holding extreme augustinian views about virtue, sin, and redemption. If Pascal can be trusted, it seems that certain writers even advanced the theory that in order for a sinful action to matter, a complete set of subjective conditions had to be met. The theory apparently developed to the point that among the subjective conditions some included the requirement that a person fully recognize that the disordered action directly opposed God's law. Pascal retorts:

> *Blessings on you, my good Father, for this way of justifying people! Others prescribe painful austerities for healing the soul; but you show that souls which may be though desperately distempered are in quite good health. What an excellent device for being happy both in this world and in the next! I had always supposed that the less a man thought of God, the more he sinned; but, from what I see now, if one could only succeed in bringing himself not to think upon God at all, everything would be pure with him in all time coming. Away with your half-and-half sinners, who retain some sneaking affection for virtue! They will be damned every one of them, these semi-sinners. But commend me to your arrant sinners--hardened, unalloyed, out-and-out, thoroughbred sinners. Hell is no place for them; they have cheated the devil, purely by virtue of their devotion to his service!*[19]

Obviously, Pascal's (imaginary?) Jesuit opponent fails to distinguish between a moral good in itself and the subjective disposition of the moral agent. To be sure, the view that one can actually know the "law proper to a human life restored

166

to its original truth" does not mean that the subjective side to morality does not exist.

Moral realism does not amount to a form of philosophical essentialism. Indeed, from the side of the subject a range of dispositions from the swift upsurge of lust to the highly personal intentions which direct acts of self-sacrifice can certainly affect the complete moral analysis of whatever moral objective. In the former case, unruly passion upsets the voluntary, as Aristotle termed the basic source for moral action in the human person. And although the disordered activity, for instance, sexual assault, still embodies its own punishment, involuntary or non-voluntary behavior does nevertheless disqualify the actor from further moral scrutiny. In the latter case, on the contrary, personal intentions can transform otherwise purposeless events, such as undergoing unjust punishment, into expressions of virtue. Nevertheless, in both instances one can identify a moral objective, for example, rape or martyrdom, whose basic goodness or badness derives from the action's conformity to the authentic goals of human and divine flourishing. Rape obviously diminishes the good of sexual congress whether the rapist be sane or not. On the other hand, martyrdom furthers the good of the Church by its witness to the truth about God and a godly life, even if both martyr and political prisoner suffer the same physical torments. Act and intention combine to make the difference.

Furthermore, the various schools of casuistry, as the different casuist models were called, also shared a common philosophical conception about human freedom. The casuists spoke about the "liberty of indifference."[20] Thus, they defined human freedom as the ability of the person to remain indifferent towards the judgment of reason about a particular good to be done or evil avoided. They held that a person should maintain this free "indifference" even when reason recognized a particular moral objective as insufficient for a life of human and divine fulfillment. Casuist freedom, then, principally refers to choosing between contraries, that is, between what the intellect presents as a reasonable moral action and its contrary. To be sure, such a conception of freedom results in the construal of free choice as exclusively the work of will or the rational appetite. As a matter of interest, this explains why in certain Roman Catholic circles we frequently hear reference made to grace and "free will." The implications of this direction for Christian doctrine, however, are serious and long-reaching. They include principally a divorce between the cognitive and the volitional powers and the subsequent limitation of right reason on human choosing. Still, the separation that the casuists make is essentially grounded in a fractured anthropology.

Thus, the casuists do not recognize either reasoned appetite or appetitive reasoning, but only naked free will choosing. Historians of philosophy generally agree that the roots of this conception of freedom lies in the *via moderna*, especially, in the teaching of the nominalist William of Ockham. In fact, the theory does reflect the nominalists' suspicion about the intellect's ability to possess any kind of universal moral knowledge and the consequent ineffectiveness of *recta ratio* for pointing the way towards moral good. On this point there exists the sharpest similarity and strongest comparison between casuist views of freedom and the conception of freedom which undergirds moral theories of personal responsibility and freedom. The New Testament, however, reminds us that in order for one to enjoy the freedom and fidelity of Christ, we must put on the mind of Christ. In this context, then, we recall that Paul VI urges us to follow the "law proper to a human life restored to its original truth." All in all, free choice involves knowing what we want as much as wanting what we know. As the theologians remind us, we find our wholeness, not in philosophical disputes but in the Lord.

A second theme associated with moral revisionism considers the consequences or end results of an action as a principal determinant in moral reasoning. A generic version of the principle of proportionate reason runs like this: Desired good results can provide legitimate grounds for performing an action, even if it does not conform to a good moral objective, provided there exists a discernible proportion between the disordered action and the good result.[21] As you know, many theologians and ethicists use some form of this argument to promote AIH, IVF and, even, AID. Thus the report of the Ethics Committee of the American Fertility Society states: "In specific instances, the use of heterologous gametes (in AID) may protect the offspring, for example, when a serious genetic disease would be conveyed by the gametes of one of the parents."[22] Obviously the focus on good results coming from bad actions makes the theory of non-moral/pre-moral/ontic evil an attractive companion theory for the principle of proportionate reason. In the example of AID, one simply regards the pre-moral adulterous conception with "creative regret."[23] Some may even complete the inversion of the moral order by calling the donation of a gamete to an infertile couple an act of charity.[24] In this connection, one recalls Nietzsche's wish that philosophers become legislators and invent new values!

Before closing this first section I want to stress that good moral theology must consider both the personal intention of the moral agent as well as the circumstances in which he or she acts. In fact, the traditional norms for formulating a moral analysis include reference to what the manualists called "object, end, and circumstance."[25] My purpose in simply concentrating on the role of moral objectives derives from the fact that ordinary moral discourse today pays very little attention to them. As a result, the revisionist platform does not easily include a plank for virtue. We should not find this surprising. As the philosopher William M. Sullivan recently remarked, "The moral problems of a predominantly utilitarian self are simply strategic or technical problems."[26] Virtue, on the other hand, ensures that the whole person, *"corpore et anima unus,"* as the Council put it, embrace the good ends of human life embodied in moral objectives.[27]

CHRIST, MORAL THEOLOGY, AND THE BLESSED TRINITY

By definition, Christian theology results from intelligent reflection upon the revealed Word of God. As such, it embraces within its range of concerns everything which has to do with God himself and the real world which he created. However, because the human person possesses the capacity for a personal relationship with the blessed Trinity, men and women hold a privileged place among theology's interests. Moral theology, in particular, comprises that part of theology which studies human action as ordered to the ultimate goal of human existence. Only the loving vision of God, the only true and complete Beatitude, satisfies both the personal desires and the natural capacities of each human person. All in all, this kind of moral life finds its specific detail and achievement only through divine grace, which includes the exercise of the moral and theological virtues as well as the practice of the Gifts of the Holy Spirit. In addition, the biblical Beatitudes contained in the Sermon on the Mount assure that the moral life of the new dispensation goes beyond the casuistic minimum sometimes suggested by forms of moral positivism.

To the extent that its development depends upon the light of divine Revelation, moral theology constitutes a science formally distinct from natural ethics. Nevertheless, moral theology, since it forms a constitutive part of the *sacra doctrina*, must adapt to human ways of knowing and speaking. Thus, the moral theologian relies upon the structures and categories of moral philosophy for the articulation of his science. Still, the starting point of moral theology always remains the words and deeds of Jesus Christ as they have been recorded in the canonical Scriptures. These *acta et gesta Christi*, as Aquinas calls them--the words and deeds of Christ--hold a unique place in the life of the Christian Church.[28] The reason is simple. Although Jesus remains a man, one like us in all things but sin, yet he also remains hypostaticly united to the divine Logos. His words, then, embody both wisdom and life.

The Christian vocation always entails the following of Christ. Nevertheless, both Christian life and theology begin in the very depths of God's own Being. For only there does the Eternal Father speak his personal Word which perfectly reflects the divine nature and the intelligibility of all creation. In fact, Jesus himself bears witness to this truth when he tells his disciples "Now they know that everything that thou hast given me is from thee; for I have given them the words thou gavest me . . . " (John 17: 7,8). Accordingly, when the Dominican theologian, Cardinal Cajetan (1469-1534), defined *sacra doctrina* as all knowledge taught us by God's grace, he affirmed something very important about Christian theology.[29] In particular, Cajetan teaches that theological wisdom forms part of the *reditus*, that is, the return of the human creature to God. Thus, *Donum vitae* rightly reminds us that "no biologist or doctor can reasonably claim, by virtue of his scientific competence, to be able to decide on people's origin and destiny."[30] No, the origin and destiny of the human person constitute subject matter for theology.

This conception of theology as derivative from the *sacra doctrina* allows us to make some general observations about the nature of theology and the place bioethical concerns hold in theological discourse. First, theology, as Aquinas reminds us, remains formally a single discipline. As a result, only purposes of organization require that one distinguish between moral and dogmatic theology. In order to provide a complete theological argument for the Church's teaching on natural family planning or any issue related to the use of reproductive technology, the moral theologian remains obliged to address so-called dogmatic issues, for example, the blessed Trinity, the passion of Christ, the Immaculate Conception and other mysteries whereby we live our faith. Christ not only teaches us the truth, but he also makes it possible for us to live it. The living out of moral truth belongs to the economy of salvation. As St. Augustine suggests, he who does the truth does so in virtue of him who is the Truth.[31]

Secondly, although the so-called "specificity of Christian ethics" debate once again has raised the question of the relationship which exists between rational ethics and moral theology, all authentic theological discourse remains a science of faith. In brief, this means that God--not the Church--ultimately guarantees the truth of divine instruction on morals. For the Christian, then, there does not exist a separate realm of moral wisdom--what some refer to as the "categorical level" of morality--which remains independent of the First Truth who is God. *Donum vitae* makes clear that judgments about reproductive technology can only stand "in reference to the dignity of the human person, who is called to realize his vocation from God."[32] Indeed, the difficult questions of the proper use of reproductive technology make it abundantly clear that attempts to identify neutral rational precepts within moral theology simply miss the point of *sacra doctrina*.

Thirdly, the *sacra doctrina* must concern itself about a kind of thing called natural law, just as it is concerned about the five ways of "proving" God's existence. However, the theologian's primary interest in natural law will be its functions *in fide,* or in the Faith (not before the Faith) as actually permeated by divine grace which alone establishes our supernatural and only final end. Such a situation requires the presence of Christ. In other words, by some ecclesiological arrangement, Christ makes it known how, concretely, union with the blessed Trinity is to be worked out in everyday ethical matters. Indeed, the Beatitudes indicate that he is not proposing any kind of casuistic minimum but criteria acceptable to God himself. One of the tasks for the theologian lies in discovering the humanistic values implied in the Gospel message. This will not be just for the sake of persuading non-believers that Catholic morality is also human morality. The theologian himself needs to discover the humanistic praeambula (natural law principles) because the Gospel ethic of love remains a bit vague when it comes to details of life in the 20th century. Thus even natural law thinking points to the truth that only a supernatural end exists for the human race.

Indeed, this realist conception of moral theology requires a strong teaching on virtue in order to implement and complete its vision of the moral life. Those of you who are familiar with Aquinas's *Summa theologiae* know that the largest section, the *secunda pars,* comprises a treatment of nearly three hundred particular virtues which concretely describe the moral life. Virtue, for Aquinas, puts flesh and blood onto his God-centered teleology. Modern forms of ethical idealism, however, have accustomed us to think that moral practice always begins and ends in the head. As the philosopher Dilthey observed, "There is no real blood flowing through the veins of the knowing subject constructed by Locke, Hume, and Kant, only the diluted juices of reason, a mere parade of thought."[33] But only a person's complete participation in the moral life measures up to the concerns of Christian anthropology.

According to the classical scheme, the cardinal virtues address the moral formation of the whole person. Since virtue engages us with the good ends of human fulfillment and divine beatitude, the virtuous man or woman exhibits all the characteristic marks of a happy person. The final section suggests ways in which the Thomist teaching on the infused virtues can serve as a practical instruction for those who take *Donum vitae* and other moral matters seriously.

VIRTUE AND BIOETHICS

We have already remarked that the project for renewal carried on by the revisionist moral theologians does not include a strong emphasis on the development of virtue, but a reductionism to *techne.* Yet, for the better part of the Christian era, except during the ascendancy of casuistry, the principal way in which the Church encouraged men and women towards a godly life was by the practice of virtue. Aquinas, for example, accepted a definition that has its remote origins in the writings of St. Augustine. Virtue is a good quality of mind, he wrote, by which one lives righteously, of which no one can make bad use, which God works in us without us.[34] This definition supposes that virtues embody a pattern of human behavior ordered towards the achievement of particular good ends (moral objectives) which the human person requires for human fulfillment. The philosophical term for this pattern is *habitus.* These qualities of soul constitute specific kinds of ability developed in an individual either by repeated practice or received directly from God as part of the life of grace. And in the Christian dispensation, it always remains the *"gratia Christi,"* the grace of Christ.

When we refer to virtue as a quality or a *habitus* we understand that virtue shapes or modifies the various capacities of the human person in a way that allows them to operate in a certain way. The Christian tradition usually refers to four cardinal moral virtues, prudence, justice, fortitude, and temperance. Thus, prudence, for example, conforms the intellect to the original truth of human life and also directs the appetites towards their proper ends. Justice shapes the rational appetite or will towards embracing the right order established for common life in society. The virtues of personal discipline, as theologians call temperance and fortitude, give a definitive shape to the sense appetites so that our emotional life fits into the whole complex of good ends whose pursual involve human passion. The saints, of course, look upon these virtues as so many different ways of experiencing conformity with the person of Jesus Christ. So in each area of human life, then, virtue enables a person to choose the moral good in conformity to right reason. All in all, this amounts to what St. Paul taught when he urged his disciples to put on the mind of Christ. Although St. Thomas Aquinas defends the legitimacy of the acquired virtues in Christian theology, the practical purposes of our discussion require a consideration of the infused virtues.

In a special work, the disputed questions *De virtutibus in communi,* St. Thomas explains the function of the infused virtues.

> *In order that we might perform acts ordered to eternal life as their proper end, God first infuses grace into the rational creature. This provides the soul with a certain (participation) in the spiritual or divine being. Then he infuses faith, hope, and charity. Faith enlightens the mind concerning*

supernatural truths which serve as principles for their own order in the same way that naturally known principles serve as the foundation for natural actions. Hope and charity provide the will with an inclination to the supernatural good to which the human will simply by its own natural operations remains inadequately ordered.

In addition, besides the natural capacities which man possesses, the human person also requires virtuous *habitus in order to achieve perfection in the created order. Thus besides the supernatural principles, God also endows the believer with certain infused virtues which perfect men and women in ordering (moral) actions towards their proper end which remains eternal life.*[35]

Admittedly, Aquinas makes it clear that the human person does not require the infused moral virtues for any activity other than that which the moral law dictates. But he also insists that the infused moral virtues account for a more perfect performance of the same activity. In other terms, the infused moral virtues make it possible for one to accomplish the good ends of human life through conformity to Christ. In this context, infused virtue spells out the "law proper to a human life restored to its original truth and conducted by the Spirit of God." Only the union of the believer with Christ makes it possible to live in accord with the truth of the moral law. To be sure, the difficulties of disordered passion, especially in the case of the virtues of personal discipline, will still be felt. But the infused virtues insure that emotional tugs and pulls will not frustrate the dynamic of virtue's goal. Actually, Aquinas himself held the opinion that God permits these remnants of disorder to remain in us for a purpose. In fact, they serve as reminders about the relationship which exists between union with Christ and the strength to accomplish the good. Actually, the unity that is Christ is capable of integrating everything.

Thus, since the infused virtues remain totally supernatural in form, they constitute a thoroughly new ordering and shaping of human activity, even if seated within the natural powers of mind and will. This new informing of human activity derives from the conscious consent of the believer to God's revealed mysteries. We might say that the virtues prepare us for heaven, since they direct our lives towards implementing the New Testament Beatitudes now. The Christian character, caught between this world and the next, remains at once incarnational and eschatological. So we expect that the Beatitudes give a degree of specificity to the moral virtues. In this way, one understands better how the mysteries of salvation remain part of moral theology in the same way that moral truths constitute an essential part of the *sacra doctrina.* The moral virtues infused by God lead the powers of the soul from their pursuits within the earthly city to a fellow-citizenship with the saints in heaven.

Virtue, then, provides a constant disposition or *habitus* for living the life of Christian faith. As a result, all the powers of the soul acting through the body become stabilized in morally good objectives. They prevent us from acquiescing to any isolationism or negative attitude. This shaping pertains principally to the psychological powers of the soul such that right reason operates effectively in the accomplishment of a good life. Virtue also produces promptness and facility in action. When our capacities conform to good moral objectives, a second nature develops. This means that the virtuous man or woman accomplishes the good in a way that may appear effortless, but actually results from a disciplined life suffused with the grace of the Holy Spirit. In this Trinitarian embrace, the Christian faithful realize their wholeness and as a result experience the joy of virtue. The saints, in fact, witness to the same.[36]

As you know, *Donum vitae* does not make direct reference to the role virtue plays in the Christian life. It seems to me, however, that issues in bioethics usually require the exercise of all the cardinal virtues in order to conform to the good objectives set forth in the Instruction. Of course, it would require a separate paper to explain the way in which prudence directs the other moral virtues. But, suffice it to say that once prudence accepts moral truth as a concrete manifestation of the Eternal law, the very wisdom of God himself, the other virtues take their cue, as it were, from this principal virtue of the moral life. So particular moral truths, such as those given in the *Instruction*, reflect how God knows the world and the order of human life to be. In turn, the virtues of personal discipline conform the appetites to embrace this truth. In particular, temperance restrains those desires which make the truth difficult to accomplish while fortitude strengthens those emotions required to support what ever suffering doing the good entails. Thus as the Church contemplates the mystery of the Incarnate Word, she also comes to understand what it means to be human. *Donum vitae* continues, "by proclaiming the Gospel of salvation, she reveals to man his dignity and invites him to discover fully the truth of his own being."[37]

Finally, the Christian gospel refrains from disclosing the full dimension of human fulfillment. Rather it affirms that what we shall be has not yet appeared. Still, our faith confirms that we shall be like God because we shall see him as he is. The dangers of reductionism lead to the narrowing of consciousness implicit in any ideology. A narrow view of human fulfillment, such as technology promotes, can only result in an eventual compromise between the authentic freedom of God's children and the illusion of liberty represented by choices made available through ever-developing *techne*. On the other hand, the ability to perceive the relation between end and appropriate means constitutes a function of holy wisdom grounded in the vision of faith. It remains a Gift of the Holy Spirit given to all those ready to receive God's word.

ENDNOTES

[1]This article is reprinted with permission of The Thomist.

[2]Paul VI, Humanae Vitae, n. 20.

[3] For a representative sample of his work, see Josef Fuchs, S.J., <u>Personal Responsibility and Christian Morality</u>, trans. William Cleves et al., (Washington, D.C.: Georgetown University Press, 1983) and a second collection of essays, <u>Christian Morality: The Word Becomes Flesh</u>, trans. Brian McNeil, (Washington, D.C.: Georgetown University Press, 1987).

[4] His three-volume <u>Free & Faithful in Christ</u> (New York: Crossroad, 1982) presents the most comprehensive and latest statement of Haring's outlook.

[5] See <u>Directions in Fundamental Moral Theology</u> (Notre Dame, University of Notre Dame Press, 1985) for a general overview of Curran's positions.

[6] Servais Pinckaers provides the best theological analysis of the casuist model in <u>Les sources de la morale chrétienne. Sa méthode, son contenu, son histoire</u> (Paris: Editions du Cerf, 1985), esp. cc. 10, 11.

[7] Curran actually argues that the presence of sin in the world requires such a "theological reality." Thus he writes that the "presence of sin may force a person to do something one would not do if there were no sin present . . . A theory of compromise does not give us a blank check to shirk our Christian responsibilities. However, there are situations in which the value sacrificed (read: "original truth of human life") is not proportionate to the demand asked of the Christian." See his essay on natural law in <u>Directions</u>, p. 124. In a later essay, "Utilitarianism, Consequentialism, and Moral Theology," Curran acknowledges that "it was a mistake to use the term the 'theory' of compromise..." ibid., p. 193. Rather, he changes the proposal to a theological reality.

[8] Commenting on the last request of the Our Father, St. Augustine wrote: "We pray to be delivered from evil, for this liberation makes of us free beings, that is, sons of God, in such a way that, thanks to the spirit of adoption, we cry out to God: Father, Father!" <u>De Sermone in monte</u>, II, 11, 38 (PL vol. 34, col 1285). Ceslaus Spicq, O.P. explicates this point in <u>Charity and Liberty in the New Testament</u> (New York: Alba House, 1965).

[9] Cf. <u>Gaudium et spes</u>, c. 2, no. 24 *in fine* makes this remark with reference to the <u>imago Dei</u> and Trinitarian indwelling. "This likeness reveals that man, who is the only creature on earth which God willed for itself, cannot fully find himself except through a sincere gift of himself."

[10] For example, John Mahoney, S.J. argues that since couples remain free to express married love in ways other than intercourse, conception need not occur only as a result of the marital act. See "Test-tube Babies," <u>Tablet</u> 232 (1978), p. 734.

[11] <u>Donum vitae</u>, Introduction, 3.

[12] See Louis Janssens, "Ontic Evil and Moral Evil," in <u>Reading in Moral Theology. No. 1. Moral Norms and Catholic Tradition</u>, edited by Charles E. Curran and Richard A. McCormick, S.J. (New York: Paulist Press, 1979), p. 67.

[13] Thomas Gilby, O.P., <u>Principles of Morality</u>. (Summa theologia Ia2ae. 18-21), Vol. 18, (New York: McGraw-Hill Book Company, 1965) provides a succinct explanation of this concept in Appendix 11, "Moral Objectives" as a commentary on Aquinas's q. 18 of the *prima-secundae*.

[14]Thus, André E. Hellegers and Richard A. McCormick, S.J., in "Unanswered Questions on Test Tube Life," America 139 (1978), pp. 74-78 argue that artificial insemination (AIH), and to that extent in vitro fertilization with embryo transfer, "cannot be analyzed in a morally decisive way by exclusive appeal to the design of the conjugal act."

[15]For example, Rabbi Seymour Siegel in the Washington Post, July 28, 1978: noted that "if nature played a trick, as it has in this case, if we can outsmart nature, that is theologically permissible."

[16]See for example, Charles E. Curran, "Sexual Ethics: Reaction and Critique," Linacre Quarterly 43 (1976), pp. 147-64.

[17]See T.C. O'Brien, Effects of Sin, Stain and Guilt. (Summa theologiae 1a2ae. 86-89), Vol. 27, (New York: McGraw-Hill Book Company, 1974), pp. 99-109.

[18]Donum vitae, II, 8.

[19]Pascal. The Provincial Letters, trans. A.J. Krailsheimer, (Baltimore: Penguin Books, 1967), pp. 64,65.

[20]Even the Dominican author, Dominic Prümmer, felt obliged to include reference to the liberty of indifference. He concludes a brief discussion of the difference between the free and the necessary: "Ex quibus declarationibus datis sequitur, ut omne liberum sit voluntarium, sed non vice versa omne voluntarium sit liberum. Ad hoc etiam, ut voluntarium sit liberum, omnino requiritur, ut accedat libertas indifferentiae." Manuale Theologiae Moralis secundum principia S. Thomae Aquinatis. Tomus I. (Fribourg, 1923), p. 39.

[21]Cf. Brian Johnstone, C.Ss.R., "The Meaning of Proportionate Reason in Contemporary Moral Theology," The Thomist 49 (1985), pp. 223-247 for a survey of the various models employed by revisionist moral theologians. For a good example of how one might employ a revisionist model to interpret Donum vitae see Thomas A. Shannon and Lisa Sowle Cahill, Religion and Artificial Reproduction (New York: Crossroads, 1988).

[22]The American Fertility Society, Fertility and Sterility, Supplement 1, 49 (1988), p. 2S.

[23]See Albert R. Di Ianni, S.M., "The Direct/Indirect Distinction in Morals," The Thomist 41 (1977), pp. 350-380.

[24]Fertility and Sterility, loc. cit.

[25]For example, see the excellent study of William E. May, "Aquinas and Janssens on the Moral Meaning of Human Acts," The Thomist 48 (1984), pp. 566-606.

[26]William F. Sullivan's address, "Religious Communities of Memory and Hope," to the 1988 assembly of the Conference of Major Superiors of Men, Origins, September 22, 1988 (Vol. 18, no. 15).

[27]Gaudium et spes c. 1, no. 14 as quoted in Donum vitae, Introduction, 3.

[28]See his introduction in <u>Summa theologiae</u> IIIa q. 27 where he enunciates the principle that all the mysteries of Christ's life compose the one act of divine salvation.

[29]See Cajetan's commentary on <u>Summa theologiae</u> Ia q. 1 printed in the Leonine edition. Special attention to <u>Summa theologiae</u> Ia q. 1, a. 5, ad 2um provides a clear statement concerning how *sacra docrina* relates to the other sciences.

[30]<u>Donum vitae</u> Introduction, 3.

[31]The celebrated conflict between Abelard and St. Bernard on this point underlines the importance of setting forth moral teaching within the context of the Mystical Body. At least in his <u>Expositio in Epistolam ad Romanos</u>, Abelard seems to intimate that Christ provides only example and encouragement for the moral life. Cf. Richard E. Weingart, <u>The Logic of Divine Love: A Critical Analysis of the Soteriology of Peter Abailard</u> (New York: Oxford University Press, 1970), esp. pp. 139-44.

[32]<u>Donum vitae</u> Introduction, 3.

[33]W. Dilthey, <u>Selected Writings</u>, trans. and ed. H.P. Rickman (London, 1976), p. 162.

[34]The definition actually represents a collation of texts from the writings of St. Augustine, probably first formulated by Peter of Poitiers in his <u>Sentences</u> II, 1 (PL 211, 1041). See Aquinas's use of this definition in <u>Summa theologiae</u> Ia-Iae q. 55, a. 4.

[35]<u>De virtutibus in commune</u> q. 1, a. 10.

[36]See <u>Summa theologiae</u> I, q. 1, a. 6, ad 3um. There Aquinas explains the wisdom given to the saints on the basis of a comparison with the way the virtuous person acts.

[37]<u>Donum vitae</u> Introduction, 1.

12

Christian Anthropology as it Applies to Reproductive and Sexual Morality

Rev. John Sheets, S.J.

INTRODUCTION: MEANING OF CHRISTIAN ANTHROPOLOGY

The purpose of this paper is to attempt to formulate answers to specific questions about human sexuality within the larger context of what is called a Christian anthropology.[1] In the context of our discussion here, there are two main questions concerning a sexual morality. One concerns the transmission of life, in particular the inseparability of the unitive and the procreative aspects of the conjugal act. This question is addressed in the Encyclical, *Humanae Vitae*.

The second has to do with the continuum of the transmission of life. Life is initiated in the conjugal act, takes place in conception, comes to term in the birth of the child, and is continued in the nurturing of the child. The "two-in-one-flesh" nature of the conjugal union describes the whole process as a unified continuum from beginning to its term and its continuation in the nurturing of the child. Questions that touch the disruption of the "two-in-one flesh" continuum of the process are addressed in the *Instruction on Respect for Human Life in its Origin and the Dignity of Procreation.*

First it is necessary to describe what is meant by the term "Christian Anthropology." It means the study of the various aspects of the human person within the context of the meaning of the whole person. According to our Christian faith, the complete meaning of the human person is found only through revelation.

In Christian Anthropology, then, the partial perspectives find their meaning in the light of the whole. Through revelation we know there is more at work in the heart of man, in the world of things, in the events of history than can be discovered by reason. Revelation is precisely that light, picked up by faith, which illumines the whole meaning of man, both his mystery as a graced person as well as his enigmatic character as carrying with him the effects of both personal as well as original sin.

At the basis of the method of approaching the answers to particular questions from the wider context of Christian anthropology are two principles. The first is: the higher cannot stand without the lower; the second, the lower, in turn, takes on new meaning as it is subsumed in the higher. Our intellectual life, for example, the higher, cannot of course stand without biological life the lower. Further the lower is enhanced when it is taken up into the higher.

Both *Humanae Vitae* and the *Instruction on Respect for Human Life* point out that the moral evaluation of these questions has to be sought within the context of a total view of human existence. In *Humanae Vitae*, for example, we read: "The problem of birth, like every other problem regarding human life, is to be considered, beyond partial perspectives--whether of the biological or psychological, demographic or sociological orders--in the light of an integral vision of man and of his vocation, not his natural and earthly, but also his supernatural and eternal vocation".[2] In a subsequent paragraph, the document uses the words of Pope Pius XII, referring to the "principle of totality" to emphasize again the need to find answers for specific questions within the context of a Christian anthropology.

In a similar way, the *Instruction on Respect for Human Life*, calls attention to the necessity of keeping in view the total view of the human person in questions that have to do with moral questions in the biomedical field. "For it is only in keeping with his true nature that the human person can achieve self-realization as a 'unified totality': and this nature is at the same time corporal and spiritual. By virtue of its substantial union with a spiritual soul, the human body cannot be considered as a mere complex of tissues, organs and functions, nor can it be evaluated in the same way as the body of animals; rather it is a constitutive part of the person who manifests himself through it".[3]

This method of argumentation might be called the argument of "intrinsic coherence." The whole network of relations that constitute the identity of the human person has its own intrinsic laws. The violation of one of these laws leads to a disequilibrium that weakens and distorts the coherence of the whole.

The next question is: "Is there an adequate Christian anthropology that can serve as the matrix of meaning in which one can contextualize the answers to the specific problems and answers presented in *Humanae Vitae* and in the *Instruction on Respect for Human Life?*'

I think the most adequate is that which is presented in the writings of Pope John Paul II. His main thoughts on these subjects are found in a series of talks given at various general audiences over the course of five years from September, 1979 to November, 1984.

They have been collected in four volumes under the titles: *Original Unity of Man and Woman: Cathechesis on the Book of Genesis; Blessed are the Pure of Heart; The Theology of Marriage and Celibacy; Reflections on Humanae Vitae.* Even though the talks were extended over such a long period, there is a remarkable continuity and steady progression in development of the theme.

However, the Holy Father's theology of the body is still waiting for some one to put it into systematic form so that it is possible to see how it all fits together.[4] He brings a freshness to these "old" questions. This comes from his own insightfulness. At the same time the doctoral work that he did on the thought of the German phenomenologist, Max Scheler, has reinforced the personalist approach that belongs to the inner spirit of the Pope.

His methodology is unique. He works out of a central insight that moves in a kind of shuttle fashion in both a horizontal and vertical direction. Along the horizontal level he pulls together various truths, where each illumines the other. At the same time on the vertical level he moves back and forth from the depths to the heights of the mystery of God and man. Thematic to all his writings is the mystery of the redemption. But it has to be admitted that, while a rich reward awaits the person who can accompany him in this shuttle movement, it is a laborious process.

It is not possible to comment on the series of talks in detail. However, before I attempt a brief summary, I would like to describe five terms which can help us organize the thoughts of the Holy Father on the meaning of the body.

SOME GUIDELINES TOWARD A CHRISTIAN ANTHROPOLOGY

First of all, I shall make use of a term used by C.S. Lewis. It is called *transposition*. By this Lewis wants to describe how there are descents of the greater into the less. It is not a difficult concept to grasp. We are constantly putting the more into the less. When we put the more of our thoughts into words on a sheet of paper, or when an artist puts his inspiration into paint or words or sound, he is putting the more into the less.

Theologically the term is useful to describe the "descents" of God into his creation: in creation, when he breathes his own image and likeness into clay, and, as Scripture says, "man becomes a human soul (or person);" in the incarnation, when the more of the Word is put into the less of our human flesh; at Pentecost, when the depths of God, the Holy Spirit, is poured into the less of our human spirit.

The tremendous mystery of the Church as making present the paschal mystery of Christ, through the apostles, and their successors, is a mystery of transposition. "'As the Father has sent me, so I send you.' He breathed on them saying, 'Receive the Holy Spirit. Whose sins you shall forgive, they stand forgiven. Whose sins you shall retain, they are retained'" (Jn. 20.21).

Here I use it to help understand the meaning of Christian anthropology. Through the gift of the Father, in the power of the Spirit, the whole network of relationships that belong to Jesus Christ is transposed into us, affecting the orientation of the whole of our lives, including the orientation of one aspect of our lives, our sexuality, which is the subject of our discussions over these days.

It is probably safe to say that the momentous meaning of this truth does not affect our Christian consciousness as it should, nor does it affect our thinking or moral judgments. An illustration might help us appreciate the significance of this transposition. In a planetarium, one sees something like a facsimile of the sky on the ceiling. If one could imagine, on the other hand, the whole of space being poured into that tiny planetarium, we might get some remote realization of the mystery of the human person as graced. The infinite God has poured himself into the limitedness of our humanity.

Secondly, it is important to recall the theological notion of *relationship*. In his book, *Introduction to Christianity,* a series of lectures given to the faculty and students of the University of Tuebingen by Professor Ratzinger about twenty years ago, he described how the modern notion of person dawned upon the world. This took place largely in the context of the theological debates concerning the Trinity and Christology. "With the perception that, seen as substance, God is one, but that there exists in him the phenomenon of dialogue, of differentiation and of relationship through speech, the category *relation* gained a completely new significance for Christian thought. To Aristotle it was among the 'accidents,' the chance circumstances of being, which are separate from substance, the sole sustaining form of the real ... It now became clear that the dialogue, the *relation,* stands beside the substance as an equally primordial form of being."[5]

The notion of relationship is key to understanding the meaning of a Christian anthropology. It means that our mode of being is a mode-of-being-related. Further, that this mode-of-being-related is Christ's own mode-of-being-related, which is his being-related to the Father. The Holy Spirit who is poured into our hearts has created within us the very same mode-of-being-related that belongs to the inner life of the Trinity.

This mode-of-being is the transposition of Christ's own mode of being into us, the more into the less. Our sexual orientation, as well as every aspect of the "lower," takes on, then, through the transposition of Christ's relationships into us, a special mode-of-being-related. The higher processes of Trinitarian life are transposed into the lower processes of life.

They form an organic whole, a genuine hierarchy. The word "hierarchy," it should be remembered in its original meaning, means a "holy order." The very holy-order that belongs to the Trinity, then, is poured into us. In theological terms, this is called the sacramental character which comes through the reshaping of all our relationships through baptism.

Thirdly, the Scriptural meaning of *fruitfulness* is important in the questions we are discussing. There is a basic law at work in the whole of reality. Life exists, grows, becomes fruitful only in relationship. All life is bonded dynamically in a mysterious kind of circulation of life: reception of life, transforming of that which is received, and the transmission of that which has been transformed. All life then leads to fruitfulness, which in turn is put back into the process to lead to greater fruitfulness.

Fruitfulness is the word used in Scripture to describe linked levels of inter-relatedness: the fruitfulness of deeper interrelatedness of husband and wife ("unitive"), the openness to the possibility of originating a new relationship in a conception of a child ("procreative"), which draws husband and wife into deeper relationship with God ("holiness"), the fruitfulness of the Holy Spirit.

This network of dynamic relationships forms an organic whole. The higher (holiness) cannot stand without the lower (unitive and procreative). And the lower is enhanced by being taken up into the higher.

In Genesis fruitfulness is described in terms of a series of transpositions in the way that God's own creativity is transposed into creatures. First of all he puts seeds into the plants, so that they cooperate with God in bringing forth fruit. Then he blesses fish, animals, and birds, with the power to be fruitful, sharing his own power to bring forth life. "Be fruitful and increase, fill the waters of the seas; and let the birds increase on land" (Gen. 1.10).

Then the climax of the shared creativity comes in the creation of man, male and female. The mystery of the creativity of God when it is transposed into man, male and female, takes the form of human sexuality. It is described as a blessing. "God blessed them and said to them, 'Be fruitful and increase...'" (Gen. 1.28).

Genesis, then, describes in a simple way the most profound truth, the multi-leveled ways in which the life of the Holy Spirit is layered within the created world: the fruitfulness of nature, the fruitfulness of the womb of a mother, the fruitfulness of love.

The words "fruit," "fruitfulness" appear so often in Scripture that their inner meaning, one might say their metaphysical meaning, is overlooked. They form as it were a "spiritual physiology" where we can see the mystery of a co-creativity that brings into the world a completely new reality. The newness of the reality comes out of a relationship and brings about a new level of relationship.

To take a few examples, Christ is called the "firstfruits" of the resurrection (1 Cor. 15.23). The Holy Spirit is given to us as the "firstfruits of the harvest to come" (Rom. 8.23). Paul speaks of the fruits of the Spirit, "love, joy, peace, patience, kindness, goodness, fidelity, gentleness, self-control" (Gal. 5.22).

The words, then, that have to do with fruitfulness bring out the intrinsic vitality of the relationships that are transposed into us, on the levels of nature and grace. Newness comes about as the fruit of a mutual gift of one to another.

Fourthly, there is the Scriptural meaning of the word *presence of God*. The word is not used simply to describe a fact. It is a way of describing a way of being present that creates communion. When Scripture speaks of man being created to the image and likeness of God, male and female, God's presence envelopes both male and female. First of all he creates a twoness, male and female, but it is a twoness that is a oneness. This mystery is a mystery of God's presence as the originating mystery of a oneness that is shared in the Trinity of persons.

In the Old Testament, God's presence is always an enveloping presence. The covenant relationship is the way he envelopes each by enveloping the whole. This symbol of this enveloping presence is the Tent of Meeting, or the Temple. In the New Testament, it will describe the enveloping presence of the Spirit who brings out new modes of fruitfulness, through new modes of relationships.

In the fifth place, there is the word *vocation*. In Scripture this word is used to describe the various levels of the processes at work that have the same source, God, the same orientation, the same ultimate fruition of God, eternal life. The word means to call. It emphasizes God's initiative in the whole process, both of creation, and salvation. He calls the world of nature into being as a pre-step in calling man, male, and female. He calls them into being as a pre-step to eternal life.

After the fall, an anti-life process enters into time and history. It is the process of dissolution of relationships, a fragmentation of the wholeness into parts which are at odds with one another.

But at the same time another entirely new process enters into time and history. It is the mystery of the redemption, of re-calling. But the re-call, however, is the revelation of a new calling in Christ. Now fruition takes on a new aspect. It will always take on the nature of *a victory* over the forces of dissolution. The unity of the network of relationships binding man and woman, mankind with one another, and the world of nature carries within itself now a kind of death-wish. Such a unity will always be fragile, vulnerable. It will need the support of all that comes from the redemptive event of Christ. Fruition now is always not simply a way of becoming, but of *over-coming* the processes of anti-life.

History, then, becomes salvation history through call or vocation. The call of Abraham, of Moses, the prophets, Christ, the apostles, and each Christian.

All of God's plans, whether in nature or history are at the service of his calling. This means that the whole of created reality is held together from above, from in front, not from below. It is somewhat in the same way as a director of a symphony holds the whole together from above and from in front.

These ideas can help us organize the Holy Father's ideas into a more systematic form. Now I shall comment briefly on each of the books which contain Pope John Paul's theology of the body.

THE CHRISTIAN ANTHROPOLOGY OF POPE JOHN PAUL II

The first series of talks is published under the title, *Original Unity of Man and Woman: Cathehesis on the Book of Genesis*.[6] He takes as his text that forms the "composition" of his thought the passage from Mt. 19.3 ff. "And some Pharisees came up to him and tested him by asking, 'Is it lawful to divorce one's wife for any cause?' He answered, 'Have you not read that he who made them from the beginning made them male and female,' and said, 'For this reason a man shall leave his father and mother and be joined to his wife, and the two shall become one flesh? So they are no longer two but one flesh. What therefore God has joined together, let not man put asunder.' They said to him, 'Why then did Moses command one to give a certificate of divorce, and to put her away?' He said to them, 'For the hardness of your heart Moses allowed you to divorce your wives, but from the beginning it was not so.'"

The Holy Father calls attention to the fact that Jesus used the expression "from the beginning" twice. Jesus not only quotes from Genesis, but draws a conclusion to which he gives the same authority as the Scripture itself. "What God has joined together, let not man put asunder." He also teaches that Moses' teaching was an accommodation of the original meaning because man had lost the original innocence which was there in the beginning.

The word "beginning" does not refer only to chronological time. It refers to a mode of being which is a mode-of-being-related. This mode of being the Holy Father calls the "nuptial meaning of the body." Creation of man and woman in the image and likeness of God is the transposition of the mystery of God's own inner communion into a mode of being that by its very nature manifests the fruitful union of one for another. The body therefore manifests the interior orientation of the persons to one another with the orientation to a threefold interrelated fruitfulness, the fruitfulness of closer union with one another, fruitfulness which issues in the life of a new human being, fruitfulness of closer union with God, which is another name for holiness.

The orientation is not only a physical instinct. "In the beginning" it was the way of becoming oneself by making the gift of oneself to another. The nuptial meaning of the body comes from the inner presence of God which envelopes man and woman to live out as image and likeness the inner mystery of God himself. In Scriptural terms it is a *shekina*, a transposition of the presence of God, a tent of meeting of two persons whose whole meaning is to be found in their fruitful relatedness.

The sense of the "wholeness" that was there in the beginning is described when the sacred author adds, "Now, both of them were naked, the man and his wife, but they felt no shame." It is a term which the Holy Father uses to describe what he calls the "radiation of life" which belongs to the inbuilt nuptial character of the body. Nakedness, which is something physical, is a way of describing the absence of a mode of existence where the body says what the person is meant for, that is, to be a gift, and to make a gift of oneself. Woman discovers herself in relationship to man. And man discovers himself in relationship to woman.

"Thus, in this dimension, there is constituted a primordial sacrament, understood as a sign that transmits effectively in the visible world the invisible mystery hidden in God from time immemorial. And this is the mystery of truth and love, the mystery of divine life, in which man participates . . . The body, in fact, and it alone, is capable of making visible what is invisible: the spiritual and the divine. It was created to transfer into the visible reality of the world the mystery hidden since time immemorial in God, and thus be a sign of it".[7]

Another name for his mode of being which is a mode-of-being-related is holiness. It is not something added to the union "at the beginning." It is identified with their initial mode-of-being. "The sacrament of the world and the sacrament of man in the world, comes from the divine source of holiness, and at the same time is instituted for holiness. Original innocence, connected with the experience of the nuptial meaning of the body, is the same holiness that enables man to express himself deeply with his own body, and that, precisely, by means of the 'sincere gift' of himself. . . in his body as male or female, man feels he is a subject of holiness".[8]

He says that it should not be strange to speak of a "theology of the body". The Incarnation is at the center of our faith. All theology finds its base in the enfleshment of the Son of God.

In the second cycle of talks, collected under the title, *Blessed are the Pure of Heart*,[9] he takes a text from the Sermon on the Mount as his point of departure, "You have heard that it was said, you shall not commit adultery. But I say to you that everyone who looks at a woman lustfully has already committed adultery in his heart" (Mt. 5.27-8).

This takes him back to the texts in Genesis which he had commented on. Lust is one aspect of the distortion in the mystery of creative-communion which belonged to man and woman at the beginning. He recalls the text from the first letter of John which speaks of the three-fold concupiscence. "If anyone loves the world, the Father's love has not place in him, for nothing that the world affords comes from the Father. Carnal allurements, enticements for the eye, the life of empty show - all these are from the world" (Jn. 2.15-6).

The fall from the graced mode-of-being-related brought about a distortion in the whole network of relationships. The higher cannot stand without the lower. And the lower loses its equilibrium if it is taken out of the higher. It brought about a rupture in man between body and spirit. "Concupiscence of the body limits and distorts the body's objective way of existing."[10] The heart becomes a battlefield of contending forces, of love and lust.

The nature of man and woman "in the beginning" as co-signs of created and creative communion became a broken and often antagonistic symbol after the fall. "On the one hand the eternal attraction of man towards femininity frees in him-- or perhaps should free--a gamut of spiritual-corporal desires of an especially personal and 'sharing' nature . . . to which a proportionate pyramid of values corresponds. On the other hand, 'lust' limits this gamut, obscuring the pyramid of values that marks the perennial attraction of male and female.[11]

Christ's words, then, call attention to the heart, the center of the person, the ethos of the interior self. "Interior man is the specific subject of the ethos of the body, with which Christ wishes to imbue the conscience and will of his listeners and disciples".[12] It is a completely new ethos compared to the Old Testament and to the moral teaching of the whole of mankind. It is already an appeal to the sensitivity that will come from the gift of the Spirit through the redemption.

The third cycle has the title, *The Theology of Marriage and Celibacy*.[13] There are two texts the Holy Father uses to develop further his ideas on the theology of the body. The first is taken from the discussion with the Sadducees. This was the group among the Jews who rejected the notion of the resurrection. Hoping to make the idea of the resurrection appear ridiculous, they presented Jesus with a hypothetical case. In keeping with the law of Levirate marriage, seven brothers married the same wife as one brother after the other died. They then asked, "Now at the resurrection to which of these will she be wife?"

Jesus said, "You are wrong, because you understand neither the scriptures nor the power of God. For at the resurrection men and women do not marry; no, they are like the angels in heaven. And as for the resurrection of the dead, have you never read what God himself said to you: 'I am the God of Abraham, the God of Isaac and the God of Jacob?' God is not the God of the dead but of the living" (Mt. 22.29-33).

The Holy Father uses this passage to show the ultimate fruitfulness that belongs to the spirituality of the body. Man keeps his psychosomatic nature. But it undergoes a spiritualization. He says that the whole of theological anthropology can be considered an anthropology of the resurrection.[14] It is a spiritualization through divinization. They will become not only like the angels but "sons of God." It is the fullness of the transposition. The human person, body and soul, takes on the very subjectivity of God himself which is to take on the fullness of communion. It is the fullness of the nuptial meaning of the body. It is the deepest revelation of the extent of God's self-communication to the world, in particular to mankind.[15] The spiritual body means the perfect sensitivity of the senses, their perfect harmonization with the activity of the human spirit in truth and in liberty.[16]

Then he returns to the text from Matthew where Jesus spoke about marriage as it was "in the beginning." Jesus' words about the indissolubility of marriage struck the disciples as a hard saying. "If that is how things are between husband and wife, it is not advisable to marry." This leads Jesus to speak about an option that is open to those who are offered a special grace: celibacy for the Kingdom of God.

It is an entirely new aspect of the nuptial meaning of the body. Celibacy for the Kingdom of God is not something negative, the putting aside of a normal relationship. It is a new way of being related to Christ. It is a mode of communion with Christ which anticipates in time the nuptial union with God described in the passage about the resurrection. It is itself a mode-of-being-in-communion, for the Kingdom of God. The fruitfulness of celibacy for the Kingdom of God was already a manifest reality in the choice of Mary and of Jesus of celibacy for the Kingdom of God in their own lives. This leads the Holy Father to speak at length about the meaning of celibacy and of continence.

Finally, he turns to the text which he sees as the perfect expression of all that has been said in the previous passages. He refers to Ephesians 5 where Jesus draws an analogy between the sacramental union of husband and wife and the union of Christ and the Church. St. Paul calls this "a great mystery."

The analogy of the nuptial union of husband and wife with the nuptial union of Christ and the Church leads the Holy Father to coin the word "bi-subjectivity." By this word he wants to describe the inwardness of presence of each of the spouses in the subjectivity of the other. He uses the word "subjectivity" to describe what is most personal in an individual.

There is then a parallel in the bi-subjectivity of Christ and the Church, and the bi-subjectivity of husband and wife. But there is more than a parallel. The more of the bi-subjectivity of the interrelationship of Christ and the Church is transposed into the bi-subjectivity of husband and wife, the more into the less. Now the bi-subjectivity of the spouses is animated by the bi-subjectivity existing between Christ and his spouse, the Church.

In the sacrament of marriage, there is found a new mystery of communion, a new dimension of the nuptial meaning of the body that goes beyond what was there "in the beginning." "This seems to be the integral significance of the sacramental sign of marriage. In that sign - through the 'language of the body' - man and woman encounter the great 'mystery' in order to transfer the light of that mystery--the light of truth and beauty, expressed in liturgical language--to the 'language of the body,' that is, the ethos rooted in the 'redemption of the body' (cf. Rm. 8.23). In this way conjugal life becomes in a certain sense liturgical".[17]

The final collection of talks, *Reflections on Humanae Vitae: Conjugal Morality and Spirituality*,[18] presuppose the "theology of the body" which the Holy Father developed in the previous talks. He applies the theological anthropology developed in those talks to support the doctrine taught in *Humanae Vitae*. Although the *Instruction on Respect for Human Life* came out three years later, the same principles developed in his talks on the theology of the body supply a foundation for the positions set forth in that document.

At this point I would like to recall the two principles I mentioned earlier: (1) the higher cannot stand without the lower, and (2) the lower finds its meaning only in what is higher. Also, the terms which I felt could be used as points around which to organize Pope John Paul's thought: (1) the notion of transposition, (2) or relationship, (3) fruitfulness, (4) presence, (5) vocation.

The book, *Reflections on Humanae Vitae: Conjugal Morality and Spirituality*, contains fifteen talks that touch on various aspects of conjugal morality and spirituality. The topics range from questions that could be called strictly moral to those which describe the highest ranges of the spirituality of married life.

The theme that runs throughout is what he calls the "language of the body." "Here we are dealing with nothing other than reading the 'language of the body.'"[19]

The expression, "language of the body," is a short-hand way which the Holy Father uses to sum up the meaning of his Christian anthropology. He says: "The human body is not merely an organism of sexual reactions, but it is, at the same time, the means of expressing the entire man, the person, which reveals itself by means of the 'language of the body'".[20] "It is necessary to bear in mind that the 'body speaks' not merely with the whole external expression of masculinity and femininity, but also with the internal structures of the organism, of the somatic and psychosomatic reaction. All this should find its appropriate place in that language in which husband and wife dialogue with each other, as persons called to the communion of the 'union of the body'".[21]

Like all language, the language of the body can take on many forms. It can be clear, meaningful, and true; or it can be obscure, garbled, and false. In other words the relationships that were there "in the beginning" are no longer there. "In the beginning" the body "spoke" spontaneously the language of what it meant to be a person whose mode-of-being was to-be-related. This is what the Holy Father means by the "nuptial" meaning of the body. The body spoke the total relatedness, of man to woman, and of man and woman to God.

But the language of the body took another form when this relationship to God was broken. The twisted desires of the heart affected the total language-system of the body. What before was the language that came from union and led to deeper union has become an ambiguous sign. The external sign which signified love can now be a sign of lust. The language of the body that spoke of the inner gift of oneself to another can become a sign of manipulation and domination of the other. As was said above, the higher cannot stand without the lower; and the lower, when taken out of what is higher, becomes distorted.

The very nature of evil, then, is to destroy life which exists only in relationship by breaking the relationship into separate parts. This is evident in many contemporary approaches to sexuality. In the first place, there is the attempt to separate in our ordinary language truth from meaning. Language has two inseparable aspects: the communication of meaning, but at the same time the communication of truthful meaning. For example, the words, "I love you," have meaning. But unfortunately they can also be a lie. To be a genuine communication, meaning and truth cannot be separated. As the Holy Father says, "The moral norm . . . arises from reading the 'language of the body' *in truth*".[22]

The nature of evil, as we have stressed, is to take the lower out of the context of the higher. It is a process of breaking a relationship by breaking the continuum that gives coherence to the whole process from beginning to end.

Up to recent times this separation has only been possible in the separation of the unitive from the procreative orientation of the conjugal act through contraception. But technology has made is possible to break down the components of the act even further. The continuum of the act which by its nature is directed to inseparable stages of fruitfulness, the fruitfulness of closer union of the spouses, the fruitfulness of the conception of a child, and the fruitfulness of growth in union with God, can be broken in ways never before anticipated. This takes place, for example, in surrogate motherhood or *in vitro* fertilization.

AN APPROACH TO UNDERSTANDING
THE THEOLOGICAL ANTHROPOLOGY
OF POPE JOHN PAUL II

I spoke above of the principles at work in a Christian anthropology: that the higher cannot exist without the lower, and that the lower finds its meaning in the higher. Also, that Christian anthropology means a new mode of being that comes from being related. The relationships that belong to Christ are transposed into us. We also spoke of the mystery of fruitfulness. The source of fruitfulness is what Pope John Paul speaks of as bi-subjectivity. A new mode of life comes into being as the fruit of the same bi-subjectivity that brought into being the fruit of a deeper union with each other through love.

Throughout all these subtle distinctions, there is the mystery of presence. The Father's presence in Christ, Christ's presence in us, and the presence of husband and wife to one another in what is called their bi-subjectivity.

But all of the interrelated aspects of these mysterious networks of relationships are held together from above. This is the meaning of vocation. It is not morally licit to thus fragment and isolate the parts of the interlocking continuum of the stages which God's vocation shows, a point I have stressed in so many different ways. Activities which disrupt the intrinsic process that have to do with the circulation of life, reception, transformation, fruitfulness are disruptive not only of an aspect of our lives but have a domino effect on the whole network of relationships that constitute our human existence. Each moment and each step of our lives are a response to the dialogue with God to be faithful to the circulation of life and love which issues in fruitfulness on so many different but related levels.

All of this is the work of the Spirit. We find that the lowest element in creation as well as the highest are united through the coordinating activity of the Holy Spirit. We find ourselves, then, at the ultimate answer, which is also the ultimate mystery. It is the mystery of the Holy Spirit. The Holy Spirit is the mystery of the bi-subjectivity of the Father and the Son. He is the mystery of the fruitfulness of the gift of Father to God, and of Son to Father. For this reason we say he "proceeds" from the Father and the Son. The Holy Spirit then is the energizing process between all levels of life. All levels of life are called to issue in the fruitfulness that belongs to their particular level. But all lower levels are called to take part in that fruitfulness which belongs to the Trinitarian love, who is a Person, the Holy Spirit.

The violation of the laws that are inbuilt in this circulation of life and love are not only morally wrong. It is also what St. Paul calls "saddening the Spirit" (Eph. 4.30), or "stifling the Spirit" (1 Th. 5.19). They block the fruitfulness of the Holy Spirit along the whole continuum of his gifts.

Ultimately, then, morality finds its norm in pneumatology. St. Paul says "The love of God has been poured into our hearts through the Holy Spirit who has been given to us" (Rom. 5.5). There is a level then where morality and spirituality meet in the mysterious bi-subjectivity of the Spirit. The Spirit who is the source of the mystery is also the only one who can give us an appreciation of the mystery. To quote St. Paul again, "A man who is unspiritual refuses what belongs to the Spirit. It is folly to him. He cannot grasp it, because it needs to be judged in the light of the Spirit" (1 Cor. 2.14).

The Holy Father uses this term "Spiritual appreciation" to describe how husband and wife have the secret and sacred power of being attuned to all of the signs that make up the mutuality of the language of the body. "This can happen only through a profound appreciation of the personal dignity of both the feminine 'I and the masculine I' in their shared life. This spiritual appreciation is the fundamental fruit of the gift of the Spirit which urges the person to respect the work of God. From this appreciation, and therefore indirectly from that gift, all the 'affectionate manifestations' which make up the fabric of remaining faithful to the union of marriage derive their true spousal meaning".[23]

CONCLUSION

Have we provided answers then to the questions about contraception and the various ways of mechanizing the process of bringing a child into the world? Yes, and no. There are some questions that are answered by explanation, e.g. scientific questions. Other questions cannot be answered by explanation. Questions like: "Why be grateful? Why be humble? What is faith, love," etc. They can be answered only within a heightened awareness of the coherence of the interrelatedness and interdependence of all the relationships.

On the other hand, one should not underestimate the need, validity, importance of arguments based on reasons coming from ethics, psychology, physiology, or any other science, which gives strong evidence against contraception, abortion, and the mechanization of the process of conception. Again, to be realistic, not everyone has the ability or the opportunity to grasp the "architectonic" picture we have described. But this "architectonic" picture, a theological anthropology, reinforces these other arguments by situating them within a morality of "intrinsic coherence" with the whole network of relationships (natural and supernatural) that constitute human existence.

If a person does not have a sense of the whole, explanations might be a contribution to understanding. Ultimately, however, answers coming out of particular perspectives are satisfactory only to the extent that a person can see how they are "demanded" by the coherence of the parts with the whole.

This kind of refinement of the sense of the "harmonics" of the network of relationships created by the spirit can come only from the refinement of a pure heart. "Blessed are the pure of heart, for they shall see God." This provides an instinctive sense of the "ought," that is, that immorality is not simply a violation of this law or that, but, a disruption of the whole network of the relationships.

In his book, *The Joy of Music,* Leonard Bernstein, in commenting on a series of notes in one of Mozart's symphonies, says, "This note, no other, simply has to be there. No other note would fit." By way of analogy the same is true in the notes that make up the network of fruitful relationships which form our lives. What Bernstein is certain of through a refined aesthetic sense, the person of faith and love is certain of on the spiritual and moral level.

Another parallel from the life of Bernstein strikes me as applicable to what we are talking about. With the great sensitivity that comes with the refinement of the aesthetic sense, there is also the sense of outrage at what distorts that beauty.

On one occasion, when Bernstein was conducting Mozart's Fortieth Symphony at Harvard, the symphony was interrupted because of a bomb scare. Everyone had to leave the hall. The symphony was resumed after a couple of hours, but not before Bernstein expressed his horror and indignation at the fact that anyone could be so inhuman, crude, uncultured, insensitive, barbaric to interrupt something so beautiful as that symphony.

The application is clear. If our spiritual sensitivities were as refined as our aesthetic, we would not have to be seeking for rational proofs for the way that contraception, abortion, the mechanization of conception disrupts the whole harmonics of the relationships which belong to us as human beings.

Faith is another name for the special power of perceiving the network of these relationships. Teilhard de Chardin calls this network of relationships "The Divine Millieu." Love is the name that describes the spiritual attunement of the heart that provides the sensitivity to all that can contribute to the deepening of these relationships or which threaten them. This sensitivity to the "symphonic" nature of our relationships is a special gift of the Holy Spirit. We should pray for it as one of the greatest needs of our time.

Bernard Lonergan describes the results of this lack of sensitivity on the social level by the term, "group scotosis," group blindness. It is an apt expression to describe the phenomenon that has affected whole segments of society in the way they perceive (or fail to perceive) the answers the Church provides to these questions, answers which also find support in the intrinsic coherence of a Christian anthropology.

ENDNOTES

[1] This article will be reproduced in a forthcoming issue of the Linacre Quarterly.

[2] Pope Paul VI, Humanae Vitae, n. 7.

[3] Instruction on Respect for Human Life in Its Origin and the Dignity of Procreation, Introduction, n. 3.

[4]Only after finishing this paper did I discover the book of Mary G. Durkin, Feast of Love: Pope John Paul II on Human Intimacy (Loyola University Press, Chicago, 1983). This was the book I was looking for to provide a systematic presentation of the richness of Pope John Paul II's theology of the body.

[5]Joseph Cardinal Ratzinger, Introduction to Christianity. A series of lectures given to the faculty and students of the University of Tuebingen about twenty years ago, p. 131.

[6]Pope John Paul II, Original Unity of Man and Woman: Catechesis on the Book of Genesis (Boston: St. Paul Editions, 1981).

[7]Ibid., pp. 143-44.

[8]Ibid., p. 145.

[9]Pope John Paul II, Blessed Are the Pure of Heart (Boston: St. Paul Editions, 1983).

[10]Ibid., p. 73.

[11]Ibid., p. 126-27.

[12]Ibid., p. 190.

[13]Pope John Paul II, The Theology of Marriage and Celibacy (Boston: St. Paul Editions, 1986).

[14]Ibid., p. 21.

[15]Ibid., p. 29.

[16]Ibid., p. 62.

[17]Ibid., p. 366.

[18]Pope John Paul II, Reflections on Humanae Vitae: Conjugal Morality and Spirituality (Boston: St. Paul Editions, 1984).

[19]Ibid., p. 5.

[20]Ibid., pp. 30-31.

[21]Ibid., p. 42.

[22]Ibid., p. 6.

[23]Ibid., p. 85.

13

The Gift of Life:
An Inspiration for Our Time
Sr. Marilyn Wallace, R.S.M., Ph.D.

Dr. Hilgers has asked that I give a few closing remarks. This is not intended as a research paper, as were the other lectures of the conference. Instead it is offered as a meditative look in symbol form at what we have tried to do during this weekend. Yesterday our introduction recalled the words of our Holy Father, Pope John Paul II telling us that reproductive technology must not proceed separated from transcendental and spiritual values.[1] In addition current ethical and medical literature asks us to search for solutions to problems faced by medicine (and technology) by developing the intellectual tools of the humanities in order to focus on the person, rather than the problems to be solved.[2] At the leading edge of medical progress the humanities can speak once more about the transcendent meaning of this human person.[3]

Thus today I will use the tools of the humanities: art, literature, and architecture, in order to establish a symbolic medium of language in which to discuss what this conference has presented. By appealing to the period of the Middle Ages, I hope to discover not only a symbol for the fullness of the human person, but a symbol of marriage renewed in the light of faith, that will offer a radical challenge for today's omniverous scientific reproductive technology. Futhermore a third symbol will situate the scientific challenges of today within the light of faith; for the human person in his drive to succeed cannot forget either who he is, as a person, or what he is called by God to become.[4] The symbol reminds him of this truth. Borrowed from the medieval world view, three symbols: the cathedral, the flower, and the quest comprise the truth of *Donum vitae,* the message our conference wishes to express.

THE CATHEDRAL

The Cathedral of Notre Dame in Paris like many of the medieval cathedrals of its time is built upon an architectural plan that was deliberately left *incomplete*. Its graceful towers, unfinished, stand as a tribute to the unending fullness of the human spirit. *Donum vitae* proclaims the inherent dignity of the human person and his/her integral vocation.[5] As the Church contemplates Christ, the Instruction says, She discovers at the same time the mystery of Man:

The mystery of who She is.[6] I would like to compare this human person (addressed in the *Instruction* as: embryo, child, parent, scientist, doctor, teacher, lawyer)--as this unfinished masterpiece: the cathedral, for all time, in us all, the transcendent grandeur of the human spirit. It is within this perspective, a vision of faith,[7] that the human person is able to accept the teaching authority of the Church and move beyond the many critics who seek to destroy the very meaning of the Church's message on bioethical questions.

Today we heard presented the extreme vulnerability of the person in face of new reproductive technologies that combat infertility.[8] Not able to achieve a desired pregnancy, suffering the physical and emotional strain of handing over this most intimate part of one's sexual relationship to the scientific laboratory, only through the sufferings of Christ can this kind of personal tragedy ever hope to be understood.[9] In addition, the fractured structure of the person's origin within a broken family unit, no longer providing security from impending dangers as it had in prior civilizations, demonstrates that a revolution is truly needed today in the understanding of human sexuality: something like a cerebrocentric approach to the multidimensional architecture of the human person. Such an approach would be at one and the same time--spiritual, physical, intellectual, creative, communicative, emotional, and psychological.[10]

Because the human person stands within a vision of faith, represented by sacred scripture and tradition, this vision can be applied by the teaching Church to the bioethical technology of today.[11] Yet the human person is not without a philosophical grounding within that tradition to help him understand just how his moral decisions can be made.[12] But it is only the virtuous person, steeped in prayer, who will be able to go beyond the natural demands of morality. Such a person is able to accept the Church's teaching because he understands specific norms to be an incorporation into the mind of Christ Himself.[13]

Thus today the cathedral of the human person, open to unending fulfillment, and buttressed by certain major choices he has made, is situated overlooking specific reproductive questions. *Donum vitae* speaks of one such choice: marriage. Explained in terms of a commitment or basic good; marriage cannot be understood as an isolated action or goal, but a major choice which frames the person's life.[14] This type of choice makes the person who he is, and such a choice abides in him.[15] The human person can determine himself through this self-determining choice, a self-created choice which transcends the material world. Although particular acts come and go, a commitment once made, determines the self, unless or until one makes another incompatible choice. Commitments are those large choices which put the person in a position of having to carry out such commitments by many small choices throughout life. The marriage commitment is one type of such basic good, which are the REASONS *prior* to any specific goal or choice. The marriage commitment provides a reason for choosing and acting, a reason that requires NO PRIOR REASON.[16] Basic goods are anything that a person can in anyway desire, those concrete terms which make up the unfinished cathedral of the person. Hence the theory of marriage as a basic good forms a rational foundation which further develops the official Church position found in teachings like *Donum vitae*.

Furthermore are also two moral principles from which the most specific norms can be deduced and by which judgments of conscience can be criticized. This conference wishes to affirm that moral decision making is more than just a question of how any person feels about a particular action; but moral decision making is what the person is called by God from creation to become. This is made known to the person in the form of certain basic goods, which in turn supply the *reasons* for his subsequent choices under the light of grace.

Unfortunately today the human person as a unity is threatened in this decision making process by a fractured anthropology of dissenting theological opinion. Such dissenting opinon has overstressed the importance of the will and by doing this, offers the human person no criteria for moral decision making other than the consequences of what the person wishes to do in the moment of choice itself. In contrast, the tradition of Catholic moral theology has always brought together the functioning of both intellect and will. Whereas dissenting theological opinion fractures this reality by creating theoretical categories like ontic evil, which take the person away from the call to virtue and to holiness. Thus dissenting theories create a minimalist perfectionism, a far cry from what Pope Paul VI called, "The law proper to human life restored to its original truth."[17] The work of Pope John Paul II on marriage and the family presents man as this original unity, incomplete it is true, and yet original, mysterious, unique. It will only be in coming to terms with this aloneness, this uniqueness, that one is capable of becoming with another in marriage--all one.[18]

Distinctions between making and doing (that which is merely an isolated choice versus that which determines the self) allows one to view major choices like marriage as a context for the evaluation of specific reproductive choices. The cathedral of the person stands open from creation to certain basic goods. One of these basic goods is marriage, spoken about in *Donum vitae*.[19] A second symbol will now be used to speak about this reality of the marriage commitment: a flower--the chevrefeuille.

THE FLOWER

The first woman poetess of France, Marie de France, presents the secular symbol of love as the story of a flower, the chevrefeuille, planted on the graves of those who have loved in life.[20] One flower searches out and entwines with the other, as a symbol of a love stronger than death.[21] It is the Church who takes over the secular symbol of love to establish marriage as a natural indissoluble monogomous union. *Donum vitae* states that marriage has two inseparable aspects: the unitive and the procreative, intertwined like two flowers, in an *eternal* union of meaning, given at creation by the Creator Himself. Likewise the *Instruction* reminds us that man and woman are called in a special way to share in the mystery of personal communion with God in His work as Creator and Father. Because of this calling, marriage possesses specific goods and values in the unitive and procreative aspects which cannot be likened to any lower forms of life.[22] So we are reminded that the flower--remains only that, a limping analogy--able to be filled with meaning only through a vision of faith that is a grace given by God Himself. Thus a moral evaluation in reference to any reproductive technology must always be weighed and measured, as the *Instruction* insists, from the vision of the cathedral of the person who is called to realize this flowering vocation of marriage: as a gift of love and life from God Himself.[23]

Furthermore, the inseparability of these two aspects of marriage: the unitive and the procreative (interiorly ordained at creation) has been the heritage of Church tradition throughout the teaching of the fathers from St. Augustine to St. Thomas Aquinas. Most recently, however, it has been the basis for the great encyclical *Humanae Vitae* whose twentieth anniversary we celebrate this year. Our present Holy Father, Pope John Paul II, also reiterates this principle in his encyclical on marriage and the family *Familiaris Consortio.* However *Donum vitae* presents the teaching on the unitive and the procreative meaning of marriage within the context of specific questions on reproductive technology.[24] Two other secondary lines of argument also emerge in this *Instruction:* 1) that generating life in a laboratory is a form of production violating the dignity of the child produced; and 2) engendering human life in this way falsifies the language of the body. This term "language of the body" is developed by John Paul II in his writings on marriage and the family.[25]

In addition, the unitive and the procreative aspects of marriage show that the gift of marriage brings with it: *munus/munera* -- duties of spouses.[26] Fatherhood and motherhood must acknowledge that in regard to the transmission of human life, they are not limited by the horizons of this life only. Thus *munus* is a duty which cannot translate into a right to be exercised. If munus is a duty more akin to a gift than to a right, then the human person cannot understand himself to have failed, if he is unable for whatever reason, to actualize the fullness of that gift.[27] Since no one has a right to a gift, no one has a right to a person. A sterility that would cause a couple to do anything to have a child would express a possessiveness which is at odds with that service required for those who would be good parents. Because every human desire is subject to scrutiny, desire to have children is no exception, and *Donum vitae* reminds us of this truth.[28]

Yet it is only within the context of the family that the development of the human person receives a context compatible with the person's human dignity. The child as fruit and sign of self-giving of the spouses, their love and their fidelity, renders certain reproductive techniques morally objectionable because they separate the unitive and the procreative meanings of the marital act and do not meet the necessary conditions for this child's coming to be. The child then is not an object, a thing, but a person and must be reared in a context compatible with this dignity.[29]

Hence the secular symbol of the flower seems not enough to sustain the open-ended aspirations of the human heart. It is only in the transcendent meaning of marriage, expression of Christ's love for the Church, which is broad enough to fulfill the true aspirations of the human person.[30] The inseparability of the unitive and the procreative aspects of marriage--as symbolized by this flower, the chevrefuille, planted on the graves of the dead--illumines from a faith perspective, the human reality of marriage, into an eternal union--a union which can still transcend the fragile, often fading reality of love in a permissive secular culture.

In addition to the meaning of marriage, specific questions in reproductive technology along with their moral and legal aspects are also addressed in this conference in order to show why such individual acts often tend to undermine the commitment of marriage and family life. Individual acts need to be situated in regard to the central truth of the conference: how the human person understands himself and appropriates the symbols of his commitment in his reproductive quest. For how the human person understands his own commitment under grace determines whether the horizon of today be on the brink of new genetic progress, or merely the beginning of a second dark age, worse than the first, marked by human gargoyles, *made*, not begotten, by the work of our own hands. Yet for the moment, the cathedral of the person stands silent--viewing love and marriage for what they really are in Christ -- pondering, *Donum vitae*, a teaching that is reasoned, but a teaching that demands reflection.

My second symbol recalls the medieval story of a flower, entertwined with another in love and planted on the graves of the dead, only a shadow of marriage, taken up by the Church as a natural institution and infused with the power of Christ into a symbol of eternal love. Christian marriage becomes a true symbol of everlasting fidelity, powerful enough to image the relationship between Christ and His Church. It is a symbol that every person is of inestimable worth, that every person is worth dying for. The teaching of the unity and inseparability of marriage is the major premise of *Donum vitae*. It is within this framework that the Church has spoken out today against certain reproductive technologies.

In relation to this inseparability of the unitive and the procreative aspects of marriage, certain reproductive technologies such as IVF, AID, AIH, TOT and GIFT are judged to be contrary to this basic principle.[31] LTOT on the other hand is seen to be morally acceptable because it aids the marriage act rather than substitutes for it.[32] In addition, the Pope Paul VI Institute with its concern for cerebrocentric human sexuality, along with advanced hormone treatment to combat infertility, supplies yet another alternative method to illicit technological practice.[33] The legal and ethical implications of the surrogate mother issue moreover prove to be one of the most destructive forces of reproductive technology in our time.[34] Surrogate motherhood requires the law to choose the basis upon which it will enforce one party against the other. In other words, it is a positive conferral of rights by the state (because they make up this right, because they say so, one has a right). Another example of such positive conferral of rights by the State would be the legal enforcement of claims, grounded solely in respect for the autonomous individual choice. In this last example, the individual will of the one, wins out over the natural right of the other. Thus the individual whose rights are recognized, treats the other as "property." In this sense surrogate motherhood can be seen as the new revival of slavery in the United States today. This is in direct opposition to the notion of basic human dignity and equality central to the traditional legal system, a fundamental threat to the United States' democratic system.[35] In order to deal with this question of reproductive technology it is necessary to invoke then a third symbol in the context of the human person, image of God--the symbol of a quest.

THE QUEST

Near the end of the middle ages there is a story in French medieval literature of Perceval and the legend of the Holy Grail.[36] Written by the first short story writer of France Chretien de Troyes who died around the end of the 12th century, his story, like the cathedral, was left unfinished. The story has been called the first piece of mystical writing, replete with eucharistic significance.[37] For this reason I choose it today, the last day of the conference, to center our focus on Christ, on prayer, and on our incorporation with him. Christ is the heart and determining factor of the moral life. Christ not only teaches the truth, but makes it possible to live it. It is God ultimately, not the Church, who guarantees the truth of divine instruction on morals. And *Donum vitae* has shown us that individual judgments about reproductive technologies cannot stand apart from the dignity of the person--what his vocation has called him to be.

As the story opens, a young boy Perceval is about to leave his aged mother to find, in his words, "fame and glory in the court of King Arthur." The mother cautions him that knighthood means holiness, honor, and service, but he departs brusquely on his way leaving her to die of a broken heart. At the court of the king, Perceval finds glory, but he hears of a Fisher King who lives only by the host brought to him in the holy grail. And one day, while riding far from Camelot, Perceval comes upon the castle of the Fisher King. Perceval is welcomed, fed, and royally treated, spending three nights with the Fisher King. While at table Perceval sees the grail--the vessel used at the last supper, pass mysteriously before him. He watches a young maiden carry past him a lance with drops of blood. And Perceval wonders too about the crippled Fisher King and whom the grail serves, but Perceval is too frightened to ask the questions in his heart. And so he rides away from the castle of the Fisher King--turning back for a brief moment to find the king, the grail, and the castle itself have mysteriously disappeared.

Later at Arthur's court, when Perceval is to receive a laurel crown for his achievements, a wretched woman in black riding a mule approaches to charge that Perceval is not worthy of honor because he has left the Fisher King whose lands have been laid waste; and all because Perceval failed to ask those questions within his heart. Perceval, the legend says, gets up immediately and rides off, never again to rest two nights in the same place, until he finds once more the Fisher King, until he sees the grail and asks whom it serves. The woman in black has stated for Perceval his Christian anthropology: the meaning of his life must be seen in the light of the whole; fame and fortune are not ultimate. She has allowed him to see that it was the Revelation of the Fisher King which could give final meaning to his quest. Moreover, the problem of birth and human life are like this. They cannot be considered from any partial perspective--be it psychological, biological, sociological because the integral vision of man's life is destined for the eternal.

This small final paper has been another exercise of C.S. Lewis--the putting of the more into the less: transposition.[38] The conference has presented how the notion of relationship reflects Christ transposing the more into the less-- being related to us, as He is related to the Father. Hence the higher processes of the trinity extend into the lower processes of our human life.[39] More- over it is through relatedness with Christ in Baptism (and with each other in every day life) which enables fruitfulness to happen. A basic principle involved here is that the higher cannot stand without the lower. The work one does cannot be truly fruitful without the corresponding holiness of life. But newness of life happens only through relationship--the giving of the one to the other, which in turn creates greater holiness: union with God. The highest form of this transposition is divinization: becoming a child of God.[40]

We learned that the Holy Father's expression for Christian anthropology is summarized in the term "language of the body." And that a moral norm arises from reading this language of the body IN TRUTH.[41] Each moment and step of our lives is a response to the dialogue with God to be faithful to the circulation of life and love which issues in fruitfulness--the lowest to the highest through the co-ordinating activity of the Holy Spirit. And the fundamental fruit of the gift of the Spirit urges the person to respect the work of God in life. Through this heightened awareness of the interrelatedness of all relationships under the light of faith, explanations can be offered on the concrete level for particular scientific questions, as we have tried to do here this weekend. But the ultimate answer must remain that mysterious process whereby the Holy Trinity energizes all the levels of human life. Yet only a deepened sensitivity born of holiness can appreciate the answers given by the Church; otherwise one can only go away blinded as Perceval was by his desire for fame and fortune. But Perceval, having achieved great things by his own power at the court of King Arthur, could not decide in the end quite what to do with such power. By turning back in search of the Fisher King, Perceval expresses in symbol what Vatican II has said in reali- ty: that the future of the world stands in peril unless wiser men are forth- coming.[42]

The Church has always believed that man is guided by both natural law and the Gospel, but neither functions in a vacuum, a spiritual illumination irrespect- ive of the incarnated presence of Christ which is mediated faithfully through the magisterium of the Church. Like the lady in black, magesterial teaching does challenge personal ambition and inordinate self-interest of 20th Century tech- nological power. Faith then does indeed cast light on everyday moral and human questions. Man is not left to experience alone. *Donum vitae* can be compared to the words of the Fisher King--a brief account of what is judged to be right, awaiting the task of scholars who will draw upon this foundation, and that of Church tradition, to explain a detailed argument for the Church's position. This is what our scholars have done at this conference. They have presented to you arguments for why the teaching of *Donum vitae* is true and good. They are faithful knights of scholarship at the table of the King. Furthermore, the testimony of the couples has witnessed to the blessing and strength that the teaching of the Church does bring in the midst of suffering. These married couples challenge theologians and all of us not to give up the difficult task of explaining the positions of the Church which bring such meaning and peace in the midst of tragedy.[43]

The tale of the Fisher King invites all to the banquet of Christian perfection, a heavenly knighthood whose code is exemplified by the Sermon on the Mount. It is the call to virtue, the fruit of good moral choice. Perceval, as we noted, was not at first cognizant of the basic good of knighthood--his vocation. He seemed to absolutize morality in his quest for fame and glory, instead of subordinating it to the wider good of human flourishing: holiness, honor, and service. Deontologically speaking perhaps, one could even say, Perceval used his conquests, or his service, as a mere means to the goal of fame and fortune, instead of defending the absolute dignity of every human person. The basic goods of truth and friendship he first passed by, because he overvalued the basic good of work to the detriment of other basic goods. And by this he lost other important basic goods besides: including harmony, that interior peace within himself, and worship before his God. Perceval had offended, if you will, the first principle of morality: choose only those possibilities compatible with integral human fulfillment, but recognize the limitations of your choosing, and regard any partial good as limited, a participation in a larger good. One might say Perceval transgressed the intermediate principle also because he unjustly limited the people he cared about and the people he was willing to defend. Perhaps he acted on hostile feelings violating still another intermediate principle; yet certainly, the lady on the mule insisted that by his walking away from the need of the Fisher King (who represents Christ,) he broke the third and last intermediate moral principle: he did evil to achieve good.[44]

Likewise, perhaps one could say Perceval resented the negative moral absolutes that this last intermediate principle generates because they were a threat to his concrete interests, as they are to many people today.[45] In any event, these intermediate principles shaped for Perceval the first principle of morality into definite responsibilities, responsibilities which he only acknowledged later in his life, responsibilities which he rode off forever into history to fulfill.

The story of the legend of the Holy Grail is therefore an unfinished story of the mystical life, a mysterious allegory of the supernatural. The allegory can be understood on many levels, and so the Fisher King can symbolize the Christ both in his person and also as mediated through the ordinary teaching authority of his Church. It is for our time in history not only a consolation (as it was for Perceval,) but also a judgment. None who claims to be Christian is free to pursue his success unaware of this teaching and its meaning. Those who are one with Christ will know by this oneness the truth of *Donum vitae* and its demands. The poor among us are indeed the helpless, those whose lands are ravaged, yes; this is true. And they are also the unborn, the elderly, the broken, The Christ, --the helpless in need wherever they are found.

But Christ and His gospel bring to each person true freedom, the freeing of the free will; not freedom or self fulfillment as ends in themselves, but the consciousness of certain basic goods. Therefore, freedom becomes not an end in itself, but a means through grace to achieve basic goods. The natural good of knighthood is brought to fulfillment in a supernatural union with the Fisher King. Thus, gospel liberation has two aspects working to build community in the Church and in the world (this is the first stage of liberation but it re- mains incomplete). There is a second stage of liberation which requires the suf- fering of the upright, and the suffering that can only find its meaning in a di- vine act--the sufferings of Christ.[46] Such suffering will be completed only in the rising up of all who die in faith. There is here no room for compromise. Either the teachings of the Church are accepted as wisdom and often as a chance for such incorporation into the sufferings of Christ (as St. Paul in the Phillip- ians recalls) or the exception becomes the norm, in a spirit of "creative re- gret", when one has not the faith to accept the principles that the Church is teaching.

The message of the conference like the legend of the Holy Grail comprises who we are, as well as what we do (as the old mother reminded her too-adventurous son). The basic goods of life are written within the human person because God created him this way, in His image. Individual goals will always find themselves subject to this fundamental truth: the basic goods of human life. Whether un- finished desires, or vanquished possibilities, "the heart is restless until it rests in Thee", as St. Augustine tells us. Basic goods then are what this rest- lessness is all about.

Our conference is finished; the middle ages is no more. Yet its symbols stand in beauty as well as in warning, lest along the road one day we meet in black a victim of our genetic manipulation. *Donum vitae* tells us it is wrong to experiment on those who cannot answer for themselves, if the experiment is nontherapeutic, or if it is harmful to the person without their consent.[47] *Donum vitae* proclaims that there is in each and everyone of us no matter how small, how weak--a dignity within.

At the National Gallery of Art in Washington there hangs a series of paintings of the Cathedral of Rouen by Claude Monet. They are several paintings of the same reality, captured in bright sunlight and in varying shades of twilight. Like the human person whether in the shadow of darkness and tragedy, the brightness of new life, the twilight of anticipation--*Donum vitae* stands as a reminder that the human person is always the masterpiece of God. This is the message of *Donum vitae:* An inspiration for our time.

ENDNOTES

[1]See Appendix, The Pope's Easter Message.

[2]Cassell, M.D., Eric, J. The Place of the Humanities in Medicine. (Hastings-on-the Hudson, New York, 1984), p. 7.

[3]Ibid.

[4]Donum vitae, Introduction n. 3.

[5]Ibid., n. 1.

[6]Ibid.

[7]Donum vitae, Conclusion.

[8]Cvetkovich, p. 15.

[9]Ibid.

[10]Hilgers, p. 43.

[11]Lawler, p. 28.

[12]Ibid.

[13]Cessario, p. 172.

[14]Grisez, p. 71.

[15]Ibid.

[16]Ibid. p. 2

[17]Cessario, p. 164.

[18]Pope John Paul II, Original Unity of Man and Woman: Catechesis on the Book of Genesis. (Boston: St. Paul Editions, 1981).

[20]Tuffaru, Paul. Ed. Les Lais de Marie de France. (l'Edition d'Art, Paris, 1963), p. v.

[21]Ibid. p. 53.

[22]Donum vitae, Part II, B, 4.

[23]Ibid.

[24]Ibid.

[25]Sheets, p. 187.

[26]Smith, pp. 55-58.

[27]Boyle, p. 25.

[28]Ibid.

[29]May, p. 85.

[30]Sheets, p. 186.

[31]May pp. 87-88.

[32]Ibid.

[33]Hilgers, pp. 128-134.

[34]Wagner, p. 116.

[35]Ibid. p. 115.

[36]Lagarde, André and Michard, Laurent Moyen age: les grands auteurs français du programme (Paris: Les Editions Bordas, n.d.), pp. 70-73.

[37]Ibid., p. 73.

[38]Sheets, p. 179.

[39]Ibid. p. 188-189.

[40]Ibid.

[41]Grisez, p. 70.

[42]Lawler, p. 27.

[43]Testimony of the Couples.

[44]Grisez, p. 70.

[45]Ibid., p. 67.

[46]Ibid., p. 73.

[47]Donum vitae.

APPENDIX

DONUM VITAE

INSTRUCTION ON RESPECT FOR HUMAN LIFE IN ITS ORIGIN AND ON THE DIGNITY OF PROCREATION

FOREWORD

The Congregation for the Doctrine of the Faith has been approached by various episcopal conferences or individual bishops, by theologians, doctors and scientists, concerning biomedical techniques, which make it possible to intervene in the initial phase of the life of a human being and in the very processes of procreation and their conformity with the principles of Catholic morality. The present instruction, which is the result of wide consultation and in particular of a careful evaluation of the declarations made by episcopates, does not intend to repeat all the church's teaching on the dignity of human life as it originates and on procreation, but to offer, in the light of the previous teaching of the magisterium, some specific replies to the main questions being asked in this regard.

The exposition is arranged as follows: An introduction will recall the fundamental principles of an anthropological and moral character which are necessary for a proper evaluation of the problems and for working out replies to those questions; the first part will have as its subject respect for the human being from the first moment of his or her existence; the second part will deal with the moral questions raised by technical interventions on human procreation; the third part will offer some orientations on the relationships between moral law and civil law in terms of the respect due to human embryos and fetuses* and as regards the legitimacy of techniques of artificial procreation.

---

* The terms *zygote, pre-embryo, embryo* and *fetus* can indicate in the vocabulary of biology successive stages of the development of a human being. The present instruction makes free use of these terms, attributing to them an identical ethical relevance, in order to designate the result (whether visible or not) of human generation, from the first moment of its existence until birth. The reason for this usage is clarified by the text (cf. I,1).

INTRODUCTION

1. Biomedical Research and the Teaching of the Church

The gift of life which God the Creator and Father has entrusted to man calls him to appreciate the inestimable value of what he has been given and to take responsibility for it: This fundamental principle must be placed at the center of one's reflection in order to clarify and solve the moral problems raised by artificial interventions on life as it originates and on the processes of procreation.

Thanks to the progress of the biological and medical sciences, man has at his disposal ever more effective therapeutic resources; but he can also acquire new powers, with unforeseeable consequences, over human life at its very beginning and in its first stages. Various procedures now make it possible to intervene not only in order to assist, but also to dominate the processes of procreation. These techniques can enable man to "take in hand his own destiny," but they also expose him "to the temptation to go beyond the limits of a reasonable dominion over nature."[1] They might constitute progress in the service of man, but they also involve serious risks. Many people are therefore expressing an urgent appeal that in interventions on procreation the values and rights of the human person be safeguarded. Requests for clarification and guidance are coming not only from the faithful, but also from those who recognize the church as "an expert in humanity"[2] with a mission to serve the "civilization of love"[3] and of life.

The church's magisterium does not intervene on the basis of a particular competence in the area of the experimental sciences; but having taken account of the data of research and technology, it intends to put forward, by virtue of its evangelical mission and apostolic duty, the moral teaching corresponding to the dignity of the person and to his or her integral vocation. It intends to do so by expounding the criteria of moral judgment as regards the applications of scientific research and technology, especially in relation to human life and its beginnings. These criteria are the respect, defense and promotion of man, his "primary and fundamental right" to life,[4] his dignity as a person who is endowed with a spiritual soul and with moral responsibility[5] and who is called to beatific communion with God.

The church's intervention in this field is inspired also by the love which she owes to man, helping him to recognize and respect his rights and duties. This love draws from the fount of Christ's love: As she contemplates the mystery of the incarnate word, the church also comes to understand the "mystery of man",[6] by proclaiming the Gospel of salvation, she reveals to man his dignity and invites him to discover fully the truth of his own being. Thus the church once more puts forward the divine law in order to accomplish the work of truth and liberation.

For it is out of goodness - in order to indicate the path of life - that God gives human beings his commandments and the grace to observe them; and it is likewise out of goodness - in order to help them persevere along the same path - that God always offers to everyone his forgiveness. Christ has compassion on our weaknesses: He is our Creator and Redeemer. May his Spirit open men's hearts to the gift of God's peace and to an understanding of his precepts.

2. Science and Technology at the Service of the Human Person

God created man in his own image and likeness: "Male and female he created them" (Gn. 1:27), entrusting to them the task of "having dominion over the earth" (Gn. 1:28). Basic scientific research and applied research constitute a significant expression of this dominion of man over creation. Science and technology are valuable resources for man when placed at his service and when they promote his integral development for the benefit of all; but they cannot of themselves show the meaning of existence and of human progress. Being ordered to man, who initiates and develops them, they draw from the person and his moral values the indication of their purpose and the awareness of their limits.

It would on the one hand be illusory to claim that scientific research and its applications are morally neutral; on the other hand one cannot derive criteria for guidance from mere technical efficiency, from research's possible usefulness to some at the expense of others or, worse still, from prevailing ideologies. Thus science and technology require for their own intrinsic meaning an unconditional respect for the fundamental criteria of the moral law: That is to say, they must be at the service of the human person, of his inalienable rights and his true and integral good according to the design and will of God.[7]

The rapid development of technological discoveries gives greater urgency to this need to respect the criteria just mentioned: Science without conscience can only lead to man's ruin. "Our era needs such wisdom more than bygone ages if the discoveries made by man are to be further humanized. For the future of the world stands in peril unless wise people are forthcoming."[8]

3. Anthropology and Procedures in the Biomedical Field

Which moral criteria must be applied in order to clarify the problems posed today in the field of biomedicine? The answer to this question presupposes a proper idea of the nature of the human person in his bodily dimension.

For it is only in keeping with his true nature that the human person can achieve self-realization as a "unified totality"; and this nature is at the same time corporal and spiritual. By virtue of its substantial union with a spiritual soul, the human body cannot be considered as a mere complex of tissues, organs and functions, nor can it be evaluated in the same way as the body of animals; rather it is a constitutive part of the person who manifests and expresses himself through it.

The natural moral law expresses and lays down the purposes, rights and duties which are based upon the bodily and spiritual nature of the human person. Therefore this law cannot be thought of as simply a set of norms on the biological level; rather it must be defined as the rational order whereby man is called by the Creator to direct and regulate his life and actions and in particular to make use of his own body.[10]

A first consequence can be deduced from these principles: An intervention on the human body affects not only the tissues, the organs and their functions, but also involves the person himself on different levels. It involves, therefore, perhaps in an implicit but nonetheless real way, a moral significance and responsibility. Pope John Paul II forcefully reaffirmed this to the World Medical Association when he said:

"Each human person, in his absolutely unique singularity, is constituted not only by his spirit, but by his body as well. Thus, in the body and through the body, one touches the person himself in his concrete reality. To respect the dignity of man consequently amounts to safeguarding this identity of the man cor- pore et anima unus,' as the Second Vatican Council says (Gaudium et Spes, 14.1). It is on the basis of this anthropological vision that one is to find the fundamental criteria for decision making in the case of procedures which are not strictly therapeutic, as, for example, those aimed at the improvement of the human biological condition."[11]

Applied biology and medicine work together for the integral good of human life when they come to the aid of a person stricken by illness and infirmity and when they respect his or her dignity as a creature of God. No biologist or doctor can reasonably claim, by virtue of his scientific competence, to be able to decide on people's origin and destiny. This norm must be applied in a particular way in the field of sexuality and procreation, in which man and woman actualizes the fundamental values of love and life.

God, who is love and life, has inscribed in man and woman the vocation to share in a special way in his mystery of personal communion and in his work as Creator and Father.[12] For this reason marriage possesses specific goods and values in its union and in procreation which cannot be likened to those existing in lower forms of life. Such values and meanings are of the personal order and determine from the moral point of view the meaning and limits of artificial interventions on procreation and on the origin of human life. These interventions are not to be rejected on the grounds that they are artificial. As such, they bear witness to the possibilities of the art of medicine. But they must be given a moral evaluation in reference to the dignity of the human person, who is called to realize his vocation from God to the gift of love and the gift of life.

4. Fundamental Criteria for a Moral Judgment

The fundamental values connected with the techniques of artificial human procreation are two: the life of the human being called into existence and the special nature of the transmission of human life in marriage. The moral judgment on such methods of artificial procreation must therefore be formulated in reference to these values.

Physical life, with which the course of human life in the world begins, certainly does not itself contain the whole of a person's value nor does it represent the supreme good of man, who is called to eternal life. However it does constitute in a certain way the "fundamental" value of life precisely because upon this

208

physical life all the other values of the person are based and developed.[13]
The inviolability of the innocent human being's right to life "from the moment of
conception until death"[14] is a sign and requirement of the very inviolability of the person to whom the Creator has given the gift of life.

By comparison with the transmission of other forms of life in the universe,
the transmission of human life has a special character of its own, which derives
from the special nature of the human person. "The transmission of human life is
entrusted by nature to a personal and conscious act and as such is subject to the
all-holy laws of God: immutable and inviolable laws which must be recognized and
observed. For this reason one cannot use means and follow methods which could be
licit in the transmission of the life of plants and animals."[15]

Advances in technology have now made it possible to procreate apart from
sexual relations through the meeting *in vitro* of the germ cells previously
taken from the man and the woman. But what is technically possible is not for
that very reason morally admissible. Rational reflection on the fundamental
values of life and of human procreation is therefore indispensable for formulating
a moral evaluation of such technological interventions on a human being from the
first stages of his development.

5. Teachings of the Magisterium

On its part, the magisterium of the church offers to human reason in this
field too the light of revelation: The doctrine concerning man taught by the magisterium contains many elements which throw light on the problems being faced
here.

From the moment of conception, the life of every human being is to be
respected in an absolute way because man is the only creature on earth that God
has "wished for himself"[16] and the spiritual soul of each man is "immediately created" by God;[17] his whole being bears the image of the Creator.
Human life is sacred because from its beginning it involves "the creative action
of God,"[18] and it remains forever in a special relationship with the Creator, who is its sole end.[19] God alone is the Lord of life from its beginning until its end: No one can in any circumstance claim for himself the right to
destroy directly an innocent human being.[20]

Human procreation requires on the part of the spouses responsible collaboration with the fruitful love of God;[21] the gift of human life must be actualized in marriage through the specific and exclusive acts of husband and wife,
in accordance with the laws inscribed in their persons and in their union.[22]

I. RESPECT FOR HUMAN EMBRYOS

Careful reflection on this teaching of the magisterium and on the evidence of
reason, as mentioned above, enables us to respond to the numerous moral problems
posed by technical interventions upon the human being in the first phases of his
life and upon the processes of his conception.

1. **What respect is due to the human embryo, taking into account his nature and identity?**

The human being must be respected - as a person - from the very first instant of his existence.

The implementation of procedures of artificial fertilization has made possible various interventions upon embryos and human fetuses. The aims pursued are of various kinds: diagnostic and therapeutic, scientific and commercial. From all of this, serious problems arise. Can one speak of a right to experimentation upon human embryos for the purpose of scientific research? What norms or laws should be worked out with regard to this matter? The response to these problems presupposes a detailed reflection on the nature and specific identity - the word *status* is used - of the human embryo itself.

At the Second Vatican Council, the church for her part presented once again to modern man her constant and certain doctrine according to which: "Life once conceived, must be protected with the utmost care; abortion and infanticide are abominable crimes."[23] More recently, the Charter of the Rights of the Family, published by the Holy See, confirmed that "human life must be absolutely respected and protected from the moment of conception."[24]

This congregation is aware of the current debates concerning the beginning of human life, concerning the individuality of the human being and concerning the identity of the human person. The congregation recalls the teachings found in the Declaration on Procured Abortion:

"From the time that the ovum is fertilized, a new life is begun which is neither that of the father nor of the mother; it is rather the life of a new human being with his own growth. It would never be made human if it were not human already. To this perpetual evidence . . . modern genetic science brings valuable confirmation. It has demonstrated that, from the first instant, the program is fixed as to what this living being will be: a man, this individual man with his characteristic aspects already well determined. Right from fertilization is begun the adventure of a human life, and each of its great capacities requires time ... to find its place and to be in a position to act."[25]

This teaching remains valid and is further confirmed, if confirmation were needed, by recent findings of human biological science which recognize that in the zygote (the cell produced when the nuclei of the two gametes have fused) resulting from fertilization the biological identity of a new human individual is already constituted.

Certainly no experimental datum can be in itself sufficient to bring us to the recognition of a spiritual soul; nevertheless, the conclusions of science regarding the human embryo provide a valuable indication for discerning by the use of reason a personal presence at the moment of this first appearance of a human life: How could a human individual not be a human person? The magisterium has not expressly committed itself to an affirmation of a philosophical nature, but it constantly reaffirms the moral condemnation of any kind of procured abortion. This teaching has not been changed and is unchangeable.[26]

Thus the fruit of human generation from the first moment of its existence, that is to say, from the moment the zygote has formed, demands the unconditional respect that is morally due to the human being in his bodily and spiritual totality. The human being is to be respected and treated as a person from the moment of conception and therefore from that same moment his rights as a person must be recognized, among which in the first place is the inviolable right of every innocent human being to life.

This doctrine reminder provides the fundamental criterion for the solution of the various problems posed by the development of the biomedical sciences in this field: Since the embryo must be treated as a person, it must also be defended in its integrity, tended and cared for, to the extent possible, in the same way as any other human being as far as medical assistance is concerned.

2. Is prenatal diagnosis morally licit?

If prenatal diagnosis respects the life and integrity of the embryo and the human fetus and is directed toward its safeguarding or healing as an individual, then the answer is affirmative.

For prenatal diagnosis makes it possible to know the condition of the embryo and of the fetus when still in the mother's womb. It permits or makes it possible to anticipate earlier and more effectively, certain therapeutic, medical or surgical procedures.

Such diagnosis is permissible, with the consent of the parents after they have been adequately informed, if the methods employed safeguard the life and integrity of the embryo and the mother, without subjecting them to disproportionate risks.[27] But this diagnosis is gravely opposed to the moral law when it is done with the thought of possibly inducing an abortion depending upon the results: A diagnosis which shows the existence of a malformation or a hereditary illness must not be the equivalent of a death sentence. Thus a woman would be committing a gravely illicit act if she were to request such a diagnosis with the deliberate intention of having an abortion should the results confirm the existence of a malformation or abnormality. The spouse or relatives or anyone else would similarly be acting in a manner contrary to the moral law if they were to counsel or impose such a diagnostic procedure on the expectant mother with the same intention of possibly proceeding to an abortion. So too the specialist would be guilty of illicit collaboration if, in conducting the diagnosis and in communicating its results, he were deliberately to contribute to establishing or favoring a link between prenatal diagnosis and abortion.

In conclusion, any directive or program of the civil and health authorities or of scientific organizations which in any way were to favor a link between prenatal diagnosis and abortion, or which were to go as far as directly to induce expectant mothers to submit to prenatal diagnosis planned for the purpose of eliminating fetuses which are affected by malformations or which are carriers of hereditary illness, is to be condemned as a violation of the unborn child's right to life and as an abuse of the prior rights and duties of the spouses.

3. Are therapeutic procedures carried out on the human embryo licit?

As with all medical interventions on patients, *one must uphold as licit procedures carried out on the human embryo which respect the life and integrity of the embryo and do not involve disproportionate risks for it, but are directed toward its healing, the improvement of its condition of health or its individual survival.*

Whatever the type of medical, surgical or other therapy, the free and informed consent of the parents is required, according to the deontological rules followed in the case of children. The application of this moral principle may call for delicate and particular precautions in the case of embryonic or fetal life.

The legitimacy and criteria of such procedures have been clearly stated by Pope John Paul II: "A strictly therapeutic intervention whose explicit objective is the healing of various maladies such as those stemming from chromosomal defects will, in principle, be considered desirable, provided it is directed to the true promotion of the personal well-being of the individual without doing harm to his integrity or worsening his conditions of life. Such an intervention would indeed fall within the logic of the Christian moral tradition."[28]

4. How is one to evaluate morally research and experimentation[*] on human embryos and fetuses?

Medical research must refrain from operations on live embryos, unless there is a moral certainty of not causing harm to the life or integrity of the unborn child and the mother, and on condition that the parents have given their free and informed consent to the procedure. It follows that all research, even when limited to the simple observation of the embryo, would become illicit were it to involve risk to the embryo's physical integrity or life by reason of the methods used or the effects induced.

---

[*] Since the terms *research* and *experimentation* are often used equivalently and ambiguously, it is deemed necessary to specify the exact meaning given them in this document.
1) By *research* is meant any inductive-deductive process which aims at promoting the systematic observation of a given phenomenon in the human field or at verifying a hypothesis arising from previous observations.
2) By *experimentation* is meant any research in which the human being (in the various stages of his existence: embryo, fetus, child or adult) represents the object through which or upon which one intends to verify the effect, at present unknown or not sufficiently known, of a given treatment (e.g., pharmacological, teratogenic, surgical, etc.).

As regards experimentation, and presupposing the general distinction between experimentation for purposes which are not directly therapeutic and experimentation which is clearly therapeutic for the subject himself, in the case in point one must also distinguish between experimentation carried out on embryos which are still alive and experimentation carried out on embryos which are dead. *If the embryos are living, whether viable or not, they must be respected just like any other human person; experimentation on embryos which is not directly therapeutic is illicit.*[29]

No objective, even though noble in itself such as a foreseeable advantage to science, to other human beings or to society, can in any way justify experimentation on living human embryos or fetuses, whether viable or not, either inside or outside the mother's womb. The informed consent ordinarily required for clinical experimentation on adults cannot be granted by the parents, who may not freely dispose of the physical integrity or life of the unborn child. Moreover, experimentation on embryos and fetuses always involves risk, and indeed in most cases it involves the certain expectation of harm to their physical integrity or even their death.

To use human embryos or fetuses as the object or instrument of experimentation constitutes a crime against their dignity as human beings having a right to the same respect that is due to the child already born and to every human person.

The Charter of the Rights of the Family published by the Holy See affirms: "Respect for the dignity of the human being excludes all experimental manipulation or exploitation of the human embryo."[30] The practice of keeping alive human embryos *in vivo* or *in vitro* for experimental or commercial purposes is totally opposed to human dignity.

In the case of experimentation that is clearly therapeutic, namely, when it is a matter of experimental forms of therapy used for the benefit of the embryo itself in a final attempt to save its life and in the absence of other reliable forms of therapy, recourse to drugs or procedures not yet fully tested can be licit.[31]

The corpses of human embryos and fetuses, whether they have been deliberately aborted or not, must be respected just as the remains of other human beings. In particular, they cannot be subjected to mutilation or to autopsies if their death has not yet been verified and without the consent of the parents or of the mother. Furthermore, the moral requirements must be safeguarded that there be no complicity in deliberate abortion and that the risk of scandal be avoided. Also, in the case of dead fetuses, as for the corpses of adult persons, all commercial trafficking must be considered illicit and should be prohibited.

5. How is one to evaluate morally the use for research purposes of embryos obtained by fertilization "in vitro?"

Human embryos obtained *in vitro* are human beings and subjects with rights: Their dignity and right to life must be respected from the first moment of their existence. *It is immoral to produce human embryos destined to be exploited as disposable "biological materials."*

In the usual practice of *in vitro* fertilization, not all of the embryos are transferred to the woman's body; some are destroyed. Just as the church condemns induced abortion, so she also forbids acts against the life of their human beings. *It is a duty to condemn the particular gravity of the voluntary destruction of human embryos obtained "in vitro" for the sole purpose of research, either by means of artificial insemination or by means of "twin fission."* By acting in this way the researcher usurps the place of God; and, even though he may be unaware of this, he sets himself up as the master of the destiny of others inasmuch as he arbitrarily chooses whom he will allow to live and whom he will send to death and kills defenseless human beings.

Methods of observation or experimentation which damage or impose grave and disproportionate risks upon embryos obtained *in vitro* are morally illicit for the same reasons. Every human being is to be reduced in worth to a pure and simple instrument for the advantage of others. *It is therefore not in conformity with the moral law deliberately to expose to death human embryos obtained in vitro.* In consequence of the fact that they have been produced *in vitro*, those embryos which are not transferred into the body of the mother and are called "spare" are exposed to an absurd fate, with no possibility of their being offered safe means of survival which can be licitly pursued.

6. What judgment should be made on other procedures of manipulating embryos connected with the "techniques of human reproduction?"

Techniques of fertilization *in vitro* can open the way to other forms of biological and genetic manipulation of human embryos, such as attempts or plans for fertilization between human and animal gametes and the gestation of human embryos in the uterus of animals, or the hypothesis or project of constructing artificial uteruses for the human embryo. *These procedures are contrary to the human dignity proper to the embryo, and at the same time they are contrary to the right of every person to be conceived and to be born within marriage and from marriage.*[32] *Also, attempts or hypotheses for obtaining a human being without any connection with sexuality through "twin fission," cloning or parthenogenesis are to be considered contrary to the moral law, since they are in opposition to the dignity both of human procreation and of the conjugal union.*

The freezing of embryos, even when carried out in order to preserve the life of an embryo - cryopreservation - *constitutes an offense against the respect due to human beings* by exposing them to grave risks of death or harm to their physical integrity and depriving them, at least temporarily, of maternal shelter and gestation, thus placing them in a situation in which further offenses and manipulation are possible.

Certain attempts to influence chromosomic or genetic inheritance are not therapeutic, but are aimed at producing human beings selected according to sex or

214

other predetermined qualities. These manipulations are contrary to the personal dignity of the human being and his or her integrity and identity. Therefore in no way can they be justified on the grounds of possible beneficial consequences for future humanity.[33] Every person must be respected for himself: In this consists the dignity and right of every human being from his or her beginning.

II. INTERVENTIONS UPON HUMAN PROCREATION

By *artificial procreation or artificial fertilization* are understood here the different technical procedures directed toward obtaining a human conception in a manner other than the sexual union of man and woman. This instruction deals with fertilization of an ovum in a test tube (*in vitro* fertilization) and artificial insemination through transfer into the woman's genital tracts of previously collected sperm.

A preliminary point for the moral evaluation of such technical procedures is constituted by the consideration or the circumstances and consequences which those procedures involve in relation to the respect due the human embryo. Development of the practice of *in vitro* fertilization has required innumerable fertilizations and destructions of human embryos. Even today, the usual practice presupposes a hyperovulation on the part of the woman: A number of ova are withdrawn, fertilized and then cultivated *in vitro* for some days. Usually not all are transferred into the genital tracts of the woman; some embryos, generally called "spare," are destroyed or frozen. On occasion, some of the implanted embryos are sacrificed for various eugenic, economic or psychological reasons. Such deliberate destruction of human beings or their utilization for different purposes to the detriment of their integrity and life is contrary to the doctrine on procured abortion already recalled.

The connection between *in vitro* fertilization and the voluntary destruction of human embryos occurs too often. This is significant: Through these procedures, with apparently contrary purposes, life and death are subjected to the decision of man, who thus sets himself up as the giver of life and death by decree. This dynamic of violence and domination may remain unnoticed by those very individuals who, in wishing to utilize this procedure, become subject to it themselves. The facts recorded and the cold logic which links them must be taken into consideration for a moral judgment on *in vitro* fertilization and embryo transfer: The abortion mentality which has made this procedure possible, thus leads, whether one wants it or not, to man's domination over the life and death of his fellow human beings and can lead to a system of radical eugenics.

Nevertheless, such abuses do not exempt one from a further and thorough ethical study of the techniques of artificial procreation considered in themselves, abstracting as far as possible from the destruction of embryos produced *in vitro*.

The present instruction will therefore take into consideration in the first place the problems posed by heterologous artificial fertilization (II, 103),[*] and subsequently those linked with homologous artificial fertilization (II, 4-6).[**]

Before formulating an ethical judgment on each of these procedures, the principles and values which determine the moral evaluation of each of them will be considered.

A. Heterologous Artificial Fertilization

1. Why must human procreation take place in marriage?

Every human being is always to be accepted as a gift and blessing of God. However, from the moral point of view a truly responsible procreation vis-a-vis the unborn child must be the fruit of marriage.

For human procreation has specific characteristics by virtue of the personal dignity of the parents and of the children: The procreation of a new person, whereby the man and the woman collaborate with the power of the Creator, must be the fruit and the sign of the mutual self-giving of the spouses, of their love and of their fidelity.[34] *The fidelity of the spouses in the unity of marriage involves reciprocal respect of their right to become a father and a mother only through each other.*

The child has the right to be conceived, carried in the womb, brought into the world and brought up within marriage: It is through the secure and recognized relationship to his own parents that the child can discover his own identity and achieve his own proper human development.

---

[*] By the term *heterologous artificial fertilization or procreation*, the instruction means techniques used to obtain a human conception artificially by the use of gametes coming from at least one donor other than the spouses who are joined in marriage. Such techniques can be of two types:

a) *Heterologous "in vitro" fertilization and embryo transfer:* the technique used to obtain a human conception through the meeting *in vitro* of gametes taken from at least one donor other than the two spouses joining in marriage.

b) *Heterologous artificial insemination:* the technique used to obtain a human conception through the transfer into the genital tracts of the woman of the sperm previously collected from a donor other than the husband.

[**] By *artificial homologous fertilization or procreation*, the instruction means the technique used to obtain a human conception using the gametes of the two spouses joined in marriage. Homologous artificial fertilization can be carried out by two different methods:

a) *Homologous "in vitro" fertilization and embryo transfer:* the technique used to obtain a human conception through the meeting *in vitro* of the gametes of the spouses joined in marriage.

b) *Homologous artificial insemination:* the technique used to obtain a human conception through the transfer into the genital tracts of a married woman of the sperm previously collected from her husband.

The parents find in their child a confirmation and completion of their reciprocal self-giving: The child is the living image of their love, the permanent sign of their conjugal union, the living and indissoluble concrete expression of their paternity and maternity.[35]

By reason of the vocation and social responsibility of the person, the good of the children and of the parents contributes to the good of civil society; the vitality and stability of society require that children come into the world within a family and that the family be firmly based on marriage.

The tradition of the church and anthropological reflection recognize in marriage and in its indissoluble unity the only setting worthy of truly responsible procreation.

2. Does heterologous artificial fertilization conform to the dignity of the couple and to the truth of marriage?

Through *in vitro* fertilization and embryo transfer and heterologous artificial insemination, human conception is achieved through the fusion of gametes of at least one donor other than the spouses who are united in marriage. *Heterologous artificial fertilization is contrary to the unity of marriage, to the dignity of the spouses, to the vocation proper to parents, and to the child's right to be conceived and brought into the world in marriage and from marriage.*[36]

Respect for the unity of marriage and for conjugal fidelity demands that the child be conceived in marriage; the bond existing between husband and wife accords the spouses, in an objective and inalienable manner, the exclusive right to become father and mother solely through each other.[37] Recourse to the gametes of a third person in order to have sperm or ovum available constitutes a violation of the reciprocal commitment of the spouses and a grave lack in regard to that essential property of marriage which is its unity.

Heterologous artificial fertilization violates the rights of the child; it deprives him of his filial relationship with his parental origins and can hinder the maturing of his personal identity. Furthermore, it offends the common vocation of the spouses who are called to fatherhood and motherhood: It objectively deprives conjugal fruitfulness of its unity and integrity; it brings about and manifests a rupture between genetic parenthood, gestational parenthood and responsibility for upbringing. Such damage to the personal relationships within the family has repercussions on civil society: What threatens the unity and stability of the family is a source of dissension, disorder and injustice in the whole of social life.

These reasons lead to a negative moral judgment concerning heretologous artificial fertilization: Consequently, fertilization of a married woman with the sperm of a donor different from her husband and fertilization with the husband's sperm of an ovum not coming from his wife are morally illicit. Furthermore, the artificial fertilization of a woman who is unmarried or a widow, whoever the donor may be, cannot be morally justified.

The desire to have a child and the love between spouses who long to obviate a sterility which cannot be overcome in any other way constitute understandable motivations; but subjectively good intentions do not render heterologous artificial fertilization conformable to the objective and inalienable properties of marriage or respectful of the rights of the child and of the spouses.

3. Is "surrogate"* motherhood morally licit?

No, for the same reasons which lead one to reject heterologous artificial fertilization: For it is contrary to the unity of marriage and to the dignity of the procreation of the human person.

Surrogate motherhood represents an objective failure to meet the obligations of maternal love, of conjugal fidelity and of responsible motherhood; it offends the dignity and the right of the child to be conceived, carried in the womb, brought into the world and brought up by his own parents; it sets up, to the detriment of families, a division between the physical, psychological and moral elements which constitute those families.

B. Homologous Artificial Fertilization

Since heterologous artificial fertilization has been declared unacceptable, the question arises of how to evaluate morally the process of homologous artificial fertilization: *in vitro* fertilization and embryo transfer and artificial insemination between husband and wife. First a question of principle must be clarified.

4. What connection is required from the moral point of view between procreation and the conjugal act?

a) the church's teaching on marriage and human procreation affirms the "inseparable connection, willed by God and unable to be broken by man on his own initiative, between the two meanings of the conjugal act: the unitive meaning and the procreative meaning. Indeed, by its intimate structure the conjugal act, while most closely uniting husband and wife, capacitates them for the generation of new lives according to laws inscribed in the very being of man and of woman".[38] This principle, which is based upon the nature of marriage and the intimate connection of the goods of marriage, has well-known consequences on the level of responsible fatherhood and motherhood. "By safeguarding both these essential

---

*By *surrogate mother* the instruction means:

a) The woman who carries in pregnancy an embryo implanted in her uterus and who is genetically a stranger to the embryo because it has been obtained through the union of the gametes of "donors." She carries the pregnancy with a pledge to surrender the baby once it is born to the party who commissioned or made the agreement for the pregnancy.

b) The woman who carries in pregnancy an embryo to whose procreation she has contributed the donation of her own ovum, fertilized through insemination with the sperm of a man other than her husband. She carries the pregnancy with a pledge to surrender the child once it is born to the party who commissioned or made the agreement for the pregnancy.

aspects, the unitive and the procreative, the conjugal act preserves in its fullness the sense of true mutual love and its ordination toward man's exalted vocation to parenthood."[39]

The same doctrine concerning the link between the meanings of the conjugal act and between the goods of marriage throws light on the moral problem of homologous artificial fertilization, since "it is never permitted to separate these different aspects to such a degree as positively to exclude either the procreative intention or the conjugal relation."[40]

Contraception deliberately deprives the conjugal act of its openness to procreation and in this way brings about a voluntary dissociation of the ends of marriage. Homologous artificial fertilization, in seeking a procreation which is not the fruit of a specific act of conjugal union, objectively effects an analogous separation between the goods and the meanings of marriage.

Thus *fertilization is licitly sought when it is the result of a "conjugal act which is per se suitable for the generation of children, to which marriage is ordered by its nature and by which the spouses become one flesh."[41] But from the moral point of view procreation is deprived of its proper perfection when it is not desired as the fruit of the conjugal act, that is to say, of the specific act of the spouses' union.*

b) The moral value of the intimate link between the goods of marriage and between the meanings of the conjugal act is based upon the unity of the human being, a unity involving body and spiritual soul.[42] Spouses mutually express their personal love in the "language of the body," which clearly involves both "spousal meanings" and parental ones.[43] The conjugal act by which the couple mutually express their self-gift at the same time expresses openness to the gift of life. It is an act that is inseparably corporal and spiritual. It is in their bodies and through their bodies that the spouses consummate their marriage and are able to become father and mother. In order to respect the language of their bodies and their natural generosity, the conjugal union must take place with respect for its openness to procreation; and the procreation of a person must be the fruit and the result of married love. The origin of the human being thus follows from a procreation that is "linked to the union, not only biological but also spiritual, of the parents, made one by the bond of marriage."[44] Fertilization achieved outside the bodies of the couple remains by this very fact deprived of the meanings and the values which are expressed in the language of the body and in the union of human persons.

c) Only respect for the link between the meanings of the conjugal act and respect for the unity of the human being make possible procreation in conformity with the dignity of the person. In his unique and irrepeatable origin, the child must be respected and recognized as equal in personal dignity to those who give him life. The human person must be accepted in his parents' act of union and love; the generation of a child must therefore be the fruit of that mutual giving[45] which is realized in the conjugal act wherein the spouses cooperate as servants and not as masters in the work of the Creator, who is love.[46]

In reality, the origin of a human person is the result of an act of giving. The one conceived must be the fruit of his parents' love. He cannot be desired or conceived as the product of an intervention of medical or biological techniques; that would be equivalent to reducing him to an object of scientific technology. No one may subject the coming of a child into the world to conditions of technical efficiency which are to be evaluated according to standards of control and dominion.

The moral relevance of the link between the meanings of the conjugal act and between the goods of marriage, as well as the unity of the human being and the dignity of his origin, demand that the procreation of a human person be brought about as the fruit of the conjugal act specific to the love between spouses. The link between procreation and the conjugal act is thus shown to be of great importance on the anthropological and moral planes, and it throws light on the positions of the magisterium with regard to homologous artificial fertilization.

5. Is homologous "in vitro" fertilization morally licit?

The answer to this question is strictly dependent on the principles just mentioned. Certainly one cannot ignore the legitimate aspirations of sterile couples. For some, recourse to homologous *in vitro* fertilization and embryo transfer appears to be the only way of fulfilling their sincere desire for a child. The question is asked whether the totality of conjugal life in such situations is not sufficient to ensure the dignity proper to human procreation. It is acknowledged that *in vitro* fertilization and embryo transfer certainly cannot supply for the absence of sexual relations[47] and cannot be preferred to the specific acts of conjugal union, given the risks involved for the child and the difficulties of the procedure. But is is asked whether, when there is no other way of overcoming the sterility which is a source of suffering, homologous *in vitro* fertilization may not constitute an aid, if not a form of therapy, whereby its moral licitness could be admitted.

The desire for a child - or at the very least an openness to the transmission of life - is a necessary prerequisite from the moral point of view for responsible human procreation. But this good intention is not sufficient for making a positive moral evaluation of *in vitro* fertilization between spouses. The process of *in vitro* fertilization and embryo transfer must be judged in itself and cannot borrow its definitive moral quality from the totality of conjugal life of which it becomes part nor from the conjugal acts which may precede or follow it.[48]

It has already been recalled that in the circumstances in which it is regularly practiced *in vitro* fertilization and embryo transfer involves the destruction of human beings, which is something contrary to the doctrine on the illicitness of abortion previously mentioned.[49] But even in a situation in which every precaution were taken to avoid the death of human embryos, homologous *in vitro* fertilization and embryo transfer dissociates from the conjugal act the actions which are directed to human fertilization. For this reason the very nature of homologous *in vitro* fertilization and embryo transfer also must be taken into account, even abstracting from the link with procured abortion.

Homologous *in vitro* fertilization and embryo transfer is brought about outside the bodies of the couple through actions of third parties whose competence and technical activity determine the success of the procedure. Such fertilization entrusts the life and identity of the embryo into the power of doctors and biologists and establishes the domination of technology over the origin and destiny of the human person. Such a relationship of domination is in itself contrary to the dignity and equality that must be common to parents and children.

Conception *in vitro* is the result of the technical action which presides over fertilization. *Such fertilization is neither in fact achieved nor positively willed as the expression and fruit of a specific act of the conjugal union. In homologous "in vitro" fertilization and embryo transfer, therefore, even if it is considered in the context of de facto existing sexual relations, the generation of the human person is objectively deprived of its proper perfection: namely, that of being the result and fruit of a conjugal act* in which the spouses can become "cooperators with God for giving life to a new person."[50]

These reasons enable us to understand why the act of conjugal love is considered in the teaching of the church as the only setting worthy of human procreation. For the same reasons the so-called "simple case," i.e., a homologous *in vitro* fertilization and embryo transfer procedure that is free of any compromise with the abortive practice of destroying embryos and with masturbation, remains a technique which is morally illicit because it deprives human procreation of the dignity which is proper and connatural to it.

Certainly, homologous *in vitro* fertilization and embryo transfer fertilization is not marked by all that ethical negativity found in extraconjugal procreation; the family and marriage continue to constitute the setting for the birth and upbringing of the children. Nevertheless, in conformity with the traditional doctrine relating to the goods of marriage and the dignity of the person, *the church remains opposed from the moral point of view to homologous "in vitro" fertilization. Such fertilization is in itself illicit and in opposition to the dignity of procreation and of the conjugal union, even when everything is done to avoid the death of the human embryo.*

Although the manner in which human conception is achieved with *in vitro* fertilization and embryo transfer cannot be approved, every child which comes into the world must in any case be accepted as a living gift of the divine Goodness and must be brought up with love.

6. How is homologous artificial insemination to be evaluated from the moral point of view?

Homologous artificial insemination within marriage cannot be admitted expect for those cases in which the technical means is not a substitute for the conjugal act but serves to facilitate and to help so that the act attains its natural purpose.

The teaching of the magisterium on this point has already been stated.[51] This teaching is not just an expression of particular historical circumstances, but is based on the church's doctrine concerning the connection between the conjugal union and procreation and on a consideration of the personal nature of the conjugal act and of human procreation. "In its natural structure, the conjugal act is a personal action, a simultaneous and immediate cooperation on the part of the husband and wife, which by the very nature of the agents and the proper nature of the act is the expression of the mutual gift which, according to the words of Scripture, brings about union 'in one flesh.'"[53] If the technical means facilitates the conjugal act or helps it to reach its natural objectives, it can be morally acceptable. If, on the other hand, the procedure were to replace the conjugal act, it is morally illicit.

Artificial insemination as a substitute for the conjugal act is prohibited by reason of the voluntarily achieved dissociation of the two meanings of the conjugal act. Masturbation, through which the sperm is normally obtained, is another sign of this dissociation: Even when it is done for the purpose of procreation the act remains deprived of its unitive meaning: "It lacks the sexual relationship called for by the moral order, namely the relationship which realizes 'the full sense of mutual self-giving and human procreation in the context of true love.'"[54]

7. What moral criterion can be proposed with regard to medical intervention in human procreation?

The medical act must be evaluated not only with reference to its technical dimension, but also and above all in relation to its goal, which is the good of persons and their bodily and psychological health. The moral criteria for medical intervention in procreation are deduced from the dignity of human persons, of their sexuality and of their origin.

Medicine which seeks to be ordered to the integral good of the person must respect the specifically human values of sexuality.[55] The doctor is at the service of persons and of human procreation. He does not have the authority to dispose of them or to decide their fate. A medical intervention respects the dignity of persons when it seeks to assist the conjugal act either in order to facilitate its performance or in order to enable it to achieve its objective once it has been normally performed.[56]

On the other hand, it sometimes happens that a medical procedure technologically replaces the conjugal act in order to obtain a procreation which is neither its result nor its fruit. In this case the medical act is not, as it should be, at the service of conjugal union, but rather appropriates to itself the procreative function and thus contradicts the dignity and the inalienable rights of the spouses and of the child to be born.

The humanization of medicine, which is insisted upon today by everyone, requires respect for the integral dignity of the human person first of all in the act and at the moment in which the spouses transmit life to a new person. It is only logical therefore to address an urgent appeal to Catholic doctors and scientists that they bear exemplary witness to the respect due to the human embryo and to the dignity of procreation. The medical and nursing staff of Catholic hospitals and clinics are in a special way urged to do justice to the moral obligations which they have assumed, frequently also, as part of their contract. Those who are in charge of Catholic hospitals and clinics and who are often religious will take special care to safeguard and promote a diligent observance of the moral norms recalled in the present instruction.

8. The suffering caused by infertility in marriage.

The suffering of spouses who cannot have children or who are afraid of bringing a handicapped child into the world is a suffering that everyone must understand and properly evaluate.

On the part of the spouses, the desire for a child is natural: It expresses the vocation to fatherhood and motherhood inscribed in conjugal love. This desire can be even stronger if the couple is affected by sterility which appears incurable. Nevertheless, marriage does not confer upon the spouses the right to have a child, but only the right to perform those natural acts which are per se ordered to procreation.[57]

A true and proper right to a child would be contrary to the child's dignity and nature. The child is not an object to which one has a right nor can he be considered as an object of ownership: Rather, a child is a gift, "the supreme gift"[58] and the most gratuitous gift of marriage, and is a living testimony of the mutual giving of his parents. For this reason, the child has the right as already mentioned, to be the fruit of the specific act of the conjugal love of his parents; and he also has the right to be respected as a person from the moment of his conception.

Nevertheless, whatever its cause or prognosis, sterility is certainly a difficult trial. The community of believers is called to shed light upon and support the suffering of those who are unable to fulfill their legitimate aspiration to motherhood and fatherhood. Spouses who find themselves in this sad situation are called to find in it an opportunity for sharing in a particular way in the Lord's cross, the source of spiritual fruitfulness. Sterile couples must not forget that "even when procreation is not possible, conjugal life does not for this reason lose its value. Physical sterility in fact can be for spouses the occasion for other important services to the life of the human person, for example, adoption, various forms of educational work and assistance to other families and to poor or handicapped children."[59]

Many researchers are engaged in the fight against sterility. While fully safeguarding the dignity of human procreation, some have achieved results which previously seemed unattainable. Scientists therefore are to be encouraged to continue their research with the aim of preventing the causes of sterility and of being able to remedy them so that sterile couples will be able to procreate in full respect for their own personal dignity and that of the child to be born.

III. MORAL AND CIVIL LAW

The Values and Moral Obligations that Civil Legislation Must Respect and Sanction in this Matter

The inviolable right to life of every innocent human individual and the rights of the family and of the institution of marriage constitute fundamental moral values because they concern the natural condition and integral vocation of the human person; at the same time they are constitutive elements of civil society and its order.

For this reason the new technological possibilities which have opened up in the field of biomedicine require the intervention of the political authorities and of the legislator, since an uncontrolled application of such techniques could lead to unforeseeable and damaging consequences for civil society. Recourse to the conscience of each individual and to the self-regulation of researchers cannot be sufficient for ensuring respect for personal rights and public order. If the legislator responsible for the common good were not watchful, he could be deprived of his prerogatives by researchers claiming to govern humanity in the name of the biological discoveries and the alleged "improvement" processes which they would draw from those discoveries. "Eugenism" and forms of discrimination between human beings could come to be legitimized: This would constitute an act of violence and a serious offense to the equality, dignity and fundamental rights of the human person.

The intervention of the public authority must be inspired by the rational principles which regulate the relationships between civil law and moral law. The task of the civil law is to ensure the common good of people through the recognition of and the defense of fundamental rights and through the promotion of peace and of public morality.[60] In no sphere of life can the civil law take the place of conscience or dictate norms concerning things which are outside its competence. It must sometimes tolerate, for the sake of public order, things which it cannot forbid without a greater evil resulting. However, the inalienable rights of the person must be recognized and respected by civil society and the political authority. These human rights depend neither on single individuals nor on parents; nor do they represent a concession made by society and the state: They pertain to human nature and are inherent in the person by virtue of the creative act from which the person took his or her origin.

Among such fundamental rights one should mention in this regard: a) every human being's right to life and physical integrity from the moment of conception until death; b) the rights of the family and of marriage as an institution and, in this area, the child's right to be conceived, brought into the world and brought up by his parents. To each of these two themes it is necessary here to give some further consideration.

In various states certain laws have authorized the direct suppression of innocents: The moment a positive law deprives a category of human beings of the protection which civil legislation must accord them, the state is denying the equality of all before the law. When the state does not place its power at the service of the rights of each citizen, and in particular of the more vulnerable, the very foundations of a state based on law are undermined. The political authority consequently cannot give approval to the calling of human beings into existence through procedures which would expose them to those very grave risks noted previously. The possible recognition by positive law and the political authorities of techniques of artificial transmission of life and the experimentation connected with it would widen the breach already opened by the legalization of abortion.

As a consequence of the respect and protection which must be ensured for the unborn child from the moment of his conception, the law must provide appropriate penal sanctions for every deliberate violation of the child's rights. The law cannot tolerate - indeed it must expressly forbid - that human beings, even at the embryonic stage, should be treated as objects of experimentation, be mutilated or destroyed with the excuse that they are superfluous or incapable of developing normally.

The political authority is bound to guarantee to the institution of the family, upon which society is based, the juridical protection to which it has a right. From the very fact that it is at the service of people, the political authority must also be at the service of the family. Civil law cannot grant approval to techniques of artificial procreation which, for the benefit of third parties (doctors, biologists, economic or governmental powers), take away what is a right inherent in the relationship between spouses; and therefore civil law cannot legalize the donation of gametes between persons who are not legitimately united in marriage.

Legislation must also prohibit, by virtue of the support which is due to the family, embryo banks, post-mortem insemination and "surrogate motherhood."

It is part of the duty of the public authority to ensure that the civil law is regulated according to the fundamental norms of the moral law in matters concernig human rights, human life and the institution of the family. Politicians must commit themselves, through their interventions upon public opinion, to securing in society the widest possible consensus on such essential points and to consolidating this consensus wherever it risks being weakened or is in danger of collapse.

In many countries the legalization of abortion and juridical tolerance of unmarried couples make it more difficult to secure respect for the fundamental rights recalled by this instruction. It is to be hoped that states will not become responsible for aggravating these socially damaging situations of injustice. It is rather to be hoped that nations and states will realize all the cultural, ideological and political implications connected with the techniques of artificial procreation and will find the wisdom and courage necessary for issuing laws which are more just and more respectful of human life and the institution of the family.

The civil legislation of many states confers an undue legitimation upon certain practices in the eyes of many today; it is seen to be incapable of guarantee-

ing that morality which is in conformity with the natural exigencies of the human person and with the "unwritten laws" etched by the Creator upon the human heart. All men of good will must commit themselves, particularly within their professional field and in the exercise of their civil rights, to ensuring the reform of morally unacceptable civil laws and the correction of illicit practices. In addition, "conscientious objection" vis-a-vis such laws must be supported and recognized. A movement of passive resistance to the legitimation of practices contrary to human life and dignity is beginning to make an ever sharper impression upon the moral conscience of many, especially among specialists in the biomedical sciences.

CONCLUSION

The spread of technologies of intervention in the processes of human procreation raises very serious moral problems in relation to the respect due to the human being from the moment of conception, to the dignity of the person, of his or her sexuality and of the transmission of life.

With this instruction the Congregation for the Doctrine of the Faith, in fulfilling its responsibility to promote and defend the church's teaching in so serious a matter, addresses a new and heartfelt invitation to all those who, by reason of their role and their commitment, can exercise a positive influence and ensure that in the family and in society due respect is accorded to life and love. It addresses this invitation to those responsible for the formation of consciences and of public opinion, to scientists and medical professionals, to jurists and politicians. It hopes that all will understand the incompatibility between recognition of the dignity of the human person and contempt for life and love, between faith in the living God and the claim to decide arbitrarily the origin and fate of a human being.

In particular, the Congregation for the Doctrine of the Faith addresses an invitation with confidence and encouragement to theologians, and above all to moralists, that they study more deeply and make ever more accessible to the faithful the contents of the teaching of the church's magisterium in the light of a valid anthropology in the matter of sexuality and marriage and in the context of the necessary interdisciplinary approach. Thus they will make it possible to understand ever more clearly the reasons for and the validity of this teaching. By defending man against the excesses of his own power, the church of God reminds him of the reasons for his true nobility; only in this way can the possibility of living and loving with that dignity and liberty which derive from respect for the truth be ensured for the men and women of tomorrow. The precise indications which are offered in the present instruction therefore are not meant to halt the effort of reflection, but rather to give it a renewed impulse in unrenounceable fidelity to the teaching of the church.

In the light of the truth about the gift of human life and in the light of the moral principles which flow from that truth, everyone is invited to act in the area of responsibility proper to each and, like the Good Samaritan, to recognize as a neighbor even the littlest among the children of men (cf. Lk. 10:29-37). Here Christ's words find a new and particular echo: "What you do to one of the least of my brethren, you do unto me" (Mt. 25:40).

During an audience granted to the undersigned prefect after the plenary session of the Congregation for the Doctrine of the Faith, the supreme pontiff, John Paul II, approved this instruction and ordered it to be published.

Given at Rome, from the Congregation for the Doctrine of the Faith, Feb. 22, 1987, the feast of the chair of St. Peter, the apostle.

Cardinal Joseph Ratzinger
Prefect

Archbishop Alberto Bovone
Secretary

ENDNOTES

[1] Pope John Paul II, Discourses to those taking part in the 81st Congress of the Italian Society of Internal Medicine and the 82nd Congress of the Italian Society of General Surgery, Oct. 27, 1980: AAS 72 (1980) 1126.

[2] Pope Paul VI, Discourse to the General Assembly of the United Nations, Oct. 4, 1965: AAS 57 (1965) 878; encyclical *Populorum Progressio*, 13: AAS 59 (1967) 263.

[3] Ibid., Homily During the Mass Closing the Holy Year, Dec. 25, 1975: AAS 68 (1976) 145; Pope John Paul II, encyclical *Dives in Misericordia*, 30: AAS 72 (1980) 1224.

[4] Pope John Paul II, Discourse to those taking part in the 35th General Assembly of the World Medical Association, Oct. 29, 1983: AAS 76 (1984) 390.

[5] Cf. Declaration *Dignitatis Humanae*, 2.

[6] Pastoral constitution *Gaudium et Spes*, 22; Pope John Paul II, encyclical *Redemptor Hominis*, 8: AAS 71 (1979) 270-272.

[7] Cf. *Gaudium et Spes*, 35.

[8] Ibid., 15; cf. also *Populorum Progressio*, 20: *Redemptor Hominis*, 15: Pope John Paul II, apostolic exhortation *Familiaris Consortio*, 8: AAS 74 (1982) 89.

[9] *Familiaris Consortio*, 11.

[10] Cf. Pope Paul VI, encyclical *Humanae Vitae*, 10: AAS 60 (1986) 487-488.

[11] Pope John Paul II, Discourse to the members of the 35th General Assembly of the World Medical Association, Oct. 29, 1983: AAS 76 (1984) 393.

[12] Cf. *Familiaris Consortio, 11*, Cf. also *Gaudium et Spes*, 50.

[13] Congregation for the Doctrine of the Faith, Declaration on Procured Abortion, 9 AAS 66 (1974) 736-737.

[14] Pope John Paul II, Discourse to those taking part in the 35th General Assembly of the World Medical Association, Oct. 29, 1983: AAS 76 (1984) 390.

[15] Pope John XXIII, encyclical *Mater et Magistra, III:* AAS 53 (1961) 447.

[16] *Gaudium et Spes*, 24.

[17] Cf. Pope Pius XII, encyclical *Humani Generis:* AAS 42 (1950) 575; Pope Paul VI, *Professio Fidei:* AAS 60 (1968) 436.

[18] *Mater et Magistra*, III; cf. Pope John Paul II, Discourse to priests participating in a Seminar on "Responsible Procreation," Sept. 17, 1983, *Insegnamenti di Giovanni Paolo II*, VI, 2 (1983) 562: "At the origin of each human person there is a creative act of God: No man comes into existence by chance; he is always the result of the creative love of God."

[19] Cf. *Gaudium et Spes*, 24.

[20] Cf. Pope Pius XII, Discourse to the St. Luke Medical-Biological Union, Nov. 12, 1944: *Discorsi e Radiomessaggi VI* (1944-1945) 191-192.

[21] Cf. *Gaudium et Spes*, 50.

[22] Cf. Ibid., 51: "When it is a question of harmonizing married love with the responsible transmission of life, the moral character of one's behavior does not depend only on the good intention and the evaluation of the motives: The objective criteria must be used, criteria drawn from the nature of the human person and human acts, criteria which respect the total meaning of mutual self-giving and human procreation in the context of true love."

[23] *Gaudium et Spes*, 51.

[24] Holy See, Charter of the Rights of the Family, 4: L'Osservatore Romano, Nov. 25, 1983.

[25] Congregation for the Doctrine of the Faith, Declaration on Procured Abortion, 12-13.

[26] Cf. Pope Paul VI, Discourse to participants in the 23rd National Congress of Italian Catholic Jurists, Dec. 9, 1972: AAS 64 (1972) 777.

[27]The obligation to avoid disproportionate risks involves an authentic respect for human beings and the uprightness of therapeutic intentions. It implies that the doctor "above all . . . must carefully evaluate the possible negative consequences which the necessary use of a particular exploratory technique may have upon the unborn child and avoid recourse to diagnostic procedures which do not offer sufficient guarantees of their honest purpose and substantial harmlessness. And if, as often happens in human choices, a degree of risk must be undertaken, he will take care to assure that it is justified by a truly urgent need for the diagnosis and by the importance of the results that can be achieved by it for the benefit of the unborn child himself" (Pope John Paul II, Discourse to participants in the Pro-Life Movement Congress, Dec. 3, 1982: *Insegnamenti di Giovanni Paolo II*, V, 3 (1982) 1512). This clarification concerning "proportionate risk" is also to be kept in mind in the following sections of the present instruction, whenever this term appears.

[28]Pope John Paul II, Discourse to the participants in the 35th General Assembly of the World Medical Association, Oct. 29, 1983: AAS 76 (1984) 392.

[29]Cf. Ibid., Address to a meeting of the Pontifical Academy of Sciences, Oct. 23, 1982: AAS 75 (1983) 37: "I condemn, in the most explicit and formal way, experimental manipulations of the human embryo, since the human being, from conception to death, cannot be exploited for any purpose whatsoever."

[30]Charter of the Rights of the Family, 4b.

[31]Cf. Pope John Paul II, Address to the participants in the Pro-Life Movement Congress, Dec. 3, 1982: *Insegnamenti di Giovanni Paolo II*, v, 3 (1982) 1511: "Any form of experimentation on the fetus that may damage its integrity or worsen its condition is unacceptable, expect in the case of a final effort to save it from death." Congregation for the Doctrine of the Faith, Declaration on Euthanasia, 4: AAS 72 (1980) 550: "In the absence of other sufficient remedies, it is permitted, with the patient's consent, to have recourse to the means provided by the most advanced medical techniques, even if these means are still at the experimental stage and are not without a certain risk."

[32]No one, before coming into existence, can claim a subjective right to begin to exist; nevertheless, it is legitimate to affirm the right of the child to have a fully human origin through conception in conformity with the personal nature of the human being. Life is a gift that must be bestowed in a manner worthy both of the subject receiving it and of the subjects transmitting it. This statement is to be borne in mind also for what will be explained concerning artificial human procreation.

[33]Cf. Pope John Paul II, Discourse to those taking part in the 35th General Assembly of the World Medical Association, Oct. 29, 1983: AAS 76 (1984) 391.

[34]Cf. *Gaudium et Spes*, 50.

[35]Cf. *Familiaris Consortio*, 14.

[36]CF. Pope Pius XII, Discourse to those taking part in the Fourth International Congress of Catholic Doctors, Sept. 29, 1949: AAS 41 (1949) 559. According to the plan of the Creator, "a man leaves his father and his mother and cleaves to his wife, and they become one flesh: (Gn. 2:24). The unity of marriage, bound to the order of creation, is a truth accessible to natural reason. The church's tradition and magisterium frequently make reference to the Book of Genesis, both directly and through the passages of the New

Testament that refer to it: Mt. 19:4-6; Mk. 10:5-8, Eph. 5:31. Cf. Athenagoras, *Legatio pro christianis*, 33:PG 6, 965-967; St. Chrysostom, *In Matthaeum homilae*, LXII, 19, 1: PG 58 597; St. Leo the Great, *Epist. ad Rusticum*, 5:PL 54, 1204; Innocent III, Epist. *Gaudemus in Domino: DS 778; Council of Lyons II, IV Session: DS 860; Council of Trent, XXIV Session: DS 1798, 1802; Pope Leo XIII, encyclical Arcanum Divinae Sapientia:* AAS 12 (1879-1880) 388-391; Pope Pius XI, encyclical *Casti Connubii:* AAS 22 (1930) 546-547; *Gaudium et Spes,* 48; *Familiaris Consortio,* 19; Code of Canon Law, Canon 1056.

[37]CF. Pope Pius XII, Discourse to those taking part in the Fourth International Congress of Catholic Doctors, Sept. 29, 1949: AAS 41 (1949) 560; Discourse to those taking part in the Congress of the Italian Catholic Union of Midwives, Oct. 29, 1951: AAS 43 (1951) 850; Code of Canon Law, Canon 1134.

[38]*Humanae Vitae*, 12.

[39]Ibid.

[40]Pope Pius XII, Discourse to those taking part in the Second Naples World Congress on Fertility and Human Sterility, May 19, 1956: AAS 48 (1956) 470.

[41]Code of Canon Law, Canon 1061. According to this canon, the conjugal act is that by which the marriage is consummated if the couple "have performed (it) between themselves in a human manner."

[42]Cf. *Gaudium et Spes*, 14.

[43]Cf. Pope John Paul II, General Audience Jan. 16, 1980: *Insegnamenti di Giovanni Paolo II, III,* 1 (1980) 149-152.

[44]Ibid., Discourse to those taking part in the 35th General Assembly of the World Medical Association, Oct. 29, 1983: AAS 76 (1984) 393.

[45]Cf. *Gaudium et Spes*, 51.

[46]Ibid., 50.

[47]Cf. Pope Pius XII, Discourse to those taking part in the Fourth International Congress of Catholic Doctors, Sept. 29, 1949: AAS 41 (1949) 560: "It would be erroneous . . . to think that the possibility of resorting to this means (artificial fertilization) might render valid a marriage between persons unable to contract it because of the *impedimentum impotentiae*."

[48]A similar question was dealt with by Pope Paul VI, *Humanae Vitae*, 14.

[49]CF. *supra*: I, 1ff.

[50]*Familiaris Consortio*, 14: AAS 74 (1982) 96.

[51]Cf. Response of the Holy Office, March 17, 1897: DS 3323; Pope Pius XII, Discourse to those taking part in the Fourth International Congress of Catholic Doctors, Sept. 29, 1949: AAS 41 (1949) 560; Discourse to the Italian Catholic Union of Midwives, Oct. 29, 1951: AAS 43 (1951) 850; Discourse to those taking part in the Second Naples World Congress on Fertility and Human Sterility, May 19, 1956: AAS, 48 (1956) 471-473; Discourse to those taking part in the Seventh International Congress of the International Society of Hematology, Sept. 12, 1958: AAS 50 (1958) 733; *Mater et Magistra*, III.

[52] Pope Pius XII, Discourse to the Italian Catholic Union of Midwives, Oct. 29, 1951: AAS 43 (1951) 850.

[53] Ibid., Discourse to those taking part in the Fourth International Congress of Catholic Doctors, Sept. 29, 1949: AAS 41 (1949) 560.

[54] Congregation for the Doctrine of the Faith, Declaration on Certain Questions Concerning Sexual Ethics, 9: AAS 68 (1976) 86, which quotes *Gaudium et Spes*, 51. Cf. Decree of the Holy Office, Aug. 2, 1929: AAS 21 (1929) 490; Pope Pius XII, Discourse to those taking part in the 26th Congress of the Italian Society of Urology, Oct. 8, 1953: AAS 45 (1953) 678.

[55] Cf. Pope John XXIII, *Mater et Magistra*, III.

[56] Cf. Pope Pius XII, Discourse to those taking part in the Fourth International Congress of Catholic Doctors, Sept. 29, 1949: AAS 41 (1949), 560.

[57] Cf. Ibid., Discourse to those taking part in the Second Naples World Congress on Fertility and Human Sterility, May 19, 1956: AAS 48 (1956) 471-473.

[58] *Gaudium et Spes*, 50.

[59] *Familiaris consortio*, 14.

[60] Cf. *Dignitatis Humanae*, 7.[*]

[*] *Origins* 16 no. 40 (March 19, 1987): 697-711.

THE POPE'S ADDRESS TO SECOND INTERNATIONAL CONGRESS ON MORAL THEOLOGY

POPE JOHN PAUL II

THE DILIGENT SEARCH FOR TRUTH REQUIRES THE TEACHING OF THE MAGISTERIUM

About 400 theologians took part in the Second International Congress on Moral Theology which was held at the Pontifical Lateran University to mark the twentieth anniversary of Paul VI's Encyclical "Humanae Vitae". The following is the text of the Holy Father's address to them when they were received in audience in the Vatican on Saturday, 12 November.

1. With great joy I address my greetings to all of you who have taken part in the International Congress on Moral Theology which has now reached its conclusion. My greetings include also Cardinal Hans Hermann Groer, Archbishop of Vienna, and the representatives of the Knights of Columbus who, through their generous contribution, have made this Congress possible. A word of appreciation also goes to the Institute for Studies on Marriage and the Family of the Pontifical Lateran University, and to the Roman Academic Centre of the Holy Cross which promoted and were responsible for the Congress.

The theme which has engaged you during these days, dear brothers, and stimulated your deep reflection was the Encyclical *Humanae Vitae* with the complex set of problems connected with it.

As you know, in the last few days, a meeting has taken place, organized by the Pontifical Council for the Family, in which, as representatives of the episcopal conferences of the whole world, bishops took part who are in charge of pastoral care of the family in the respective countries. This by no means fortuitous coincidence immediately offers me the opportunity to stress the importance of collaboration between pastors and theologians and, more generally, between pastors and the world of science, in order to ensure an effective and adequate support for married persons who are committed to fulfilling the divine plan for marriage in their lives.

All are well aware of the explicit invitation in the Encyclical *Humanae Vitae* to all men of science and, in a special way, to Catholic scientists so that through their studies, they may contribute towards clarifying more and more deeply the different conditions which favor a lawful regulation of human procreation (cf. n.24). I, too, have renewed that invitation on various occasions because I am convinced that an interdisciplinary effort is indispensable for an adequate approach to the complex problems pertaining to this delicate area.

2. The second opportunity offered to me is to acknowledge the reassuring results already achieved by many experts who over these years, have furthered research in this matter. Thanks also to their contribution, it has been possible to set out clearly the depth of truth and indeed the enlightening and almost prophetic value of Paul's Encyclical, towards which persons of the most diverse cultural extraction are turning their attention with growing interest.

Some signs of rethinking can also be perceived even in those sectors of the Catholic world which were initially somewhat critical of the important document. Progress in biblical and anthropological reflection has in fact enabled its premises and meaning to be clarified better.

In particular, the witness offered by the bishops in the 1980 Synod must be recalled: "This Sacred Synod, gathered together with the Successor of Peter in the unity of faith, firmly holds what has been set forth in the Second Vatican Council (cf. *Gaudium et Spes, 50)* and afterwards in the Encyclical *Humanae Vitae,* particularly that love between husband and wife must be fully human, exclusive and open to new life (*Humanae Vitae* 11; cf. 9, 12)" (Proposition 22).

I myself then gathered together that witness in the post-Synodal Exhortation *Familiaris Consortio* and, in the broader context of the vocation and mission of the family, I presented the anthropological and moral perspective of *Humanae Vitae,* as well as the resulting ethical norm which must be drawn from it for the lives of married people.

3. It is not, in fact, a doctrine invented by man: it was stamped on the very nature of the human person by God the Creator's hand and confirmed by him in Revelation. Calling it into question, therefore, is equivalent to refusing God himself the obedience of our intelligence. It is equivalent to preferring the dim light of our reason to the light of divine Wisdom, thereby falling into the darkness of error and resulting in the undermining of other fundamental principles of Christian doctrine.

In this regard, it must be remembered that the ensemble of truths entrusted to the ministry of the Church's preaching constitutes a unitary whole, a kind of symphony, as it were, in which each truth is harmoniously integrated with the others. The past twenty years have demonstrated this intimate harmony by the argument from the contrary, that is to say, hesitation and doubt about the moral truth taught in *Humanae Vitae* has also involved other fundamental truths of reason and faith. I know that this fact was the object of careful consideration during your Congress, and I would now like to draw your attention to it.

4. As the Second Vatican Council teaches: "Deep within his conscience man discovers a law which he has not laid upon himself but which he must obey . . .

For man has in his heart a law inscribed by God. His dignity lies in observing this law, and by it he will be judged" (Constitution *Gaudium et Spes. 16*).

During these years, following the contestation about *Humanae Vitae*, the Christian doctrine on moral conscience itself has been questioned by accepting the idea of creative conscience of the moral norm. In this way, that bond of obedience to the holy will of the Creator, in which the very dignity of man consists is radically broken. Conscience, in fact, is the "place" where man is illuminated by a light which does not come to him from his created and always fallible reason, but from the very Wisdom of the Word in whom all things were created. "Conscience", as Vatican II again admirably states, "is man's most secret core, and his sanctuary. There he is alone with God whose voice echoes in his depths." (ibid).

From this some consequences are drawn which are to be stressed.

Since the *Magisterium of the Church* was created by Christ the Lord to enlighten conscience, then to appeal to that conscience precisely to contest the truth of what is taught by the Magisterium implies rejection of the Catholic concept both of the Magisterium and moral conscience. To speak about the inviolable dignity of conscience without further specification, runs the risk of grave errors. There is a great difference between the person who falls into error after having used all the means at his or her disposal in the search for truth, and the situation of one who, either through simple acquiescence to the majority opinion, often deliberately created by the powers of the world, or through negligence, takes little pains to discover the truth. The clear teaching of Vatican II reminds us of this: "Yet it often happens that conscience goes astray through ignorance which it is unable to avoid, without thereby losing its dignity. This cannot be said of the man who takes little trouble to find out what is true and good, or when conscience is by degrees almost blinded through the habit of committing sin" (ibid).

The Church's Magisterium is among the means which Christ's redeeming love has provided to avoid this danger of error. In his name it has a real teaching authority. Therefore, it cannot be said that the faithful have embarked on a diligent search for truth if they do not take into account what the Magisterium teaches, or if, by putting it on the same level as any other source of knowledge, one makes oneself judge, or if in doubt, one follows one's own opinion or that of theologians, preferring it to the sure teaching of the Magisterium.

To continue speaking in this situation about the dignity of conscience without adding anything else does not correspond to what is taught by Vatican II and by the whole Tradition of the Church.

THE MORAL NORM OF "HUMANAE VITAE" DOES NOT ADMIT EXCEPTIONS

5. Closely connected with the theme of moral conscience is *the theme of the binding force of the moral norm taught by Humanae Vitae*.

By describing the contraceptive act as intrinsically illicit, Pope Paul VI meant to teach that the moral norm is such that it does not admit exceptions. No personal or social circumstances could ever, can now, or will ever, render such an act lawful in itself. The existence of particular norms regarding man's way of acting in the world, which are endowed with a binding force that excludes always and in whatever situation the possibility of exceptions, is a constant teaching of Tradition and of the Church's Magisterium which cannot be called in question by the Catholic theologian.

Here *a central point* of Christian doctrine concerning God and man is involved. If one looks closely at what is being questioned by rejecting that teaching, one sees that *it is the very idea of the Holiness of God.* In predestining us to be holy and immaculate in his sight, he created us "in Christ Jesus for good works . . . that we should walk in them" (Eph. 2:10). Those moral norms are simply the demand--from which no historical circumstance can dispense--of the Holiness of God which is shared in the *concrete*, no longer in the abstract, with the individual human person.

Furthermore, such negation *renders the Cross of Christ meaningless* (cf. 1 Cor. 1:17). By becoming incarnate, the Word entered fully into our daily existence which consists of concrete human acts. By dying for our sins, he recreated us in the original holiness which must be expressed in our daily activity in the world.

Moreover, such negation implies, as a logical consequence, that there is no truth about man which is outside the course of historical evolution. To render void the Mystery of God results, as always, in rendering void the mystery of man, and the non-recognition of God's rights results, as always, in the negation of man's dignity.

6. The Lord grants us the celebration of this anniversary so that each one may examine himself before God and pledge himself for the future, according to his ecclesial responsibility to defend and deepen the ethical truth taught in *Humanae Vitae*.

Your responsibility in this area, dear professors of moral theology, is great. Who can measure the influence your teaching will exercise both in the formation of the faithful's conscience and in the formation of the future pastors of the Church? During the course of these twenty years, unfortunately, there have been forms of open dissent from what Paul VI taught in his Encyclical, on the part of a certain number of professors.

This anniversary can provide the impulse for a courageous rethinking of the reasons which led those scholars to adopt such positions. Then it will probably be discovered that, at the root of the "opposition" to *Humanae Vitae*, there is an erroneous or at least an insufficient understanding of the very foundations on which moral theology rests. The uncritical acceptance of postulates pertaining to some philosophical views, and the unilateral "utilization" of data offered by science may have led astray some interpreters of the papal document, despite good intentions. A generous effort is required from all in order to clarify better the basic principles of moral theology, taking care--as the Council recommended--that "its scientific presentation should draw more fully on the teaching of holy Scripture and should throw light upon the exalted vocation of the believers in Christ and their obligation to bring forth fruit in charity for the life of the world" (*Optatam Totus, 16*).

7. In this undertaking a notable impulse can come from the Pontifical Institute for Studies on Marriage and the Family, whose objective is precisely that "the truth about marriage and family may be given ever closer attention and study", and to offer the possibility to lay people, religious and priests "to receive scholarly formation in the study of marriage and the family both in the philosophical-theological and in the human sciences", so as to make them competent to work effectively in the service of the pastoral care of the family (cf. Apostolic Constitution *Magnum Matrimonii, 3*).

However, if the moral issue related to *Humanae Vitae* and *Familiaris Consortio* is to find its correct place in that important sector of the Church's work and mission, which is the pastoral care of the family, and encourage the responsible response of lay people, the protagonists of an ecclesial action, that concerns them directly, then Institutes like this one will have to be established in various countries. Only in this way will it be possible to make progress in in-depth study of the truth, and provide for initiatives of a pastoral nature adequate to the emerging needs in the different cultural and human environments.

Above all, the teaching of moral theology in seminaries and institutes of formation must conform to the directives of the Magisterium so that they may produce ministers of God who "shall speak as with one voice" (HV, 28) and "omit nothing from the saving doctrine of Christ" (HV, 29). This concerns the sense of responsibility of professors, who must be the first to give their students the example of "that sincere obedience, inward as well as outward, which is due to the Magisterium of the Church" (HV, 28).

8. Seeing so many young students--priests and others--present at this meeting, I wish to conclude with a special greeting addressed to them.

One of the great experts of the human heart, St. Augustine, wrote: "Our freedom consists in our subjection to the truth" (*De libero arbitrio, 2, 13, 37*). Always seek the truth; venerate the truth discovered; obey the truth. There is no joy beyond this search, this veneration and obedience.

In this wonderful adventure of your spirit, the Church is not an obstacle to you: on the contrary, she is a help. By departing from the Magisterium, you risk the vanity of error and the slavery of opinions: they are seemingly strong but, in reality, fragile because only the Truth of the Lord remains forever.

In invoking divine help for your noble work as seekers of truth and its apostles. I wholeheartedly impart my Blessing to all.[*]

[*] This article is a translation taken from the English edition. *L'Osservatore Romano* no. 51-52 (19-26 December, 1988): 6-7.

ON THE DOCTRINAL AUTHORITY OF "DONUM VITAE"

POPE JOHN PAUL II

Almost two years after the publication of the *Instruction on Respect for Human Life in it Origins and on the Dignity of Procreation* of 22 February 1987, the theological debate aimed at deepening its principles and arguments continues with growing interest. Studies, essays, reviews, and comments published in the Catholic and non-Catholic world number well over a hundred. Meanwhile, bio-medical research in the field of assisted procreation continues its apparently relentless course, refining ever more the techniques already tested and proposing new methods, with the intention of overcoming the problems and negative consequences encountered up to this point.

The Church's intervention, "inspired . . . by the love which she owes to man, helping him to recognize and respect his rights and duties" *(Donum vitae*, Introduction, 1), continues however, to meet determined resistance in the widespread technological and efficiency mentality that cannot be convinced how it could not be licit to use a technology that has already succeeded in producing several hundred human beings.

The impact of the successes obtained and widely publicized indeed has a dazzling effect, to the point that many are not able to understand adequately the inhuman logic of the fabricated child. Thus it happens that even among those who admit that not everything technologically possible is automatically acceptable from the moral point of view, there are those who candidly ask what is wrong in the attempt to obtain human conception in a manner other than the sexual union of a man and woman.

The hesitations and clash of opinions in the Catholic world have also contributed to make this question still more complex. Most of all, we cannot underrate the seriousness of the decision of some Catholic university clinics to continue, under certain conditions, the practice of homologous *in vitro* fertilization. After the clear condemnation contained in the document of the Congregation for the Doctrine of the Faith, such a decision, since it has been made public, has also become a challenge.

Those responsible for this most serious rebellion, although it was probably not within their intentions, now seek to justify themselves, claiming to respect the *Roman Instruction,* but not to understand the reasons and therefore, to be unable to achieve the certainty of conscience about the illicit nature of the use of homologous FIVET which they consider necessary before suspending the use of such a technique.

Even in these difficult circumstances there have not however been lacking those who have promptly and courageously expressed their clear adherence to he teaching of *Donum vitae,* thus pointing out that the case was all the more serious in that it implied public opposition to the Church's Magisterium. Indeed, the question could not be interpreted merely as an attempt to form a personal judgment of conscience in regard to a practical decision. The statements of the authorities of some universities, reported by the mass media, constitute rather the elaboration of a moral doctrine that holds as licit under certain conditions precisely what the Church's Magisterium has declared illicit under the same conditions. Such doctrinal dissent is therefore contrary to the right ordering of Catholic communion (cf. CIC 754).

Perhaps foreseeing these and other difficulties, the final part of *Donum vitae* contained "an invitation with confidence and encouragement to theologians and above all to moralists, that they study more deeply and make ever more accessible to the faithful the contents of the teaching of the Church's Magisterium" *(Donum vitae,* Conclusion). These words certainly reflect a deep-felt and realistic concern not about the logical clarity of the proposed argumentation, nor even less about the truth of the preceding magisterial teaching, but about the readiness to accept its teaching in the individual and most varied circumstances. This concern is well founded if one thinks of the recent history, known to all, of the reception of other documents of the Roman Magisterium on similar subjects, from the Encyclical *Humanae Vitae,* whose twentieth anniversary we commemorate this year, to the letter "On the Pastoral Care of Homosexual Persons" published on 1 October 1986.

However, the appeal quoted above also reveals a deep awareness on the part of the Magisterium of having reproposed in an explicit, organic, and authoritative manner, doctrinal points--on the dignity of the person, the value of human life, and the nobility of conjugal love--the teaching of which seems to be absolutely essential to the accomplishment of the Church's salvific mission. The Church feels, perhaps as never before, the responsibility, not only for the eternal salvation of the person, but also for the temporal common good from the point of view of conscience. This common good is indeed seriously endangered, both by the arms race as well as by the frenzy of an ever greater domination over mankind which occurs through the control and technological manipulation of the very sources of life. Thus, as contraception ended up by promoting abortion, it is becoming evident that artificial procreation posits the operative premises for a discriminatory cultural choice in regard to the children procreated (eugenics).

The *Instruction on Respect for Human Life in Its Origins and the Dignity of Procreation* could not have chosen a more meaningful title. However, it seems that some people have not realized that, perhaps unilaterally struck by the document's severe condemnation in regard to the techniques of artificial procreation most extolled by the media. *Donum vitae,* indeed, being the up-to-date expression of Catholic doctrine, condemns heterologous artificial fertilization--that is, with the use of gametes obtained from a third person--in that it is "contrary to the unity of marriage, to the dignity of the spouses, to the vocation proper to parents, and to the child's right to be conceived and brought into the world in marriage and from marriage" *(Donum vitae,* Part II, 2). For the same reasons surrogate motherhood is also declared illicit.

As for homologous artificial fertilization and insemination, although recognizing that they are not marked by "all that ethical negativity found in extra-conjugal procreation" *(Donum vitae,* Part II, 5), nevertheless the fact that the conception occurs in virtue of technological intervention, objectively results in the fact that the procreation of the human person--independently of the intentions of the spouses and doctors--is not the outcome and result of a conjugal act. In consequence it is separated from its most natural and specific perfection, since sexual union is the way chosen by God so that spouses may cooperate with him in the transmission of life for new human persons.

For this reason the *Instruction* unhesitatingly declares that "the Church remains opposed from the moral point of view, to homologous *in vitro* fertilization. Such fertilization is in itself illicit and in opposition to the dignity of procreation and of the conjugal union, even when everything is done to avoid the death of the human embryo" *(Donum vitae,* Part II, 5).

The *Instruction of the Congregation for the Doctrine of the Faith* profoundly and radically draws attention to the intimate connection between conjugal love and the begetting of children, between human and divine fertility. Human procreation cannot be considered merely as a physiological consequence, as it were, of love, but as something that is dynamically a part of the spousal giving and which therefore participates in the two-fold corporal and spiritual dimension of the human persons.

Truth to tell, such an affirmation--reproposed in the historic moment in which *procreation without sexual intercourse* has become a reality--cannot be considered as absolutely new. It is found in the Church's doctrinal tradition and has been recalled several times in this century by the papal Magisterium. *Donum vitae* most opportunely, in its conclusion, points out that "the precise indications which are offered in this present *Instruction* therefore are not meant to halt the effort of reflection, but rather to give it a renewed impulse" *(Donum vitae,* Conclusion), but immediately adds "in unrenounceable fidelity to the teaching of the Church" (ibid.).

If one departs from this principle of good theological methodology, and assumes a position contrary to a moral doctrine already unequivocally and authoritatively proposed by the Church's Magisterium, then one is confronted with the dilemma: either one does not recognize the specific jurisdiction of the Magisterium in *re morali,* or one does not accept the magisterial character of the document in question. Now, the first alternative is clearly in error, on the basis of what the same Magisterium has declared several times concerning its own authority in *moribus* (Vatican Council II, *Lumen Gentium*, n. 25; Paul VI, *Humanae Vitae*, n. 4; Congregation for the Doctrine of the Faith, *Mysterium Ecclesiae*, 24 June 1973: AAS 65 [1973], p. 401), and it is theologically certain that the Magisterium is competent to judge whether or not a matter falls within the sphere of its competence.

As for the second possibility, the magisterial nature of the *Instruction on Respect for Human Life in Its Origin and on the Dignity of Procreation* is inferred both from its form and its contents. *Donum vitae* is indeed a document of a doctrinal nature on moral questions, approved by the Pope and legitimately published by the Congregation for the Doctrine of the Faith. In fact, it is written in it that "during an audience granted to the undersigned Prefect after the plenary session of the Congregation for the Doctrine of the Faith, the Supreme Pontiff, John Paul II, approved this *Instruction*, and ordered it to be published" (*Donum vitae*, Conclusion).

The Congregation for the Doctrine of the Faith is the first among the Congregations which constitute the Roman Curia, through which "the Supreme Pontiff usually conducts the business of the universal Church . . . and which fulfills its duty in his name and by his authority for the good and service of the Churches" (CIC, 360). To it particularly belongs the safeguarding of the doctrine of faith and morals. It is also "in filling its responsibility to promote and defend the Church's teaching" *(Donum vitae*, Conclusion), that it has drafted the document, signed by the Prefact of the Congregation, Cardinal Ratzinger, as well as by the Secretary, Archbishop Bovone.

The style of *Donum vitae* also corresponds to a document of the authentic Magisterium: it continually speaks in the Church's name and with her authority (e.g., these significant expressions are used: *the Church's intervention,* [Introduction, 1]; *the Church once more puts forward* [ibid.]; *the Church offers* [Introduction, 5]; *the Church remains opposed* [Part 2, 5]; *the Church reminds . . . [man].* [Conclusion]) and, from the very foreword declares that it "does not intend to repeat all the Church's teaching on the dignity of human life as it originates and on procreation, but to offer in the light of the previous teaching of the Magisterium, some specific replies to the main questions being asked in this regard" *(Donum Vitae*, Foreword). In fact, as we pointed out before, the previous teaching is continually recalled, thus consolidating a continuous and homogenous doctrinal line.

In this sense, two statements in the Introduction appear particularly significant. "The Church's Magisterium", says *Donum Vitae*, thereby specifying its own magisterial nature, "does not intervene on the basis of a particular competence in the sphere of the experimental sciences; but having taken account of the data of research and technology, it intends to put forward, by virtue of its evangelical mission and apostolic duty, the moral teaching corresponding to the dignity of the person and to his or her integral vocation" (*Donum vitae*, Introduction, 1).

A little further on the document's ultimate scope is indicated: "The Church once more puts forward the divine law in order to accomplish the work of truth and liberation" (*Donum vitae,* Introduction, 1), that is, because promoting respect for the moral norms proposed forms an essential part of her salvific mission.

At this point one cannot therefore see how one can objectively deny to the *Instruction on Respect for Human Life in Its Origin and on the Dignity of Procreation* the obedience of judgement and practice that the faithful are obliged to give to the legitimate authority of the Church when she proposes doctrine or proscribes erroneous opinions (cf. CIC, 754).[*]

---

[*] This article is a translation taken from the English edition. *L'Osservatore Romano* no. 4 (23 January, 1989): 8-9.

EASTER'S GIFT OF LIFE

POPE JOHN PAUL II

"Grant that the man of the technological age may not reduce himself to a mere object, but may respect from its very beginning the unrenounceable dignity that is proper to him." Pope John Paul II said on Easter, April 19. In his "urbi et orbi" message - to the city and the world - given in St. Peter's Square, he called for a rediscovery of "life as the gift which in all its manifestations reveals the Father's love." Do not let "reverent wonder at the mystery of love" surrounding the Lord's coming into the world die out in contemporary society, he exhorted those who heard his message. The Vatican's English text of the message follows.

1. *"Victimae paschali laudes immolent Christiani."* "Praise and glory to the paschal victim, Christians." Let us join together in this hymn! Christians of Rome and of the world! Let us join together in adoration of the paschal victim, in adoration of the risen Lord!

2. *"Agnus redemit oves":* "The sheep are ransomed by the Lamb; and Christ, the undefiled, has reconciled sinners to his Father."

Behold Christ! Behold our Redeemer! The Redeemer of the world! He has given his life for the sheep. Let us join together in adoration of that death which brings us life, for love is more powerful than death: See how the death accepted out of love conquers death! See how the death accepted out of love reveals God, the lover of life, who wishes us to have life and to have it abundantly (cf. Ja. 10:10)--to have the same life that is in him.

To the paschal victim all glory and highest praise! In his death there is reconciliation with the Father. This is the reconciliation of sinners with God, the reconciliation of man, who because of sin dies to God and no longer has in himself the life which is in God and only in God. In God alone.

The death of Christ is a new beginning. The beginning of life which has no end. It is without end because it is of God and in God. Although the creature dies, God lives! When Christ dies, all of creation is reborn; blessed are you, life-giving death! Blessed is the day given us by the Lord.

3. Blessed are you, O Christ, Son of the living God! Blessed are you, Son of Man, son of Mary, blessed because you entered the history of man and of the world, even to the boundaries of death: *"Mors et vita duello conflixere mirando":* "Death with life contended: Combat strangely ended! Life's own champion, slain, yet lives to reign."

Yes, the history of man and of the world is marked by the mystery of death, marked with the stamp of dying, from end to end. You have taken this stamp upon yourself, eternally begotten Son, Son consubstantial with the Father: Life from life, and you have carried it through the boundaries of death, the death which oppresses creation, through the boundaries of our human death, in order to reveal in that death the Spirit who gives life.

4. All of us who came into the world bearing death within us, we who are born of our earthly mothers marked by the inevitability of dying, live by the power of the Spirit. And in the power of this Spirit, who is given to us by the Father, by the power of your death, O Christ, we cross the boundaries of the death that is in us, and we rise from sin to the life revealed in your resurrection!

You are the Lord of life, you who are consubstantial with the Father, who is life itself, together with you, in the Holy Spirit who is love itself--and truly love is life! In your death, O Christ, death appeared defenseless before love. And life triumphed. *"Mors et vita duello conflixere mirando dux vitae mortuus, regnat vivus."*

5. You who are the Risen One and "live to reign" forever, remain at the side of man, the man of today whom death, with its dark allure, in a thousand ways tempts and seeks to ensnare. Grant that man may rediscover life as the gift which in all its manifestations reveals the Father's love: when it is poured into those who are reborn at the baptismal font, or courses through every fiber of the body that moves, breathes and rejoices; when it reveals itself in the vast variety of the animal world or clothes the land with trees, grass and flowers. Every form of life has its inexhaustible source in your Father. From him it flows without ceasing, and to him it inevitably returns; to him, the generous giver of every perfect gift (cf. Jas. 1:17).

6. In God the life of the human being has its eternal source in a unique way, the human being whom he himself fashions in his own image when he quickens in the mother's womb. May reverent wonder for the mystery of love that surrounds his coming into the world not die out in contemporary man! We beseech you, Lord of the living! Grant that the man of the technological age may not reduce himself to a mere object, but may respect, from its very beginning, the unrenounceable dignity that is proper to him. Grant that, in harmony with the divine plan, he may live according to the only way worthy of him, the way of giving, from person to person, in a context of love expressed through the flesh in an act which from the very beginning God willed as a seal of the giving.

Grant, O Lord, that people may always respect the transcendent dignity of all their fellow human beings, whether they be poor or hungry, imprisoned, sick, dying, wounded in body or mind, beset by doubt or tempted to despair. They always remain children of God, for God's gift knows no regrets. Everyone is offered forgiveness and resurrection. Each one deserves respect and support. Deserves love.

8. *"Dic nobis Maria, quid vidisti via":* "Tell us, Mary, what you have seen upon the way." Visiting the tomb at dawn on the third day, the place where he was buried, tell us, Mary of Magdala, you who loved so much. Behold, you found the tomb empty: *"Sepulcrum Christi viventis, et gloriam vidi resurgentis"* The Lord lives! I have seen the Risen One. *"Angelicos testes, sundarium et vestes."* Who could testify to this? What human tongue? Only the angels could explain the meaning of that empty tomb and discarded shroud. The Lord lives! I have seen his glory, full of grace and truth (cf. Jn. 1:14). I have seen the glory. *"Surrexit Christus Spes mea":* Christ, my hope, has risen: He goes before you into Galilee."

9. Yes, first of all there, in the land which gave him as Son of Man. In the land of his infancy and youth. In the land of the hidden life. First of all there, in Galilee to meet the apostles. And then . . . and then, through the testimony of the apostles, in so many places, among so many nations, peoples and races!

Today the voice of this Easter message, echoing in Jerusalem at the empty tomb, seeks to reach everyone: *"Scimus Christum Surresisse a mortuis vere."* Yes, we are certain of it: Christ is truly risen.

"And you, victorious king, your salvation bring us." Amen, alleluia!*

*Origins 17 no. 46 (April 30, 1987): 804-805.

HEALTH CARE: MINISTRY IN TRANSITION

POPE JOHN PAUL II

Dear brothers and sisters, leaders in Catholic health care,

1. In the joy and peace of our Lord Jesus Christ I greet you and thank you for your warm welcome. This meeting gives us the opportunity to honor and give thanks to God for one of the most extensive and fundamental works of the Catholic Church in the United States--all that is embraced in the term "Catholic health care." I am pleased to be able to express to you who represent so many of your country's health care organizations the esteem, support and solidarity of the whole church. In you, Jesus Christ continues his healing ministry, "curing the people of every disease and illness" (cf. Mt. 4:23).

This is the high dignity to which you and your collegues are called. This is your vocation, your commitment and the path of your specific witness to the presence of God's kingdom in the world. Your health care ministry, pioneered and developed by congregations of women religious and by congregations of brothers, is one of the most vital apostolates of the ecclesial community and one of the most significant services which the Catholic Church offers to society in the name of Jesus Christ. I have been told that membership in the Catholic Health Association extends to 620 hospitals and 300 long-term care facilities; that Catholic hospital beds number 11 percent of the total number in the country; that Catholic institutions administer approximately 17 percent of the health care throughout the nation, and that they cared for nearly 46 million people last year. I am grateful to Sister Mary Eileen Wilhelm and to your president, Mr. Curley, for illustrating to us this immense network of Christian service.

2. Because of your dedication to caring for the sick and the poor, the aged and the dying, you know from your own daily experience how much illness and suffering are basic problems of human existence. When the sick flocked to Jesus during his earthly life, they recognized in him a friend whose deeply compassionate and loving heart responded to their needs. He restored physical and mental health to many. These cures, however, involved more than just healing sickness. They were also prophetic signs of his own identity and of the coming of the kingdom of God, and they very often caused a new spiritual awakening in the one who had been healed.

The power that went out from Jesus and cured people of his own time (cf. Lk. 6:19) has not lost its effect in the 2,000 year history of the church. This power remains, in the life and prayer of the church, a source of healing and reconciliation. Ever active, this power confirms the identity of the church today, authenticates her proclamation of the kingdom of God and stands as a sign of triumph over evil.

With all Catholic health care, the immediate aim is to provide for the well-being of the body and mind of the human person, especially in sickness or old age. By his example, Christ teaches the Christian "to do good by his or her suffering and to do good to those who suffer" (John Paul II, Apostolic Exhortation on Human Suffering, 30). This later aspect naturally absorbs the greater part of the energy and attention of health care ministry.

Today in the United States Catholic health care extends the mission of the church in every state of the union, in major cities, small towns, rural areas, on the campuses of academic institutions, in remote outposts and in inner-city neighborhoods. By providing health care in all these places, especially to the poor, the neglected, the needy, the newcomer, your apostolate penetrates and transforms the very fabric of American society. And sometimes you yourselves, like those you serve, are called to bow, in humble and loving resignation, to the experience of sickness--or to other forms of pain and suffering.

3. All concern for the sick and suffering is part of the church's life and mission. The church has always understood herself to be charged by Christ with the care of the poor, the weak, the defenseless, the suffering and those who mourn. This means that as you alleviate suffering and seek to heal you also bear witness to the Christian view of suffering and to the meaning of life and death as taught by your Christian faith.

In the complex world of modern health care in industrialized society, this witness must be given in a variety of ways. First, it requires continual efforts to ensure that everyone has access to health care. I know that you have already examined this question in the report of your task force on health care of the poor. In seeking to treat patients equally, regardless of social and economic status, you proclaim to your fellow citizens and to the world Christ's special love for the neglected and powerless. This particular challenge is a consequence of your Christian dedication and conviction, and it calls for great courage on the part of Catholic bodies and institutions operating in the field of health care. It is a great credit to your zeal and efficiency when, despite formidable costs, you still succeed in preventing the economic factor from being the determinant factor in human and Christian service.

Similarly, the love with which Catholic health care is performed and its professional excellence have the value of a sign testifying to the Christian view of the human person. The inalienable dignity of every human being is, of course, fundamental to all Catholic health care. All who come to you for help are worthy of respect and love, for all have been created in the image and likeness of God. All have been redeemed by Christ and, in their sufferings, bear his cross. It is fitting that our meeting is taking place on the feast of the Triumph of the Cross. Christ took upon himself the whole of human suffering and radically transformed it through the pascal mystery of his passion, death and resurrection. The triumph of the cross gives human suffering a new dimension, a redemptive value (cf. ibid., 24). It is your privilege to bear constant witness to this profound truth in so many ways.

The structural changes which have been taking place within Catholic health care in recent years have increased the challenge of preserving and even strengthening the Catholic identity of the institutions and the spiritual quality of the services given. The presence of dedicated women and men religious in hospitals and nursing homes has ensured in the past, and continues to ensure in the present, that spiritual dimension so characteristic of Catholic health care centers. The reduced number of religious and new forms of ownership and management should not lead to a loss of a spiritual atmosphere or to a loss of a sense of vocation in caring for the sick. This is an area in which the Catholic laity, at all levels of health care, have an opportunity to manifest the depth of their faith and to play their own specific part in the church's mission of evangelization and service.

4. As I have said, Catholic health care must always be carried out within the framework of the church's saving mission. This mission she has received from her divine founder; and she has accomplished it down through the ages with the help of the Holy Spirit, who guides her into the fullness of truth (cf. Jn. 16:13; Dogmatic Constitution on the Church, 4). Your ministry therefore must also reflect the mission of the church as the teacher of moral truth, especially in regard to the new frontiers of scientific research and technological achievement. Here too you face great challenges and opportunities.

Many times in recent years the church has addressed issues related to the advances of biomedical technology. She does so not in order to discourage scientific progress or to judge harshly those who seek to extend the frontiers of human knowledge and skills, but in order to affirm the moral truths which must guide the application of this knowledge and skill. Ultimately, the purpose of the church's teaching in this field is to defend the innate dignity and fundamental rights of the human person. In this regard the church cannot fail to emphasize the need to safeguard the life and integrity of the human embryo and fetus.

5. The human person is a unique composite--a unity of spirit and matter, soul and body, fashioned in the image of God and destined to live forever. Every human life is sacred, because every human person is sacred. It is in the light of this fundamental truth that the church constantly proclaims and defends the dignity of human life from the moment of conception to the moment of natural death. It is also in the light of this fundamental truth that we see the great evil of abortion and euthanasia.

Not long ago, in its' *Instruction on Respect for Human Life in Its Origin and on the Dignity of Procreation,* the Congregation for the Doctrine of the Faith once more dealt with certain vital questions concerning the human person.

Once more it defended the sanctity of innocent human life from the moment of conception onward. Once again it affirmed the sacred and inviolable character of the transmission of human life by the procreative act within marriage. It explained that new technologies may afford new means of procreation, but "what is technically possible is not for that very reason morally admissible" (Introduction, 4). To place new human knowledge at the service of the integral well-being of human persons does not inhibit true scientific progress but liberates it. The church encourages all genuine advances in knowledge, but she also insists on the sacredness of human life at every stage and in every condition. The cause she serves is the cause of human life and human dignity.

6. In the exercise of your professional activities you have a magnificent opportunity, by your constant witness to moral truth, to contribute to the formation of society's moral vision. As you give the best of yourselves in fulfilling your Christian responsibilities, you will also be aware of the important contribution you must make to building a society based on truth and justice. Your service to the sick enables you with great credibility to proclaim to the world the demands and values of the Gospel of Jesus Christ, and to foster hope and renewal of heart. In this respect, your concern with the Catholic identity of your work and of your institutions is not only timely and commendable, it is essential for the success of your ecclesial mission.

You must always see yourselves and your work as part of the church's life and mission. You are indeed a very special part of the people of God. You and your institutions have precise responsibilities toward the ecclesial community, just as that community has responsibilities toward you. It is important at every level-- national, state and local--that there be close and harmonious links between you and the bishops, who "preside in place of God over the flock whose shepherds they are, as teachers of doctrine, priests of sacred worship and officers of good order" (Dogmatic Constitution on the Church, 20). They, for their part, wish to support you in your witness and service.

7. I have come here today to encourage you in your splendid work and to confirm you in your vital apostolate. Dear brothers and sisters: For your dedication to meeting the health care needs of all people, especially the poor, I heartily congratulate you. You embody the legacy of those pioneering women and men religious who selflessly responded to the health care needs of a young and rapidly expanding country by developing an extensive network of clinics, hospitals and nursing homes.

Today you are faced with new challenges, new needs. One of these is the present crisis of immense proportions which is that of AIDS and AIDS-related complex. Besides your professional contribution and your human sensitivities toward all affected by this disease, you are called to show the love and compassion of Christ and his church. As you courageously affirm and implement your moral obligation and social responsibility to help those who suffer, you are individually and collectively living out the parable of the good Samaritan (cf. Lk. 10:30-32).

The good Samaritan of the parable showed compassion to the injured man. By taking him to the inn and giving of his own materials means, he truly gave of himself. This action, a universal symbol of human concern, has become one of the essential elements of moral culture and civilization. How beautifully the Lord speaks of the Samaritan! He "was neighbor to the man who fell in with the robbers" (Lk. 10:36). To be "neighbor" is to express love, solidarity and service, and to exclude selfishness, discrimination and neglect. The message of the parable of the good Samaritan echoes a reality connected with today's feast of the Triumph of the Cross: "The kindness and love of God our Savior appeared . . . that we might be justified by his grace and become heirs, in hope, of eternal life" (Ti. 3:4-7). In the changing world of health care, it is up to you to ensure that this "kindness and love of God our Savior" remains the heart and soul of Catholic health services.

Through prayer and with God's help, may you persevere in your commitment, providing professional assistance and selfless personal care to those who need your services. I pray that your activities and your whole lives will inspire and help all the people of America, working together, to make this society a place of full and absolute respect for the dignity of every person from the moment of conception to the moment of natural death. And may God, in whom we live and move and have our being" (Acts 17:28), sustain you by his grace. God bless you and your families and your contribution to America!*

*Origins 17 n.17 (October 8, 1987): 291-294.

PROMOTE AN AUTHENTIC CIVILIZATION OF LIFE

POPE JOHN PAUL II

The necessity and urgency to promote a "civilization of life" was stressed by the Pope during the audience on Friday, 10 June, to those taking part in the Plenary Assembly of the Pontifical Council for the Family. The following is a translation of the discourse which was delivered in French.

Your Eminence,
Dear Brothers in the Episcopate,
Dear Friends,

1. I am pleased to receive you here during these days in which you are meeting in Plenary Assembly. I greet all the Members, and especially those who are taking part for the first time in the work of the Pontifical Council for the Family and are thereby taking up a new form of responsibility for pastoral care of the family.

You have chosen for the central theme of your reflections, "The Family in the Mission of the Laity", with a special reference to a "pro-life civilization". This theme links the last Synod of Bishops with the 1980 Synod on the Family. For my part, I would like to stress the importance of the family in civil society as well as in the Church, the family which lay people constitute and defend, the family which is responsible for the evangelization of the new generations.

2. In reflecting on the vocation and mission of the laity in the Church and in the world, the last Synod of Bishops studied the teaching of the Second Vatican Council in depth and analyzed the ecclesial experiences of the last two decades. Two important aspects of the laity's vocation were emphasized; the laity's active and responsible belonging to the common mission of the Church, and the personal call to holiness which is addressed to everyone.

A great deal has been done during these years to make the Conciliar teachings known. It is necessary to continue studying them and making all the faithful aware of the essential aspects of their vocation. Our configuration to Christ --the fact that we have been baptized and are all children of God--is the common basis of the diversity of functions which fall upon the members of the People of God under the influence of the Holy Spirit. The mission of the laity in the Church is exercised not only within ecclesial structures. Faithful lay people, the salt of the earth and light of the world, contribute toward "transfiguring the whole of existence through the dynamism of grace and freedom" (cf. John Paul II, *Angelus*, 1 March 1988).

The family is a privileged area in which the Christian laity must "seek the kingdom of God by engaging in temporal affairs and directing them according to God's will" *(Lumen Gentium, 31)*. The family is the natural source from which a pro-life civilization springs, the centre where all the values that protect life converge, and the basic social unity of all civilization at the service of life.

3. From the fact that the family is the primordial cell of society and of the Church, all Christians participate in one way or another in this institution. Furthermore, the sacrament of marriage sanctifies Christians' mutual conjugal self-giving and confirms them in their role as fathers and mothers. These are the created realities which the Church's Magisterium has the mission of clarifying in the light of Christian Revelation. The exercise of the Church's Magisterium in a sphere so important for society and for the Church of Christ herself constitutes one of the bishops' ongoing pastoral concerns. The place which the Second Vatican Council gave to marriage and the family attests to this. For the subsequent period, it is well to recall what the reflection of the 1980 Synod and the doctrine presented in the Apostolic Exhortation *Familiaris Consortio* have been for the Church. Particular attention is to be given to Paul VI's Encyclical *Humanae Vitae,* of which the twentieth anniversary is being celebrated, and which represents and continues to represent a resolute "Yes" to life, to the Creator, a positive acceptance of the laws he has given to humanity for transmitting and protecting life.

4. Marriage and the family, however, are not exclusively Christian institutions. They belong to the heritage which God gave to humanity: "God created man in the image of himself, in the image of God he created him, male and female he created them" (Gen. 1:27). These natural realities were established and structured according to laws and values that, far from limiting and restricting human freedom, permit personal and social progress.

With the awareness that the sacrament of marriage elevates and sanctifies these realities of nature, Christians must appreciate and recognize the values which are at the basis of the great mystery of conjugal love between the spouses. In fact, as the Second Vatican Council recalls: "All that goes to make up the temporal order: personal and family values, culture, economic interests . . . all these are not merely helps to man's last end; they possess a value of their own, placed in them by God . . . " *(Apostolicam Actuositatem, 7)*. The values of life and of the family are therefore one of the components of the temporal order which the faithful laity must not only defend, but promote and develop, in union with all other men of good will. Society itself benefits from such action.

These values belong to the very order of creation. Also, by nature, man's heart ought to seek them and grow in them. However, pride, selfishness and all the disorder introduced by sin often hinder discovering and, above all, admitting and observing the moral laws which guarantee these values. Now, Christians perceive them in the light of Revelation and grace helps to conform to them.

5. In this sense, Christian lay people can accomplish an apostolate of evangelical preparation. By placing their expertise at the service of the values pointed out by the Magisterium, they contribute to making them better recognized by persons and social groups. Their action will aim at making these basic values respected so that they will be upheld even by governments.

The witness of family life led by Christian spouses can be a valuable contribution by making clear to the whole of society what the family really is: "in what it is and what it does as an 'intimate community of life and love'" *(Familiaris Consortio, 50)*. The richness of the communion of persons, in their fidelity, will make it better understood that divorce and instability of self-giving are in reality seeds of death since the indissoluble personal bond is the source of life.

Attitudes contrary to life, its acceptance and transmission lead to acts such as abortion, sterilization or contraception. This brings about a distorted vision of marriage; it limits the meaning of the mutual self-giving between spouses. "The ultimate reason for these mentalities is the absence in people's hearts of God, whose love alone is stronger than all the world's fears and can conquer them" (FC, 30). When a child is not regarded as a gift of God, when conjugal love becomes like a selfish turning in upon oneself, when the laws of marriage are considered as an unbearable obstacle, when civil powers do not support the family in its structure and needs, then promotion of an authentic pro-life civilization becomes especially necessary. It is the laity--men and women of all generations--who can make known in their surroundings, by a daily apostolate beginning with education, the values and riches involved in human needs.

"The family is the first and fundamental school of social living . . . the communion and sharing that are part of everyday life in the home at times of joy and at times of difficulty are the most concrete and effective pedagogy for the active, responsible and fruitful inclusion of the children in the wider horizon of society" (FC, 37).

6. Through you, dear friends, I address myself to all Christian spouses. Make the social significance of your vocation as Christian spouses and parents understood. Your activity does not belong to an area extraneous to the good of all society. Respect for life, concern about human and Christian formation, the virtues of honesty, moderation and hospitality, education to chastity and self-control, the ability to love beyond one's own self-centeredness, care for the aged and the sick--these are all part of a whole set of values that people need in order to live up to their full dignity.

I therefore encourage all groups which, in fidelity to the Church's Magisterium, help Christian spouses to affirm their spirituality and develop their apostolate.

Promoting the family so that it will respond fully to its vocation is an apostolic concern common to all Christians. Everyone must be attentive to what clarifies or strengthens the values of marriage, fatherhood and motherhood. At the crossroads of the generations, marriage takes on a special missionary dimension in the Church. Living and solid, it is a primary place for a wider spreading of the kingdom of God in the present world.

7. I express my best wishes for your work, for all your activities, together with all those who have the responsibility for pastoral care of the family in the local Churches. I ask the Lord to fill you with his Blessings as well as the families to whose service you are dedicated.*

* This article is a translation taken from the English edition. *L'Osservatore Romano* N. 28 (11 July, 1988): 14.

POPE JOHN PAUL II DEPARTURE CEREMONY
DETROIT, SEPTEMBER 19, 1987

Mr. Vice President, dear friends, dear people of America,

1. Once again God has given me the joy of making a pastoral visit to your country --The United States of America. I am filled with gratitude to him and to you. I thank the Vice President for his presence here today, and I thank all of you from my heart for the kindness and warm hospitality that I have received everywhere.

I cannot leave without expressing my thanks to all those who worked so hard to make this visit possible. In particular I thank my brother bishops and all their collaborators, who for many months have planned and organized all the details of the last 10 days. My gratitude goes to all those who provided security and ensured such excellent public order. I thank all those who have worked to make this visit above all a time of fruitful evangelization and prayerful celebration of our unity in faith and love.

I am also grateful to the people of other churches and creeds and to all Americans of good will who have accompanied me in person or through the media as I traveled from city to city. A particular word of thanks goes to the men and women of the media for their constant and diligent assistance in bringing my message to the people and in helping me to reach millions of those with whom otherwise I would have had no contact. Most important, I am grateful to all those who supported me by their prayers, especially the elderly and the sick, who are so dear to the heart of Jesus Christ.

As I leave, I express my gratitude to God also for what he is accomplishing in your midst. With the words of St. Paul, I too can say with confident assurance "that he who has begun the good work in you will carry it through to completion, right up to the day of Christ Jesus" (Phil 1:6-7). And so I am confident too that America will be ever more conscious of her responsibility for justice and peace in the world. As a nation that has received so much, she is called to continued generosity and service toward others.

2. As I go, I take with me vivid memories of a dynamic nation, a warm and welcoming people, a church abundantly blessed with a rich blend of cultural tradition. I depart with admiration for the ecumenical spirit that breathes strongly throughout this land, for the genuine enthusiasm of your young people and for the hopeful aspirations of your most recent immigrants. I take with me an unforgettable memory of a country that God has richly blessed from the beginning until now.

America the beautiful! So you sing in one of your national songs. Yes, America, you are beautiful indeed and blessed in so many ways:

· In your majestic mountains and fertile plains.
· In the goodness and sacrifice hidden in your teeming cities and expanding suburbs.
· In your genius for invention and for splendid progress.
· In the power that you use for service and in the wealth that you share with others.
· In what you give to your own and in what you do for others beyond your borders.
· In how you serve and in how you keep alive the flame of hope in many hearts.
· In your quest for excellence and in your desire to right all wrongs.

Yes, America, all this belongs to you. But your greatest beauty and your richest blessing is found in the human person: in every man, woman and child, in every immigrant, in every native-born son and daughter.

3. For this reason, America, your deepest identity and truest character as a nation is revealed in the position you take toward the human person. The ultimate test of your greatness is the way you treat every human being, but especially the weakest and most defenseless ones.

The best traditions of your land presume respect for those who cannot defend themselves. If you want equal justice for all and true freedom and lasting peace, then, America, defend life! All the great causes that are yours today will have meaning only to the extent that you guarantee the right to life and protect the human person.

· Feeding the poor and welcoming refugees.
· Reinforcing the social fabric of this nation.
· Promoting the true advancement of women.
· Securing the rights of minorities.
· Pursuing disarmament, while guaranteeing legitimate defense.

All this will succeed only if respect for life and its protection by the law are granted to every human being from conception until natural death.

Every human person - no matter how vulnerable or helpless, no matter how young or how old, no matter how healthy, handicapped or sick, no matter how useful or productive for society - is a being of inestimable worth created in the image and likeness of God. This is the dignity of America, the reason she exists, the condition for her survival--yes, the ultimate test of her greatness; to respect every human person, especially the weakest and most defenseless ones, those as yet unborn.

With these sentiments of love and hope for America, I now say goodbye in words that I spoke once before: "Today, therefore, my final prayer is this: that God will bless America, so that she may increasingly become--and truly be--and long remain--'one nation, under God, indivisible. With liberty and justice for all'" (Oct. 7, 1979).

May God bless you all.

God bless America![*]

*_Origins_ 17, No. 18 (October 15, 1987)

GLOSSARY *

A

Amelioration - improvement, as of the condition of a patient

Amniocentesis - surgical transabdominal perforation of the uterus, to obtain amniotic fluid

Anovulation - absence of ovulation

Architectonic - the formal scheme, structural design, or method of elucidation of a system.

Augustinianism - thoughts of St. Augustine's on grace

Axiomatic - self evident truth; established principle

Azoospermia - lack of spermatozoa in the semen

B

Bioethicist - one who studies the ethical problems arising from scientific advances, especially in biology or medicine

C

Casuistry - the science of determining cases of conscience

Cerclage - encirclement of the incompetent cervix

Concupiscence - desire for pleasure of delight of the senses

Congenital anomalies - birth defects

263

Consubstantial - theological notion, rejected by the Catholic Church, that in the Eucharist the body and blood of Christ become present but coexist with the substance of bread and wine which remains in an absolute sense - not merely in species.

Copernicus - astronomer who theorized that the planets revolve around the sun and that the turning of the earth on its axis accounts for the apparent rising and setting of the stars; basis of modern astronomy

Corona Radiata - a layer of elongated follicle cells surrounding the zona pellucida of an ovum

Culpability - guilt; liability to blame; sinfulness,

Cumulus mass - a solid mass of follicular cells surrounding the ovum in the side of a developing ovarian follicle

D

De Facto - in fact; in reality; existing (regardless of legal or moral considerations)

Defeasance - a rendering void; the annulment of a contract or deed

Deontological - relating to the theory of duty or moral obligation; ethics

DES - (Diethylstilbestrol), a synthetic estrogenic compound

Divine Logos - understanding of God as the cosmic being who gives order and intelligibility to the world

Dogma - a proposition to be believed with divine and Catholic faith; a proposition which the Church expressly teaches in her ordinary magisterium as divinely revealed

E

Empiricist - one who believes in the philosophical theory that sensory experience is the only source of knowledge

Endometriosis - a condition in which tissue resembling the uterine mucous membrane (the endometrium) occurs in various locations in the pelvic cavity

Ensoul - to endow with a soul

Epistemological - having to do with the theory or science that investigates the origins, nature, methods and limits of science

Eschatological - related to that part of theology dealing with the last things, namely, death, judgment, heaven, hell and the end of the world

Excursus - a digression; a dissertation containing a fuller exposition of some important point or topic

Exigent - to drive out or drive forth; urgent; demanding

Ex parte - relating to only one part or side; one-sided

Extracorporeal - situated or occurring outside the body

Extrude - to force out or to occupy a position distal to that normally occupied

F

Fallopian tube - a pair of slender tubes by which the ova are carried from the ovaries to the uterus

Fecundity - fertility; fruitfulness; the ability to produce offspring

Follicle (ovarian) - the ovarian cyst which contains the egg (ovum)

Fractioned - separated chemically into fractions by distillation, crystallization

G

Gamete - a reproductive element; one of two cells, male (spermatozoon) and female (ovum), whose union is necessary in sexual reproduction to initiate the development of a new individual

H

Hypospadias - a malformation of the penis in which the opening of the urethra is along the under side

I

Immanent - present throughout the universe; said of God

Indefeasible - not to be defeated; not to be made void

Inextricable - cannot be disentangled or untied; so complicated or involved as to be insolvable

Intestate - not disposed of by will; a person who has died without having made a valid will

Intuitionalist - one who believes in the philosophical doctrine that absolute truth or any given truth can be perceived by intuition

Inviolable - not to be injured, broken or treated with irreverence; indesructible

K

Kantianism - the philosophy of Immanuel Kant (1724-1804), also called the critical philosophy, criticism, transcendentalism, or transcendental idealism. Its roots lay in the Enlightment, but it sought to establish a comprehensive method and doctrine of experience which would undercut the rationalistic metaphysics of the 17th and 18th centuries.

M

Meiotic division of the oocyte - the process of nuclear division of the female germ cells in which the number of chromosomes is reduced from the diploids or double, number found in somatic cells to the haploid, or halved, number found in gametes

Metaphysics - the branch of philosophy that deals with first principles and seeks to explain the nature of being or reality and of the origin and structure of the world

Mosaics - in genetics, an indivudal having two or more cell lines that are karotypically or genotypically distinct and are derived from a single zygote

N

Neo-Platonism - a school of philosophy established perhaps by Saccus in the second century in Alexandria, ending at a formal school with Proclus in the fifth century

Neuroendocrinology - study of the hormonal interactions of the brain

Nominalism - a doctrine of the late Middle Ages that all universal or abstract terms are mere necessities of thought or convenience of language and therefore exist as names only and have no realities corresponding to them

Noncommensurable - not having a common measure

Noumenal - pertaining to the philosophy of anything perceived; in Kantian philosophy an object understood by intellectual intuition, without the aid of the senses

O

Objectification - the act of giving objective form to; materialization

Occlusion - a blockage or closing

Oligoasthenospermia- a condition of few and weak spermatozoa

Opprobrium - disgrace attached to shameful conduct; anything bringing shame

P

Parthenogenesis - virgin birth; a modified form of sexual reproduction by the development of an egg without its being fertilized

Perspicuous - transparent, translucent; easily understood

Phenomenology - the science dealing with any fact, circumstance, or experience that is apparent to the senses and that can be scientifically described or appraised

Pneumatology - the doctrine of the Holy Ghost

Polar body - one of the minute cells which separate from the ovum at maturation

Polyandry - the state or practice of having two or more husbands at the same time

Polygyny - the state or practice of having two or more wives at the same time

Praxis - established practice, custom; distinguished from theory

Preparturient adoption - adoption prior to birth of the child

Pronuclei - the center of growth and development of the male or female reproductive cells

Prostaglandin - a group of naturally occurring, chemically related, long-chain hydroxy fatty acids that stimulate contractility of the uterine and other smooth muscle and have the ability to lower blood pressure and to affect the action of certain hormones

Psychogenic - having an emotional or organic basis; caused by mental conflicts

S

Spermatogenesis - the production and development of spermatozoa

T

Techne - the set of principles, or rational method, involved in the production of an object or the accomplishment of an end; the knowledge of such principles or method

Teleology - a thing which has its own constituent essence and yet is temporal and historical

Thomism - the teaching of St. Thomas Aquinas and his school which interprets his teaching in various ways and seeks to keep it alive.

Tubo-peritoneal - pertaining to a uterine tube and the peritoneum

*This glossary is intended only for use in quick reference and if the reader desires or needs greater explanation, the reader should use the various major dictionaries of the disciplines represented: anthropology, ethics, law, medicine, philosophy, theology, etc.